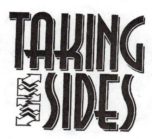

Clashing Views
on Controversial Issues
in Health and Society

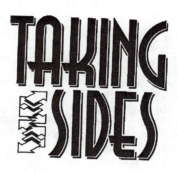

Clashing Views
on Controversial Issues
in Health and Society

Edited, Selected, and with Introductions by

Eileen L. Daniel
State University of New York
College at Brockport

The Dushkin Publishing Group, Inc.

To Mom and Dad, and to Joe Balog, with thanks

Photo Acknowledgments

Part 1   United Nations/John Isaac
Part 2   Bermuda News Bureau
Part 3   Drug Enforcement Agency
Part 4   Win McNamee/Sipa Press
Part 5   Minnesota Department of Economic Development
Part 6   New York State Department of Commerce
Part 7   Pamela Carley/The Dushkin Publishing Group

Library of Congress Cataloging-in-Publication Data

Main entry under title:
   Taking sides: clashing views on controversial issues in health and society
   1. Health. 2. Public Health. I. Daniel, Eileen L., *comp.*
   RA773   306.461
   ISBN: 1–56134–220–3   92–74290

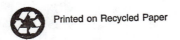 Printed on Recycled Paper

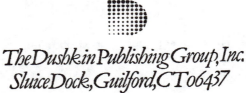

The Dushkin Publishing Group, Inc.
Sluice Dock, Guilford, CT 06437

PREFACE

This book contains 36 articles arranged in 18 *pro* and *con* pairs. Each pair addresses a controversial issue in health and society, expressed in terms of a question in order to draw the lines of debate more clearly.

Most of the questions that are included here relate to health topics of modern concern, such as AIDS, abortion, environmental health, and drug use and abuse. The authors of these articles take strong stands on specific issues and provide support for their positions. While we may not agree with a particular point of view, each author clearly defines his or her stand on the issues.

This book is divided into seven parts, each containing related issues. Each issue is preceded by an *introduction,* which sets the stage for the debate, gives historical background on the subject, and provides a context for the controversy. Each issue concludes with a *postscript,* which offers a summary of the debate and some concluding observations and suggests further readings on the subject. The postscript also raises further points, since most of the issues have more than two sides. At the back of the book is a listing of all the *contributors to this volume,* which gives information on the physicians, professors, journalists, theologians, and scientists whose views are debated here.

Taking Sides: Clashing Views on Controversial Issues in Health and Society is a tool to encourage critical thought on important health issues. Readers should not feel confined to the views expressed in the articles. Some readers may see important points on both sides of an issue and may construct for themselves a new and creative approach, which may incorporate the best of both sides or provide an entirely new vantage point for understanding.

This first edition of *Taking Sides: Clashing Views on Controversial Issues in Health and Society* presents up-to-date, opposing views on sensitive and complex issues. Although readers may approach this book with their own ideas on the debated issues, in order to achieve a good grasp of one's own viewpoint, it is important to understand the arguments of those with whom one may not agree.

Supplements An *Instructor's Manual With Test Questions* (both multiple-choice and essay) is available through the publisher for instructors using *Taking Sides* in the classroom. Also available is a general guidebook, *Using Taking Sides in the Classroom,* which discusses teaching techniques and methods for integrating the pro-con approach of *Taking Sides* into any classroom setting.

Acknowledgments Special thanks to my family, who frequently did without my company during the preparation of this book. Also, thanks to the staff at the Drake Memorial Library, State University of New York College at Brockport, for all their assistance. Finally, I appreciate the assistance of Mimi Egan, program manager, of The Dushkin Publishing Group.

Eileen L. Daniel
State University of New York College at Brockport

CONTENTS IN BRIEF

CONTENTS

Professor Vicente Navarro maintains that health care is a basic human right
and must be made available to all through a government-provided national
health insurance program similar to the Canadian system. Physician John K.
Iglehart argues that although the Canadian system is admired by much of
the Western world, it faces escalating problems, such as financial constraints
and inadequate consumer access to high-technology medicine.

Physician Timothy E. Quill, who describes a physician-assisted suicide,
believes that doctors have roles other than healing and fighting against
death. Physician Leon R. Kass argues that the weakening of the taboos against
physician-assisted suicide is a bad idea whose time must never come.

Hastings Center director Daniel Callahan believes that medical care for
elderly people at the end of their natural life expectancy should consist only

of pain relief rather than expensive health care services, which serve only to forestall death. Author Nat Hentoff argues that it is immoral to limit health care services to any one segment of the population.

Writer Michael Fumento points out that Congress continues to allocate substantial amounts of money for research and the treatment of AIDS, which he feels is disproportionate to the number of people who die annually from the disease. Medical professor Timothy F. Murphy argues that the AIDS epidemic is still fairly new and that AIDS is a lethal, contagious disease affecting thousands of Americans; thus, current funding is justified.

Professor of physics Albert L. Huebner believes that practicing healthy behaviors could both prevent and decrease the incidence of cancer. Professors Lenn E. Goodman and Madeleine J. Goodman argue that the ability to prevent disease, especially cancer, is exaggerated and limited.

Writer and editor Bernard Dixon discusses studies indicating that stress negatively impacts the immune system and, conversely, that a positive mental attitude can prevent illness. Physician Marcia Angell argues that there is no proof that a positive mental attitude can slow or prevent disease.

Policy analyst B. Bruce-Briggs believes that the war on passive smoking, which he argues is based on inaccurate data relating passive smoking with a myriad of health problems, is both a campaign against smokers and a trial run for a larger program of social manipulation. Professor of political and moral philosophy Robert E. Goodin argues that the health of nonsmokers suffers when they are forced to breathe tobacco smoke and that nonsmokers should have the right to a smoke-free environment.

Physician George E. Vaillant maintains that since alcoholism is genetically transmitted, it should be treated as a disease and not as a character flaw. Philosophy professor Herbert Fingarette argues that alcohol consumption is voluntary behavior, within the drinker's control, and that the role of heredity and genes in alcoholism is limited.

Richard J. Dennis, chairman of the Advisory Board of the Drug Policy Foundation, believes that the war on drugs has failed to reduce substance abuse or crime and argues that legalizing marijuana and cocaine would reduce the social and economic costs of drug abuse. Professors James A. Inciardi and Duane C. McBride maintain that the legalization of drugs would cause an increase in crime and produce an even greater number of addicts.

Biochemist Linus Pauling argues that taking megadoses of vitamins, particularly vitamin C, can help people achieve superior health. The editors of the *Harvard Medical School Health Letter* acknowledge that humans have a need for vitamin C; however, they argue that claims that megadoses will prevent colds, prevent cancer, and will prolong life are unsubstantiated.

American Health editor Joel Gurin claims that there is conclusive evidence that regular exercise will increase longevity. Cardiologist Henry A. Solomon argues that longevity is based on a complex interaction of genetics and lifestyle and that claims that exercise is a major variable in increasing longevity are exaggerated, unsubstantiated, and based on conflicting data.

Pesticide researchers Lawrie Mott and Karen Snyder maintain that the very foods consumers are trying to eat more of—fresh fruits and vegetables—are those most contaminated with harmful pesticide residues. Professor of biochemistry and molecular biology Bruce Ames argues that risks, if any, from pesticides in foods are minimal and such fears are greatly exaggerated.

Science writer Jon R. Luoma believes that there is convincing evidence implicating acid rain as a long-term threat to some aquatic ecosystems, forests, and public health. William M. Brown, director of energy and technological studies at the Hudson Institute in Indianapolis, argues that the dangers of acid rain have been greatly exaggerated and that scientists do not know what has caused the decline of some forests and waterways.

Health writer Royce Flippin argues that since measles and some other potentially dangerous childhood diseases are making a comeback, all children should be immunized against them. Health journalist Richard Leviton maintains that many vaccines are neither safe nor effective and that parents should have a say in whether or not their children receive them.

Associate professor of journalism Ellen Ruppel Shell maintains that chiropractors should continue to provide care for the millions who have back pain. The editors of the *Harvard Medical School Health Letter* argue that although some people may be helped by chiropractic treatment, many chiropractors adhere to a philosophy that is unproven at best, and harmful at worst.

INTRODUCTION

Dimensions and Approaches to the Study of Health and Society
Eileen L. Daniel

WHAT IS HEALTH?

Traditionally, being healthy meant being absent of illness. If someone did not have a disease, then he or she was considered to be healthy. The overall health of a nation or specific population was determined by numbers measuring illness, disease, and death rates. Today, this rather negative view of assessing individual health and health in general is changing. A healthy person is one who is not only free from disease but also fully well.

Being well, or wellness, involves the interrelationship of many dimensions of health: physical, emotional, social, mental, and spiritual. This multifaceted view of health reflects a holistic approach, which includes individuals taking responsibility for their own well-being.

Our health and longevity are affected by the many choices we make everyday: Medical reports tell us that if we abstain from smoking, drugs, excessive alcohol consumption, fat, and cholesterol, and get regular exercise, our rate of disease and disability will significantly decrease. These reports, while not totally conclusive, have encouraged many people to make positive life-style changes. Millions of people have quit smoking; alcohol consumption is down, and more and more individuals are exercising regularly and eating low-fat diets. While these changes are encouraging, many people who have been unable or unwilling to make these changes are left feeling worried and/or guilty over continuing their negative health behaviors.

But disagreement exists among the experts about the exact nature of positive health behaviors, which causes confusion. For example, some scientists claim that Americans should make efforts to reduce their serum cholesterol in order to lower their risk of heart disease. Other researchers claim that lowering serum cholesterol has no significant effect on heart health. Who do you believe? Experts also disagree on the risks of acid rain, whether or not sex education prevents unwanted pregnancy, and the role of exercise in increasing longevity.

Health status is also affected by society and government. Societal pressures have helped pass smoking restrictions in public places, mandatory safety belt legislation, and laws permitting condom distribution in public schools. The government plays a role in the health of individuals as well, although it has failed to provide minimal health care for many low-income Americans.

Unfortunately, there are no absolute answers to many questions regarding health and wellness issues. Moral questions, controversial concerns, and individual perceptions of health matters all can create opposing views. As you evaluate the issues in this book, you should keep an open mind toward both sides. You may not change your mind regarding the morality of abortion or the limitation of health care for the elderly, but you will still be able to learn from the opposing viewpoint.

WELLNESS, BEHAVIOR, AND SOCIETY

The issues in this book are divided into seven parts. The first deals with health care and society. The topics addressed in Part 1 include a debate on the U.S. versus the Canadian health care system. (The Canadian system has been seen by some as a model for Western nations, particularly the United States.) Issue 2 deals with whether or not physicians should intervene in the deaths of terminally ill patients. While many Americans agree that we cannot and should not prolong the deaths of terminally ill patients, do the elderly deserve special consideration? In Issue 3, Daniel Callahan, the director of the Hastings Center, believes that the increasing proportion of health care dollars that is going to the elderly cannot be allowed to continue. Nat Hentoff disagrees with Callahan and asks, "Who decides when someone is too old for medical treatment? Daniel Callahan?" The fourth controversy in this section is about the AIDS epidemic. The number of cases of AIDS both in the United States and throughout the world has been increasing, and there does not appear to be any indication that this trend will not continue. But some social critics nevertheless argue that other diseases (heart disease and cancer, for example) are just as serious as AIDS and should not be neglected. How should the government set priorities for funding for research and treatment for AIDS?

MIND-BODY ISSUES

Part 2 discusses two important issues related to the relationship between mind and body. Will practicing positive health behaviors and emphasizing prevention improve health, and can a positive mental attitude overcome disease? Over the past 10 years, both laypeople and the medical profession have placed an emphasis on the prevention of illness as a way to improve health. Not smoking, for instance, certainly reduces the risk of developing lung cancer. Unfortunately, the current U.S. health care system places an emphasis on treatment rather than prevention, even though prevention is less expensive, less painful, and more humane. Albert Huebner claims that the emphasis on treatment has been partially responsible for increasing cancer rates. Professors Lenn and Madeleine Goodman disagree with Huebner; they argue that prevention campaigns are often based on scanty or conflicting evidence.

As Huebner claims, we can be responsible for much of our own well-being by practicing positive health behaviors. Bernard Dixon, in Issue 6, argues that we can also control our health by maintaining a positive mental attitude. Dixon claims that the mind can influence the body by affecting the immune system. A positive mental attitude can boost the immune system, which, in turn, can help fight disease. Marcia Angell counters that there is absolutely no concrete proof that people can prevent or slow a disease's progress by maintaining a positive mental state. Blaming people for causing their own diseases through negative states of mind, she argues, is counter-productive and ignores the real causes of disease.

SUBSTANCE USE AND ABUSE

Part 3 introduces current issues related to drug use and abuse in the United States. Millions of Americans use and abuse drugs that alter their minds and affect their bodies. These drugs range from illegal substances, such as crack cocaine and opiates, to the widely used legal drugs alcohol and tobacco. Use of these substances can lead to physical and psychological addiction and the related problems of family dysfunction, reduced worker productivity, and crime. Particularly because of drug-related crime involving illegal drugs, many experts have argued for the legalization of drugs, particularly mari-juana. If drugs were legalized, law enforcement could focus on other areas, since the enormous profits would not exist.

The American drug crisis is often related to changes in or a breakdown of traditional values. The collapse of strong family and religious influences may affect drug usage, especially among young people. It has been argued, however, that some people, regardless of societal or familial influences, will use drugs based on some inherent need or inherited factor. This is partic-ularly true in relation to alcoholism. For some time, experts have maintained that alcoholism is an inherited disease because it appears to run in families. Other experts disregard the disease model of alcoholism and argue that drinking is voluntary behavior that is within an individual's control.

Also in this section is a debate on passive smoking. The individual's right to smoke in public is set against the nonsmoker's health risks when forced to breath tobacco smoke.

SEXUALITY

As the incidence of AIDS and other sexually transmitted diseases rises among teenagers and the number of adolescent pregnancies increases, will sex education in the classroom help control these problems? Unfortunately, most current sex education programs in the United States do not appear to slow the rate of teenage pregnancy, increase condom use, or prevent sexual experimentation. Is this an indication that sex education does no good? In Issue 10, Michael Carrera and Patricia Dempsey argue that while many current programs are ineffective, sex education programs characterized by multiple intervention strategies have decreased teenage pregnancy rates.

Although teenage pregnancy continues to be a major concern, is abortion an acceptable means to end an unwanted pregnancy? Mary Gordon believes that abortion is acceptable and argues in Issue 11 that it is not an immoral choice for women. Jason DeParle, in opposition, discusses why liberals and feminists do not like to talk about the morality of abortion. The abortion issue continues to cause major controversy. More restrictions have been placed on the right to abortion as a result of the political power wielded by the pro-life faction. Pro-choice followers, however, argue that making abortion illegal again will force many women to obtain dangerous "back alley" abortions.

NUTRITION, EXERCISE, AND HEALTH

Will taking megadoses of vitamins, particularly vitamin C, improve health? Can diet prevent illnesses such as cancer and heart disease? Will exercise prolong life? These questions are discussed in Part 5, which deals with nutrition and exercise. Millions of Americans are restricting their intake of cholesterol and fats in an effort to lower their serum cholesterol. Although there is a correlation between high serum cholesterol and heart disease, the evidence is less convincing for dietary manipulation as a means to lower serum cholesterol. Other myths and facts regarding this controversy are debated in Issue 12.

If reducing cholesterol will not significantly reduce the incidence of disease, will taking megadoses of vitamins help? This question is debated in Issue 13. New research indicates that the current recommendations for many vitamins are inadequate for our changing life-styles. People today are under considerable stress, are exposed to increasing amounts of environmental pollutants, often use drugs, and frequently eat away from home. These factors may make it impossible for individuals to meet their needs for vitamins via diet alone. While vitamins prevent deficiency diseases, it appears that specific vitamins may also be beneficial in the treatment and prevention of certain illnesses, such as cancer and heart disease, and may prolong life by several years. Experts warn, however, that the large doses recommended to prevent disease can have side effects and/or be toxic and that it is still safest simply to eat a balanced diet that includes plenty of fruits and vegetables.

In addition to a healthy diet, it also makes sense to get plenty of exercise to ward off the diseases that could shorten one's life expectancy. In Issue 14, health writer Joel Gurin claims that even modest amounts of exercise will substantially reduce a person's risk of heart disease or cancer and, therefore, reduce the risk for a shortened life expectancy. Cardiologist Henry Solomon disagrees, claiming that exercise is not a panacea and that longevity is affected by a myriad of behaviors, as well as heredity.

ENVIRONMENTAL HEALTH

Debate continues over the two fundamental issues surrounding the environment: human needs and the future of the environment. The debate becomes more heated as the environmental issues move closer to human concerns, such as health, economic interests, and politics. Issue 15, for example, discusses the safety of pesticide usage on fruits and vegetables. The recent Alar (a chemical growth regulator for apples) scare convinced many Americans that the apple supply was not safe and that an apple a day could cause cancer. At the same time, nutritionists as well as the Department of Agriculture were urging people to eat more fruits and vegetables to help prevent cancer.

The question of whether or not environmental changes are having a serious impact on the health of the lakes and forests is debated in Issue 16. Acid rain has many implications, including political, health, economic, and environmental. It is produced when sulphur and nitrogen oxides from burning coal are released into the upper atmosphere where they change into sulfuric and nitric acids. These acids become part of the rain and snow, which falls on lakes and forests. Since so many problems appear to be related to acid rain, why is there a controversy regarding whether or not it is a risk? One could point to reports claiming that fears regarding the dangers of acid rain have not been realized and that acid rain is not such a serious problem. This view conflicts with environmentalists, who feel that acid rain is one of the major environmental issues of the decade.

CONSUMER HEALTH ISSUES

Part 7 introduces questions about particular issues related to choices about health care services. The questions here include (1) Should All Children Be Immunized Against Childhood Diseases? and (2) Are Chiropractors Legitimate Health Providers?

At the turn of the century, millions of American children developed childhood diseases such as tetanus, polio, measles, and pertussis (whooping cough). Many of these children died or became permanently disabled because of these illnesses. Today, vaccines exist to prevent all of these conditions; however, not all children receive their recommended immunizations. Some do not get vaccinated until the schools require them, and others are allowed exemptions. More and more, parents are requesting exemptions for some or all vaccinations based on fears over their safety and/or their effectiveness. The pertussis vaccination seems to generate the biggest fears. Reports of serious injury to children following the pertussis vaccination (usually given in a combination of diphtheria, pertussis, and tetanus, or DPT) have convinced many parents to forgo immunization. As a result, the rates of measles and pertussis have been climbing after decades of decline. Is it safer to be vaccinated than to risk getting pertussis? Most medical societies and physicians believe so, but Richard Leviton argues that many vaccines are neither safe nor effective.

Current views of chiropractors and the practice of spinal manipulation are discussed in Issue 18. Due to demand by the public, chiropractors are achieving new legitimacy, despite the efforts of traditional medicine to discredit them. Traditionalists view chiropractors as a notch above quacks, but, at the same time, more and more people are turning to spinal manipulation for relief of their backaches, headaches, and other conditions.

Will the many debates presented in this book ever be resolved? Some issues may resolve themselves because of the availability of resources. For instance, funding for health care for the elderly may become restricted in the United States, as it is in the United Kingdom, simply because there are increasingly limited resources to go around. An overhaul of the health care system to provide care for all while keeping costs down (which may or may not be based on the Canadian model) seems inevitable, as most Americans agree that the system must be changed. Other controversies may require the test of time for resolution. Several more years may be required before it can be determined whether or not acid rain is really a serious environmental hazard. The debates over the effectiveness of megadoses of vitamins may also require years of research.

Other controversies may never resolve themselves. There may never be a consensus over the abortion issue, sex education in the classroom, or the disease model of alcoholism. This book will introduce you to many ongoing controversies on a variety of sensitive and complex health-related topics. In order to have a good grasp of one's own viewpoint, it is necessary to be familiar with and understand the points made by the opposition.

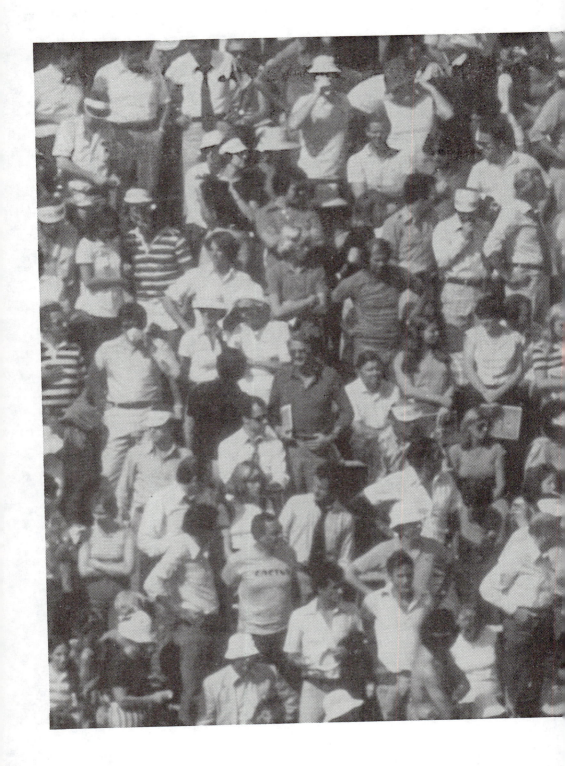

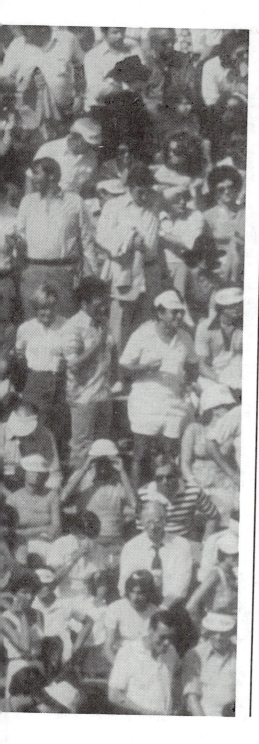

PART 1

Health Care and Society

The United States currently faces many frightening health problems, including an aging population and a lack of health care insurance for millions of people. Soceity must confront the enormous financial burden of providing health care to a growing elderly population. At the same time, the government has not been able or willing to meet the health care needs of low-income Americans. Furthermore, some people maintain that the government has allocated too much precious money and time for AIDS research. Medical and financial resources remain limited, while demands increase. To further complicate the problem, public policy and medical ethics have not always kept pace with rapidly growing technology and scientific advances. This section discusses some of the major controversies concerning the role of society in health concerns.

Should the United States Adopt a
   National Health Insurance Program?

———

Should Doctors Ever Help Terminally
   Ill Patients Commit Suicide?

———

Should Health Care for the Elderly Be
   Limited?

———

Is AIDS Getting More Than Its Share
   of Resources and Media Attention?

ISSUE 1

Should the United States Adopt a National Health Insurance Program?

YES: Vicente Navarro, from "A National Health Program Is Necessary," *Challenge* (May/June 1989)

NO: John K. Iglehart, from "Canada's Health Care System Faces Its Problems," *The New England Journal of Medicine* (February 22, 1990)

ISSUE SUMMARY

YES: Professor of social policy Vicente Navarro maintains that health care is a basic human right and must be made available to all through a government-provided national health insurance program similar to the Canadian system.

NO: Physician John K. Iglehart argues that although the Canadian system is admired by much of the Western world, it faces escalating problems, such as financial constraints, oversupply of physicians, and inadequate consumer access to high-technology medicine.

Health care in the United States is handled by various unrelated agencies and organizations and through a number of programs, including private insurance, government-supported Medicaid for the needy, and Medicare for the elderly. Currently there are 38 million people, or 16 percent of the population, who cannot afford any health insurance and who do not qualify for government-sponsored programs. These people must often do without any medical care at all. As a result, this population experiences higher rates of disability, unemployment, and infant mortality.

The United States is the only industrialized nation other than South Africa that does not provide government-sponsored health care to all its citizens. The problem does not appear related to lack of resources: The United States spends more on health care than any other nation in the world. Despite these expenditures, millions of U.S. citizens are still without basic medical coverage.

Until 1966, Canada and the United States had similar ways of financing and organizing health care costs. The Canadian insurance companies operated in the same manner as those in the United States, and most hospitals and doctors in Canada were organized in nearly the same way as their

American counterparts. Even the indicators of health and the percentages spent on health care were similar.

In 1966, Canada initiated a national health program. The basic national health insurance program in Canada includes comprehensive medical coverage for all Canadians and public nonprofit administration. This system allows physicians to bill the government for the fees allowed for the services performed. Patients can select their own doctors, but treatments by specialists require referrals from primary care physicians.

While health costs are currently increasing in Canada, the Canadian health care budget is about 20 percent less than in the United States, and the health of its citizens is comparable to that of Americans. Canadians save money while providing health care to all by a variety of means: In Canada, less is spent on administration, research, physicians' salaries, and malpractice insurance. An additional cost-saving measure involves the rationing of technologically advanced equipment and procedures. Although rationing of certain procedures does occur, since all Canadians are automatically insured in the health system, it is impossible for anyone to be denied basic medical treatment. This compares to millions of Americans who are denied access to any health care because of their inability to pay.

There are critics of the Canadian system, however. A major concern is the length of time Canadians must wait for treatment, particularly treatment involving rationed technology. Delays of several weeks and even months are not uncommon for certain procedures. While wealthy Canadians can travel to the United States and pay for operations and technologically advanced treatments, the majority must wait until services become available in their country. Rising costs may also threaten health care services in Canada and increase the waiting time even further. In addition, some critics claim that the quality of Canadian medical education is deteriorating because of government restrictions on university funding.

In the following selections, Vincente Navarro argues that Canada's federally funded health care is more efficient and less inflationary than the current American system. He feels that health care is a basic human right that should be available to all Americans as it is to all Canadians. John K. Iglehart argues that the Canadian system has serious flaws and that, although it supplies universal health care to its citizens, the rationing of services may be responsible for unnecessary deaths and disabilities.

YES
Vicente Navarro

A NATIONAL HEALTH PROGRAM
IS NECESSARY

The United States is the only Western industrialized nation (besides South Africa) without a national health program that assures access to health care as a basic right for all. Yet, as a nation, we spend more on health care than any other country on earth: 11.2 percent of our GNP goes to health care. And it is estimated that this will go up to 15 percent of GNP by the year 2000. In spite of these large expenditures, we still face problems that no other country faces.

In 1986, 38 million Americans did not have any form of health insurance coverage, public or private; 36 percent of them were children. Consequently, 200,000 people are refused care each year at private hospital emergency rooms because they cannot pay and are uninsured; another 800,000 families are denied other than emergency care each year.

The problem of coverage, however, includes not only the uninsured but also the underinsured. The majority of Americans are insufficiently covered, but they are not aware of it. For example, a recent poll showed that 62 percent of Americans felt that they could cope with the expenses incurred in long-term care if a member of the family needed it. They were wrong.

Long-term care is not covered in most health insurance benefits, and the cost of such care averages $25,000 per year—far above the possibilities of most people. Our health benefits coverage, both in the public and the private sectors, does not compare favorably with that in most other industrialized nations. We pay higher out-of-pocket expenses for medical care than in any other industrialized nation.

The situation worsened during 1980–1988. The number of people without health insurance coverage increased by 4 million; out-of-pocket expenditures for the average American increased; the percentage of Americans who do not have a regular source of care increased by 65 percent; and our elders saw Medicare premiums increase by 38 percent. People are getting less coverage, and they are paying more.

A further problem with our health care coverage is the broad range of coverage among different sectors of the labor force. The majority of Americans are covered at their workplace through employer-employee contributions. Where unions are strong, as in manufacturing, coverage is much more extensive than in sectors where unions are weak, such as services and sales (see Table 1). Thus, the kind of health benefits that families or individuals get depends on their type of work and bargaining power. A sales worker has, on average, 53 percent less coverage than a manufacturing worker.

Relating health benefits to work creates other problems. First, there is the enormous fear of job loss. Seventy-five percent of workers over 45 years of age who lost their jobs in the 1982 recession lost their health insurance as well. A related consequence is workers' resistance to labor mobility, based on their fear that their health benefits may change and be reduced.

Second, the current shift of employment in the United States from manufacturing to retail and services, the increase in part-time employment, and the high number of newly created low wage jobs lead to an increased number of under insured, uninsured, and uninsurable workers. Between 1982 and 1984, for example, 5.5 million jobs were added to the workplace, but the number of workers with employer-paid health benefits coverage fell by 1 million.

Third, when we tie health benefits to the workplace, we add an extra cost to production that burdens employers more than in any other country. Ford, for example, pays $5,000 per employee compared with $1,200 for Honda in Japan. Ford Canada is less concerned about the health benefits of its employees than its

Table 1

Percentage of Workers Who Are Unionized in Certain Types of Employment and Percentage of Coverage in Specific Types of Health Insurance

Industry	Percentage unionized	Percentage uninsured all year	Dental service coverage	Vision or hearing
Manufacturing	46%	4.8%	30.9%	15.6%
Personal services	13	16.0	17.0	5.0

Sources: Bureau of Labor Statistics; Directory of National Unions and Employment Associations, 1975; Employment and Earnings, January 1979.

United States counterparts. Canadian workers have a national health program funded by general revenues.

AN EXCESSIVE RISE IN HEALTH CARE COSTS

Besides spending the most on health care, the United States also is the country where health expenditures grow fastest (8.9 percent in 1987 compared with no growth or lower growth in most other countries). The rate of growth of these expenditures is higher than the rate of growth of our GNP. Medical care expenditures are among the fastest growing expenditures in our economy, and a major reason is the very fast growth of health care costs.

During the 1980s, the Reagan Administration and Congress tried to control the enormous growth of these costs by stimulating "competition" in the medical care sector. With hospitals and other providers competing for patients, the price and overall costs of health services were supposed to decline. They have not.

The rate of growth of national health expenditures (corrected for the overall inflation rate) has been larger in the 1980s (the "competitive" years) than in the 1970s. Costs have increased, as have out-of-pocket expenditures for the average American.

In 1985, high costs of health care were considered by the majority of Americans to be among their top five concerns in the health sector. Also, 73 percent of Americans thought that medical and hospital fees had risen too high, and 20 percent feared that they would not have been able to pay for necessary health care. As a consequence of this large growth of prices and costs, health benefits coverage declined further.

"Competition" has not only increased costs and reduced health care benefits coverage, it also has stimulated an economic behavior among providers in which patients are evaluated for their profitability. Many providers are selecting "profitable" cases and discharging prematurely or refusing "unprofitable" cases (such as AIDS patients, whose average cost per case is $120,000).

In 1986, 78 percent of admitting physicians reported pressure from their hospitals to discharge patients and lower their length of stay, particularly patients considered unprofitable. A major nursing home chain—ManorCare—refused to serve unprofitable Medicaid patients at its 147 nursing homes. In Austin, Texas, Hospital Corporation of America purchased a hospital and closed the rehabilitation unit that served about 400 severely impaired patients—the only such unit in the city—because the unit was not profitable.

PREVENTION IS WHAT'S NEEDED

The World Health Organization defines health as "the physical, mental, and social well-being of mankind, not just the absence of disease." The road to good health is not only through health care services, but through improvement of living and working conditions. And the goal of the health care system should be not only to cure but, most importantly, to prevent the acquisition of disease and disability and promote the full development of a joyful and healthy life.

These goals and the roads to achieve them require major changes in our priorities, both in our society and in our approach to medical care. For example: Poverty is a major cause of poor health, disease, and death. The medical care system tries to solve this problem with high-technology interventions. North Carolina, for example, has about the same number of babies born per year as Sweden, but has twice as many low birth weight babies and neonatal deaths, due to poverty and malnutrition. North Carolina, however, has twice as many highly expensive ventilator-equipped neonatal intensive care unit beds as Sweden, with further expansion proposed.

It would be much more humane and cost-effective to provide food, social services, and prenatal care to expectant mothers. The Neonatal Intensive Care Unit costs more than $1,000 per day, often amounting to $100,000 per infant, while adequate prenatal care costs only $800 per infant. This example shows how our medical care system can place excessive emphasis on curative, high technology medicine rather than on cheaper, and more humane, preventive health care.

The root of the problem is the system of funding and organizing health care in the United States. Of all the Western industrialized nations, the United States spends the least public funds in the health sector (4.5 percent of GNP compared with 8.8 percent in Sweden, 6.6 percent in West Germany, 6.6 percent in France, and 6.2 percent in Canada). Most of the medical care funds are private and are administered primarily by 1,550 private insurance companies that reimburse providers for delivery of services.

Considering that there are 1.7 billion hospital admissions and physician visits per year provided by 369,200 physicians and 1,047,438 hospital beds, and that providers are paid by diagnosis, visits, or admissions, we can see that an enormous administrative apparatus is required to sustain such a system. Private insurance companies consume about 8 percent of revenue for overhead, while the Canadian health care program has overhead costs of only 3 percent.

Moreover, medical care is a commodity that must be advertised and sold and that must generate profits—as in any industry—to be able to reproduce itself. Consequently, we have developed a health care bureaucracy (public and private) unmatched by any other country. A lot of funds are spent in pushing around bits of paper rather than providing health care.

A large majority of Americans—72 percent—want to see major changes in the way we fund and organize our health care. The frustrating reality is that these problems of high costs and limited coverage are avoidable.

Until 1966, Canada and the United States had similar ways of financing and organizing health care. The insurance companies in Canada operated like those in this country. The majority of hospitals were—like ours—voluntary hospitals, and the majority of physicians were paid on a fee-for-service basis. Even the health indicators were similar. And both countries spent the same percentage of their GNP on health care.

CANADA TAKES AGGRESSIVE ACTION

In 1966, however, Canada introduced a national health program that gave to a federal-provincial partnership the responsibility to insure the population. Private insurance could only sell benefits not provided in the national health program. In 1966, the Canadian Medical Care Act (Medicare) introduced federal funding into a health care system that is administered by the provinces.

In order to receive matching federal tax dollars, the provincial health programs must adhere to five health care principles: (1) comprehensive coverage; (2) universal application of the program; (3) ability to transfer coverage to other provinces; (4) speedy accessibility to the system; and (5) public nonprofit administration.

In 1984, the Canadian Parliament passed the Canada Health Act, holding back federal funding from provinces that allow doctors to "extra-bill" above normal negotiated rates or charge user fees for special services.

The United States spent about $500 billion on health services in 1987; that is about 11.2 percent of GNP, a 5.6 percent increase over 1986. Health costs consistently outrace the cost of living.

Though health costs are increasing in Canada, the Canadian health care budget for 1985 was 8.6 percent of GNP, about 20 percent less than in the United States (see Figure 1). Dollar for dollar, Canada's universal system, which is 80 percent publicly owned and operated, is more efficient and less inflationary than ours, 60 per-

Figure 1

**Health Expenditure as a Percent of GNP
United States and Canada, 1960–1985**

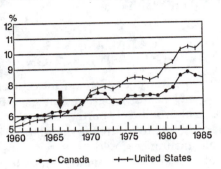

—•— Canada   —+— United States

Source: Author's own calculations.

cent of which is financed and administered by the private sector. Ironically, Canada spends relatively more on public health and capital expenditures but only one-third as much on administration.

Canadians also save in other areas, some of which are matters of contention. In 1985, Canada spent less than half of what we spend on research. Some observers suggest this is because the publicly administered system is unable to absorb high-technology advances quickly enough. Others suggest that too much high-technology medicine is overpriced, limited in use, and ineffective.

Canadian physicians receive about 80 to 85 percent of the income of their U.S. counterparts. Doomsayers once suggested that this would lead to a doctor shortage, but the desertion has not yet happened. Provincial medical societies are calling for an increase in the size of medical schools, where tuition costs less than a tenth of what is charged in the United States. Also, Canadian doctors pay only about 10 percent of what U.S. physicians dole out for malpractice insurance.

Also, since all Canadians are automatically insured in the health system, it is impossible for anyone to be denied proper medical treatment.

Ironically, the publicly administered Canadian program greatly reduces the paperwork that chokes our system. In the United States, a hospital or doctor bills a patient, who then attempts to recover the costs from a public or private insurer (if she or he is insured). In Canada, doctors and hospitals directly bill the province to reimburse fees that have been set by the government through negotiation with representatives of the medical profession.

And Canada spends virtually nothing on the advertising and marketing of basic medical services. In the United States, the recent trend toward underutilized hospital beds has led to multi-million dollar advertising campaigns in which hospitals are merchandised like fast food outlets.

Then there is the quality of care and the state of public health. Generally, infant mortality and life expectancy rates are the common indicators of a nation's medical well being. Canada, which trailed the United States until it introduced the national health program, now leads in both categories.

In 1982, the infant mortality rate in the United States was 20 percent greater than that in Canada—11.5 deaths per 1,000 live births compared with 9.1. Canada's citizens outlive their southern neighbors by more than a year on the average. As for quality of care, U.S. certifying agencies readily accept Canadian medical credentials as equal to ours, and there are constant and frequent exchanges of medical information and techniques between the two nations.

WHY COSTS ARE LOWER
IN CANADA

Canada has a federal-provincial health insurance system that contracts with the private sector for the delivery of services. Government is practically the only purchaser of services. This simplifies matters enormously. About one-half of one percent of GNP in the United States is accounted for by the excess costs (relative to the Canadian system) of paying for the reimbursement system itself.

Canadian physicians' fees are negotiated between the provincial government and the physicians' representatives. Consequently, for the past 20 years, Canada has kept the growth of fees at a pace similar to that for the rest of the economy; in the United States (as in Canada before the national health program), these fees have consistently escalated faster than general inflation rates.

Canadian hospitals are paid on a prospective budget basis rather than by diagnosis. Consequently, administrative costs are much lower than in U.S. hospitals. As an average, U.S. hospitals have 23 employees in charge of billing. Canadian hospitals have one, usually to bill U.S. citizens who use their facilities.

While the number of hospital admissions per thousand population is practically the same on both sides of the border, and the case mix of patients is similar, overall hospital costs in Canada are 20 percent lower than those in the United States. These lower costs are partly due to the reduction of administrative costs; partly due to the use of government muscle to rationalize and better plan and organize the private delivery system.

In the United States on a given day, there are 349,146 empty, staffed hospital beds—over one-third of the total staffed beds. And if we add the beds that are built but not staffed, almost half the beds in this country are unused.

As Pete Stark, Chairman of the House Ways and Means Subcommittee on Health, put it:

> In addition to empty beds, virtually every city boasts underused specialized services, such as cardiac surgery, where not enough work is done to maintain competency. And because of this amount of waste we face an approximate 11 percent increase in hospital costs year after year. Canada, on the other hand, enjoys a hospital occupancy rate of 84 percent. The reason for this significantly higher rate is clear. The Canadians do not hand their hospitals a blank check and allow them to build facilities whether they are needed or not, as we do. Canada establishes a capital budget each year at the provincial government level and carefully plans how to allocate resources within that budget so that each community has the health care facilities that it needs and that the nation can afford.

The Canadian experience shows that the reason our system does not provide comprehensive coverage is not money but the channels through which that money is spent. In 1985, we spent $1,500 per capita in personal health expenditures, whereas Canada spent $1,010 while providing universal and comprehensive coverage. Something is profoundly wrong in the way we organize and fund our health services. Seventy-five percent of Americans want major changes in the way we pay for our health services, 61 percent would prefer a system like Canada's, and 75 percent want government to establish a national health program.

Will we ever get it?

NO

John K. Iglehart

CANADA'S HEALTH CARE SYSTEM FACES ITS PROBLEMS

Canada's provincial health insurance plans have demonstrated an impressive capacity to operate successfully despite a basic policy conflict that says health care funding must be public and universal, physicians must retain their professional autonomy, consumers must have free choice of doctors and first-dollar coverage, and provincial governments must control their budgets. But now provinces are finding it increasingly difficult to maintain this equation, because a variety of factors are perturbing its balance. In the face of a large budget deficit, the national government continues to reduce its financial commitment to the plans, patients and practitioners are demanding better access to the latest forms of medical technology, the supply of physicians continues to increase at a rate outstripping the growth of the population, and doctors are restive as provinces work more aggressively to stem the rise in health expenditures.

Among industrialized nations, such conflicts are certainly not unique. Indeed, every major Western country grapples with similar issues to one degree or another. But when tax-financed programs in most nations are stretched to the limit, their stewards usually turn to private funding for relief. What is unique to Canada is the virtual absence of private-sector involvement in health insurance and the unwillingness of policy makers to encourage the development of such alternatives, which could ease the financial pressure on the provincial health plans. These plans account for 75 percent of the nation's total expenditure for medical care, which amounted to $50.4 billion (Canadian) in 1988, or 8.7 percent of the gross domestic product. The remainder of the health expenditure purchases services not covered by the plans, such as outpatient prescription drugs, dental care, cosmetic surgery, optometry, and physiotherapy.

Canada designed its provincial health insurance plans this way because of a strong belief that all citizens should have equal access to medical care, regardless of ability to pay. In essence, Canadian policy says that simply because people can afford to pay, they should not be able to purchase care

From John K. Iglehart, "Canada's Health Care System Faces Its Problems," *The New England Journal of Medicine*, vol. 322, no. 8 (February 22, 1990), pp. 562–568. Copyright © 1990 by The Massachusetts Medical Society. Reprinted by permission.

that is better or more readily available than that available to the less well off. Canada has further discouraged private payment by requiring physicians who bill patients directly to leave the provincial health insurance plans altogether. As a result, such doctors are few.

Canada's refusal to allow private health insurance to be sold, except for incidental items not covered by the provincial plans, arises from "deep-rooted suspicion of class-based systems of any kind," economist Robert G. Evans wrote recently.[1] Private schools are only a small part of Canada's educational system before college, private universities do not exist, and in public transportation only a single class of travel is usually available, except in some air and train travel. As Evans put it, "equality before the health care system" in Canada is a political principle similar to equality before the law.

This policy contrasts markedly with the method by which the bulk of care is financed in the pluralistic system of the United States and is contrary to the direction in which the socialized health schemes of Sweden and the United Kingdom are moving. Most U.S. policy makers and representatives of private-sector interests believe that except in the case of poor people, consumers should be directly responsible for a portion of the cost of care. The board of trustees of the American Medical Association (AMA), in a 1989 report to its House of Delegates about Canadian health care, characterized the absence of a direct economic link between payer and patient in the provincial health plans as "a structural defect which leads directly to an excessive demand for services, and will be a growing source of conflict between government and consumers."[2]

Whether Canada, faced with a budget deficit, general opposition to higher taxes, and real resistance to reducing the scope of covered medical benefits, can maintain a health care policy that relies on public expenditures and strongly discourages the infusion of private resources is a question asked more frequently there. At this point there is certainly no clamor for major change among private corporations; they seem well satisfied with letting government finance the bulk of medical care and limiting their involvement to paying for part of it through taxation.[3] The Progressive Conservative government of Prime Minister Brian Mulroney has shown no disposition to propose that Canadian medical care be made more readily available through private alternatives, but in other spheres of the economy it has demonstrated a philosophical preference for private investment. For example, 18 crown corporations have been privatized since Mulroney assumed office in 1984. Thus far, Canada has been able to finance its system of universal access to health care by constraining medical expenditures in various ways, as Evans outlined recently in the [New England Journal of Medicine]: keeping its insurance overhead low through the administrative simplicity of its provincial plans, controlling payments to physicians and hospitals through negotiated fees and global budgets, and restraining the diffusion of forms of technology.[4]

In this report, I cover some of the major issues that are enlivening Canada's health care debate, particularly as they apply to Ontario, which is the most populous province (with 9 million residents), the seat of the nation's capital (Ottawa), and the place where the largest number of physicians practice (about 40 percent). For a variety of reasons, conflict between provincial governments and organized medicine is more pronounced in Ontario, British Columbia, and Quebec than in the seven other provinces. As I have pointed out elsewhere,[2] some American health policy makers have become fascinated with Canada's ability to balance a host of conflicting interests and objectives of behalf of the provision of medical care to its entire population. These cross-national pursuits are not necessarily welcomed by many physicians in either country. The AMA has made it clear that philosophically, Canada's model is repugnant to its leadership and probably most of its members. Dr. David K. Peachey, director of professional affairs of the Ontario Medical Association, provided a Canadian perspective on the subject in a speech last October [1989] to the Roanoke (Va.) Academy of Medicine: "The managed care component of American medicine is being held like a Damocles' sword over the heads of Canadian physicians, while our universal health insurance is held like a Damocles' sword over you."

THE PRINCIPLES OF CANADIAN HEALTH INSURANCE

Canada's debate has not prompted many second thoughts about the basic conditions that Parliament established in 1965 when it created the framework of the provincial health insurance plans. To qualify for federal support, the plans must provide universal access to care with equal terms and conditions for all, cover all medically necessary services as determined by physicians, provide portable benefits (those that are in effect throughout the country), and be publicly administered on a nonprofit basis. The insured services of physicians include all medically required services rendered by licensed practitioners in hospitals, clinics, and doctors' offices. The insured services of hospitals include all inpatient services provided at the standard ward level, unless private or semiprivate accommodation is considered medically necessary, and all necessary drugs, biologic products, supplies, and diagnostic tests, as well as a broad range of outpatient services. The services of psychiatrists and mental hospitals are fully covered. There are no upper limits to the provision of care, as long as it is deemed medically necessary.

Despite Canada's universal coverage, the life expectancy of its citizens continues to vary according to income, although the disparity has decreased over the past 15 years. All industrialized countries report a similar phenomenon, underscoring the fact that life expectancy is derived from a variety of factors, including wealth, lifestyle, social policy, and access to medical care. In 1971, the difference in life expectancy at birth between earners of the highest and lowest incomes in Canada was 6.3 years for men, and 2.8 years for women. By 1986, according to a new study produced by the government, these differences had decreased to 5.6 years for men and 1.9 years for women.[5]

In sharp contrast to the United States, where the federal government holds far more authority over the financing of medical care than the states, Canadian health care is dominated by the provinces. The provincial medical associations are more influential than the Canadian Medical Association. In both domains, governmental and professional, the provincial entities strive to guard their prerogatives. The provinces have a broad constitutional authority to tax their citizens and private corporations. In consequence, they spend more in total tax revenues than the national government. Increasingly, the proportion (ranging from one fifth to one third) of tax revenues expended by the provinces is consumed by the provincial health insurance plans.

When Parliament established the conditions for the financing of Canadian medical care, government prohibited private insurers from paying for care already covered by the provincial plans. Thus, all funding for covered services flows through the provincial plans, which wield their monopsony powers (power of one buyer) to constrain expenditures. In this regard, the contrast with the United States is obvious, but as Evans recently pointed out, the comparison with the United Kingdom is more instructive.[1] The British National Health Service (NHS) is a public program, funded from tax revenue, and accessible to all. But if they so choose, people can seek care from a private system, to which about 8 percent of England's citizens have access—usually through their employers—as a way to avoid queues and receive care provided with more amenities.

In most Canadian provinces, it is not prohibited for patients to pay privately for medical or hospital care. What is prohibited is for physicians or hospitals to treat both patients whose care is financed by the provincial plans and patients who pay directly, as is the case in Britain. Evans views this prohibition as a critically important constraint. He writes:

> The British private consultant can use his dual role to select and steer patients according to their resources and the nature of their problems. He can even use his position within the NHS to manipulate waiting lists and other aspects of access so as to ensure that private care will be preferable to those who can afford it. The Canadian physician who decides to "go private" must go all the way. He cannot use a strategic position within the public system to cream off only the profitable patients for his private services.[1]

Canada's capacity to protect all its citizens against the economic consequences of illness at a cost that is socially acceptable has been widely admired, but its resistance to private funding makes it an exception in the Western world. Even in Sweden, a generous welfare state and one of the world's most highly taxed nations, the governing Social Democrats are promoting health care alternatives in the private sector and lower taxes. Kjell-Olof Feldt, Sweden's minister of finance and a leading advocate of private-sector alternatives to the nation's welfare state, said recently: "The squeeze in funds for the public sector has forced people to think in new ways."[6]

At both the national and the provincial levels, Canada's medical associations have been cautious in advocating multiple-source funding out of concern that such a stance would be seen more as promoting their members' self-interest than as bringing financial relief to the stressed provincial plans. One outspoken physician, Dr. John O'Brien-Bell, did express this view in 1989 in his farewell speech as president of the Canadian Medical Association. He said, "In a country that now spends 35 cents of every [tax] dollar servicing its debt, we have to ask ourselves whether we can maintain our high standards of health care without any involvement from the private sector." O'Brien-Bell suggested that an infusion of private resources would allow the provinces to raise "sorely needed" revenues to finance the strong patient demand for service.

CANADA'S STRUGGLE OVER CONFLICTING IMPERATIVES

As I suggested at the outset, Canada's provincial health insurance plans face an increasing financial struggle because of conflicting imperatives built into them at their creation. One source of tension is the moderation of support for the plans from the national government. As medical costs escalated in the 1970s, Ottawa concluded that it would have to abandon its practice of making an open-ended financial contribution to the plans. The original formula by which the provinces were encouraged to create their plans were based on an agreement that no matter how rapidly medical expenditures grew, Ottawa and the provinces would share the costs equally. This formula was incorporated into the Hospital Insurance and Diagnostic Services Act of 1957 and again in the Medical Care Act of 1971—the original federal laws on which the provincial plans were based.

Since 1977, through the enactment of the Federal–Provincial Fiscal Arrangements and Established Programs Act, the provincial governments have been placed at higher risk for increases in the cost of medical care. This change came about because the 1977 law linked the annual increase in the federal contribution to the provincial health insurance plans to the growth of the gross national product, leaving the provinces to absorb more of the health care costs when the aggregate outlays for health grew faster than the economy as a whole; health costs have increased more rapidly than the growth of Canada's economy in 8 of the past 13 years.

In 1986 and again in 1989, as Mulroney's government has sought to reduce an annual budget deficit of $30.5 billion (Canadian) on federal tax revenues of $112.4 billion, the Progressive Conservatives have altered the formula for the federal transfer of funds in ways that reduce the growth of Ottawa's contribution to the provincial plans (as well as to the costs of post-secondary education). Instead of a transfer formula based on the growth rate of a three-year running average of the gross national product, the formula is now based on this same prescription minus 3 percentage points of the gross national product. In the years 1987, 1988, and 1989, Canada's gross national product grew at rates of 9.4 percent, 9.2 percent, and 7.1 percent, respectively. The 3 percentage point reduction may seem small, but its cumulative effect on the provincial health budgets will amount to billions of dollars by the early 1990s.

To illustrate, data from Health and Welfare Canada show that Ottawa provided 44.6 percent of the total revenues of $14.1 billion expended by the provincial health insurance plans in fiscal 1979 and 1980. A decade later, Health and Welfare Canada estimates that the provincial plans will spend $39.2 billion in 1989 and 1990, only 36.7 percent of which will have been provided by the national government. In future years, officials in Ottawa anticipate that federal transfers, as a proportion of provincial health expenditures, will drop to percentages in the low 30s, although the precise projections are kept confidential. This trend, buried in the minutiae of federal–provincial transfer payments, has provoked little opposition from the provincial governments or the medical profession, although it is certain to intensify pressures on the health insurance plans.

One of the interesting aspects of Canadian health care is that the public is remarkably uninvolved in the ongoing struggles over resource allocation that pit the provincial governments against providers of care. An official of the Ontario Medical Association characterized this conflict as "tuxedo warfare," and with good reason. As political scientists would say, it engages the "elite" interest of government and medicine. Except for the occasional consumer who encounters an obstacle in obtaining access to care, the average citizen is not concerned about allocations of medical resources because government has insulated citizens time and again from worrying about the rising cost of care. Although Canadians pay the bill through general taxation (and in addition residents of Alberta and British Columbia pay legislated monthly premiums), the relation between the financing of care and the citizens to whom it is delivered is not tightly drawn, because patients do not pay at the point of service. Effective January 1 [1990], Ontario's provincial government abolished monthly premiums, which had been paid in roughly equal amounts by workers and employers, in favor of a payroll tax strictly on employers. In so doing it reinforced its policy that all possible obstacles to access should be removed. The income from premiums totaled about 13 percent of the current annual expenditure of $13.9 billion by the Ontario plan. One consequence of the overriding preference of policy makers to insulate consumers from paying for care directly is that the level of public support for the provincial plans remains very high. For example, a survey conducted in Decem-

ber 1987 for the Ontario Medical Association of attitudes toward the health care system in Ontario found that the vast majority of people (87 percent) were "very" (39 percent) or "somewhat" (48 percent) satisfied.

The outstanding recent example of government's commitment to safeguard unlimited access by patients to medical care came in 1984, when Parliament unanimously approved the Canada Health Act. In essence, this measure forced the provinces to ban the practice of extra billing by physicians (the charging of fees to patients in excess of those allowed by the provincial benefit schedule) and the practice of hospitals' charging fees directly to inpatients. Over the strong opposition of organized medicine, every province enacted legislation implementing the ban, because a failure to do so would have meant the loss of federal grants, dollar for dollar, in proportion to the amount of extra billing and user fees imposed on patients by providers. In Ontario, the provincial legislature's action provoked the longest strike by physicians in the nation's history—25 days—and ruptured relations between the provincial government and the Ontario Medical Association, which characterized the new policy as a "mortal attack on our professional freedom." The passions stirred by the strike were not altogether matched by the actions of the province's physicians; most continued to treat their patients, as data compiled by the provincial plan show. The numbers of bills submitted to the plan by physicians during the strike (from June 12 through July 6, 1986), expressed as a percentage of the average billing for each day of the week from May 1 through July 31, were: Sunday, 93.5 percent; Monday, 69.0 percent; Tuesday, 76.1

percent; Wednesday, 82.0 percent; Thursday, 82.4 percent; Friday, 80.1 percent; and Saturday, 88.1 percent.

CONSTRAINING THE DIFFUSION OF MEDICAL TECHNOLOGY

An important feature of Canada's approach to hospital budgeting is the separation of operating expenses and capital spending. Every year, Canada's 1243 hospitals (all but 9 of which are nonprofit institutions) must negotiate their annual operating budgets with the provincial government. They must apply separately for the approval and funding of new capital acquisitions. Thus, the provincial ministries have two major levers with which to control hospital growth. In some instances, hospitals raise private funds for new technological services through contributions from the community and philanthropic donors, but if an acquisition has not previously been approved by the government, the provincial plans often deny the necessary operating funds.

Through this process, the provincial plans have successfully contained the growth of hospital resources, including labor, supplies, and equipment. In three separate studies, Detsky and colleagues have documented the success of this strategy as applied by the Ontario Health Insurance Plan.[7-9] A central feature of the strategy, used by all the provincial plans, is to distribute forms of medical technology according to region in a fashion that compels physicians to judge carefully which patients would profit from their use. Virtually all the most sophisticated forms of technology are diffused in teaching hospitals only. One consequence of this effort to restrain the use of modern techniques is that such techniques are far less available in Canada than in the United States. For example, a recent study by Rublee showed that in comparison with the Federal Republic of Germany and the United States, Canada has appreciably slowed the diffusion of six major forms of technology: open-heart surgery, cardiac catheterization, organ transplantation, radiation therapy, extracorporeal shock-wave lithotripsy, and magnetic resonance imaging (MRI).[10] Key comparisons between Canada and the United States reveal that there are nearly eight times more MRI and radiation-therapy units per capita in the United States, more than six times as many lithotripsy centers, roughly three times as many cardiac catheterization and open-heart surgery units, and slightly more organ transplantation units. Rublee, a researcher affiliated with the AMA, conceded that "the differences in levels of major technology, in themselves, indicate little about the overall effectiveness, achievements, and weaknesses of the health care systems of any of the three countries studied."[10]

For the visitor to Canada, the growing conflict over the availability of technology is most readily seen in the newspaper articles and televised news accounts that report obstacles to the system's vaunted access to care, usually in a hospital setting. As the provincial plans restrain the use of technology, physicians increasingly face the difficult choice of providing care on the basis of medical need rather than rendering it to all who could benefit. Some forms of technology are more valuable than others, as is the case in all countries, but most have not been subjected to clinical trials. Recognizing the need for more information, in early December the federal, provincial, and territorial health ministers announced the creation of a Canadian

NO John K. Iglehart / 17

Coordinating Office for Health Technology Assessment.

The prime illustration of the problems provincial plans and providers are encountering in their efforts to match available resources with an effective system of triaging patients was provided by the case of Charles Coleman, a 63-year-old man who died shortly after a heart operation in a Toronto hospital. Coleman's operation had been postponed 11 times. *Maclean's*, a Canadian weekly magazine, ran a cover story[11] about the case that provoked the Ontario Health Insurance Plan to investigate the cardiac-surgery program at St. Michael's Hospital in Toronto.

The three investigators identified various problems at St. Michael's and eight other Ontario teaching hospitals that offer adult cardiac-surgery programs for the province's 9 million citizens.[12] The team found a substantial increase in the length of the waiting lists and of the wait for cardiac surgery at St. Michael's; the number of patients waiting had increased from 38 in 1984 to 232 by 1989, and the wait had increased from two to three weeks to three to five months. These trends were consistent with conditions in other Toronto-area hospitals; in the same period, the total number of patients waiting increased from 356 in 1984 to 848 by 1989, and the length of the wait increased from two to three weeks to three to nine months. Although the waiting lists have grown, the number of cardiovascular surgical procedures performed at St. Michael's and some of the other hospitals began to decline in 1986. The number of cardiac surgeons performing operations has remained about the same.

A number of problems combined to lengthen the waiting lists and times and reduce the total number of cases that could be accommodated, the investigators found. An older patient population (the average age increased from 51 to 61 over the past decade) requiring longer hospitalizations was having cardiac operations and staying longer in the intensive care unit; a pronounced shortage of nurses trained in cardiac care forced a closure of beds in the cardiovascular ward, which in turn reduced the number of planned discharges from intensive care; and new methods of treating patients who have had heart attacks increased the number of patients requiring cardiac catheterization and ultimately cardiac surgery. Dr. Martin Barkin, the deputy minister of health, commented in an interview:

> We clearly did fall behind on cardiovascular surgery, and we're now quickly moving to bring that back up to standard. But that was not a deliberate withholding of funding because we wanted to have a queue there, it's because we couldn't respond fast enough to certain changes in practice patterns.[13]

Barkin's comment points up one aspect of a planned health care system. Although it has a greater capacity at first for rational allocation of resources, its strictly planned nature inhibits needed adjustments as circumstances change. Since the circumstances of Coleman's death triggered action, Ontario's health ministry has appointed a coordinator of cardiovascular services for the province, approved additional funding to expand the capacity of St. Michael's Hospital, and created Toronto's fourth cardiovascular-surgery unit as Sunnybrook Medical Centre—a project that had been planned for almost a decade. But these actions have not alleviated the problem totally. The head of St. Michael's cardiovascular division, Dr. Tom Salerno, put it simply in a recent telephone interview: "In reality, we are still going through a lot of hardship."

Because of the problems Canadians have had in gaining rapid access to some services (cardiac care, lithotripsy, radiotherapy, and renal dialysis), there has been an assumption, reinforced by news coverage, that patients in increasing numbers are turning for treatment to American medical facilities across the border. These reports were discussed last summer by the Pepper Commission in a meeting partly devoted to a review of Canadian health care. Representative Willis D. Gradison, Jr. (R-Ohio), asked the committee's staff members to investigate the reports. They surveyed 10 institutions—Buffalo General Hospital, the Cleveland Clinic, the Detroit Medical Center, Henry Ford Hospital, Johns Hopkins Medical Center, Massachusetts General Hospital, the Mayo Clinic, the Memorial Sloan–Kettering Cancer Center, the University of Rochester Medical Center, and the University of Washington Medical Center. Only two of the institutions provided evidence that they had treated a substantial number of Canadians. Buffalo General reported that 3 percent of its patients were Canadian and that 50 of the 100 patients receiving monthly lithotripsy treatments were doing so under a formal agreement with the province of Ontario. The University of Washington Medical Center reported that 125 of the 250 in vitro fertilization procedures it performed annually involved Canadians, who paid about $5,000 out of pocket for each procedure. On the basis of these findings, the commission's staff reported to Gradison on August 10 that there was "no evidence that substantial numbers of Canadians are seeking care at American medical centers." In the vast number of cases, Canadians normally travel only to medical institutions adjacent to the border for treatment, so the survey was somewhat skewed because of the inclusion of hospitals located farther away. More recently, patients in western Ontario who have needed cardiac surgery have been sent to St. John's Hospital in Detroit under an agreement initiated by physicians in Windsor, Ontario, and accepted by the provincial health insurance plan.

SUPPLY AND INCOMES OF PHYSICIANS

In 1986, I noted that most Western nations have a common problem of public policy: they are training more physicians than they seem prepared to accommodate, but few have decided how many physicians are enough.[14] That is certainly the case in Canada, where neither the federal nor the provincial government, organized medicine, nor the Association of Canadian Medical Colleges has adopted a definitive policy on the matter. In its most recent comment on the subject, in 1989, the Canadian Medical Association declared cautiously that it was "committed to working with governments, the medical profession, hospital associations and other parties" to strike "the best balance of physician resources to realize the objective of improving health status."[15]

The pool of Canadian physicians has grown faster than the population every year since 1965, and medicine remains an attractive profession despite the problems doctors encounter. The number of physicians leaving Canada each year, presumably to practice elsewhere, has decreased from 663 to 1978 to 386 in 1985;

more stringent U.S. immigration policies may influence this trend. For each of the 1759 first-year positions filled by students in Canada's 16 medical schools in the academic year 1988–1989, there was an average of four applicants, as compared with a ratio of 1:1.6 in the United States. Eva Ryten, director of the Office of Research and Information Services of the Association of Canadian Medical Colleges, said in an interview: "On average, we have a more able applicant pool today than we had a decade ago. So medical schools are rejecting more highly qualified applicants now." There were 7124 medical school students (44.4 percent of whom were women) enrolled in Canadian universities in 1988–1989, as compared with 7492 in the peak year of 1982–1983. The total number of postdoctoral residency training positions in Canadian teaching hospitals has remained largely stable (7621 in 1989, as compared with 7633 in 1985 and 6870 in 1981), although more positions (an increase from 625 in 1981 to 1262 in 1989) are being funded by sources other than the health ministries (internal funds of the medical faculties, foreign governments, charitable foundations, and organizations established to combat a single disease), particularly in Ontario. This development saves the health ministries some money, but it does not alter the number of new doctors being produced.

As of December 1988, there were 48,706 active civilian physicians, excluding interns and residents, as compared with 35,432 a decade earlier and 25,656 in 1970. The population per practicing physician has declined over this period, from 837 in 1970 to 525 in December 1988; it ranges from a high of 766 people per physician in New Brunswick to a low of 490 in British Columbia and Quebec. In

sharp contrast to the United States, where the number of primary care physicians is dwindling in proportion to the total supply, general and family practitioners represent 52.5 percent of all doctors in Canada; in most of Canada's urban areas, the demand for general practitioners is saturated. The medical specialties generally deemed to be in short supply are general surgery, psychiatry, medical and radiation oncology, and neonatology and the other pediatric subspecialties. In 1987, 16.8 percent of all practicing Canadian physicians were women. The rapidly increasing numbers of women will influence the availability of care, because in that same year male generalist physicians reported working 49.1 hours per week, and their female counterparts 38.6 hours. Male medical specialists reported working 50.1 hours per week in 1987, and their female counterparts 43.6 hours.

There are various reasons that medicine remains, on balance, an attractive profession in Canada. One is that physicians are held in high esteem even though their public image has diminished a bit over the years. Another reason is that because the 16 medical schools are public, university-based institutions, they are subsidized heavily by the federal and provincial governments. In 1988–1989, medical students paid school fees ranging from approximately $750 a year in Quebec to $3,000 a year in British Columbia. Thus, very few Canadian medical students begin their professional careers heavily in debt, in contrast to students in the United States.

Another important reason for the continued appeal of medicine as a career is that despite the growing number of practicing doctors, physicians remain Canada's highest-paid professionals, according to the reports of the Department

Table 1

Average Practice Expenses and Net Incomes of Self-Employed Physicians in Ontario and the United States in 1986, According to Specialty*

Specialty	Ontario		United States	
	Expenses	Income	Expenses	Income
		thousands of U.S. dollars		
General practice	54.6	78.6	119.9†	84.3†
Family practice	54.9	74.7		
Internal medicine	57.3	121.9	110.5	118.6
Anesthesia	24.4	106.4	96.7	160.6
Psychiatry	35.0	91.0	46.7	98.3
Pediatrics	63.9	103.4	93.2	90.8
General surgery	63.3	109.7	112.3	152.8
Orthopedic surgery	68.4	130.4	210.3	212.8
Urology	28.2	136.1	125.5	136.6
Ophthalmology	90.6	116.4	152.3	163.5
Otolaryngology	80.2	132.5	159.6	154.2
Obstetrics and gynecology	75.7	114.9	149.5	144.5
Pathology	100.0	106.1	67.8	177.8

*The sources of these data are the Ontario Medical Association, which bases its data on information provided by Revenue Canada, and the American Medical Association's Socioeconomic Monitoring System. Income figures for Ontario are based on data for physicians whose income is derived soley from self-employment. U.S. physicians cited are nonfederal patient care practitioners.

†Figures for general practice and family practice are combined in the AMA data.

of National Health and Welfare last October, based on taxation data from Revenue Canada. Expressed in U.S. dollars, the average net income of physicians was $84,700 in 1987, as compared with $70,800 for dentists, $63,500 for lawyers and notaries, and $49,300 for accountants. A decade ago, the corresponding figures were $41,500 for physicians, $35,500 for dentists, $34,200 for lawyers and notaries, and $29,400 for accountants. For the sake of comparison, I asked the Center for Health Policy Research of the AMA how U.S. physicians' incomes compared with those of other professional groups. Although no precisely comparable survey was available, the data showed that U.S. physicians in private practice earned an average net income of $132,300 in 1987. Dentists in

independent private practice earned an average of $88,000 in the same year, according to the American Dental Association. The Bureau of Labor Statistics reported that lawyers working in the private sector had an average net income of $57,300, whereas those working in firms with two or more attorneys earned an average of $120,000.[16] The average income of men over the age of 25 working full-time who have had four years of college was $40,962.

Ontario's physicians are the highest-paid practitioners in Canada, on average. Table 1 compares their incomes with those of doctors in the United States, according to specialty. As the number of Canadian physicians has increased, the number of services they have provided to their patients has risen even more rapidly. This development has prompted 5 of Canada's 10 provinces—British Columbia, Saskatchewan, Manitoba, Ontario, and Quebec—to incorporate some method of accounting for increases in the use of services into their negotiations with the provincial medical associations about fee schedules.[17]

On the other hand, physicians themselves are less concerned about the effect of their increasing numbers on the financial accounts of the provincial plans than about what they regard as governments' contradictory efforts to squeeze spending while promoting universal access. Concern over the current trends has been expressed by physicians in academic medicine and organized medicine, as well as by individual practitioners who do not participate in medical politics. Dr. Frederick H. Lowy, a professor of psychiatry at the University of Toronto and former dean of its faculty of medicine, who recently chaired the Pharmaceutical Inquiry of Ontario, a commission established by the Ontario Ministry of Health to study the rapid rise in the cost of prescription drugs, summarized the sentiment in an interview:

> My physician colleagues are increasingly dissatisfied. Medical incomes are really quite good, that's not the central problem. It is more psychological. Physicians feel they are being increasingly conscripted by administrators and government. The cost containment methods allow government to negotiate from great strength. The playing field is quite unequal. There are significant restrictions on the availability of technology and hospital beds. Physicians are being asked to make unusual sacrifices compared to other segments of society.

A survey in 1989 of 608 physicians randomly selected from all parts of Ontario, conducted for the Ontario Medical Association, agreed with Lowy's view. When the physicians were asked whether they approved of the provincial government's handling of rising costs, 94 percent said they disapproved, and only 3 percent approved. Half the physicians polled said that they were finding it increasingly difficult to have patients admitted to hospitals; in Ontario, hospitals have an average occupancy of 90 percent.

CONCLUSION

In 1986, I reported that Canada's provincial health insurance plans resembled a pressure cooker building up steam on a hot stove.[18] Three and a half years later, the analogy holds, but the heat has been turned up. Canada's health care system is buffeted by conflicting forces—its strong commitment to universal access, of which Canadians are justifiably proud; the accelerating efforts of the provinces to control costs while they continue to expand the scope of covered benefits; and the increasing frustration of practicing physicians and hospital stewards who are caught in the middle. Until recently, these tensions have remained within manageable bounds throughout Canada, but whether that will continue, without a new accommodation, particularly if the national economy slows, is an open question. Most of the provinces have created blue-ribbon working groups in the past several years to seek solutions to identified problems, and these exercises have eased some of the tension temporarily. But it seems inevitable that Canada will eventually reopen the question of how care is financed. The provinces will jeopardize their capacity to support other social priorities if they continue to rely on tax revenues to finance unlimited access to most health services, and to produce more physicians than can be accommodated. At the same time, private investment could endanger the egalitarian nature of Canadian health care. Revising the current formulation of policy will require a more meaningful dialogue than exists at present among the federal and provincial governments, organized medicine, and other major stakeholders in the system. Without such dialogue, Canadians place at risk the future of their provincial health insurance plans, social enterprises that are admired throughout the Western world. The medical profession faces an additional challenge: to examine more rigorously the appropriateness and efficacy of the clinical care it renders.[19]

REFERENCES

1. Evans RG. "We'll take care of it for you" health care in the Canadian community. Daedalus 1988; 117(4):155–89.
2. Iglehart JK. The United States looks at Canadian health care. N Engl J Med 1989; 321:1767–72.
3. Doherty K. Is the Canadian system as good as it looks for employers? Bus Health 1989; 7(7):31–4.
4. Evans RG, Lomas J, Barer ML, et al. Controlling health expenditures—the Canadian reality. N Engl J Med 1989; 320:571–7.
5. Wilkins R, Adams O, Brancker A. Changes in mortality by income in urban Canada from 1972 to 1986; findings of a joint study undertaken by the Policy, Communications and Information branch, Health and Welfare Canada, and the Canadian Centre for Health Information, Statistics Canada, 1989.
6. Greenhouse S. Sweden's social democrats veer toward free market and lower taxes. New York Times, October 27, 1989:A3.
7. Detsky AS, Stacey SR, Bombardier C. The effectiveness of a regulatory strategy in containing hospital costs: the Ontario experience, 1967–1981. N Engl J Med 1983; 309:151–9.
8. Detsky AS, Abrams HB, Ladha L, Stacey SR. Global budgeting and the teaching hospital in Ontario. Med Care 1986; 24(1)89–94.
9. Detsky AS, O'Rourke K, Naylor DC, Stacey SR, Kitchens JM. Containing Ontario's hospital costs under universal insurance in the 1980s:

what was the record? Can Med Assoc J (in press).
10. Rublee DA. Medical technology in Canada, Germany, and the United States. Health Aff (Millwood) 1989; 8(3):178–81.
11. The crisis in health care: sick to death. Maclean's. February 13, 1989:32–5.
12. Kaminski VL, Sibbald WJ, Davis EM. Investigation of cardiac surgery at St. Michael's Hospital, Toronto, Ontario: final report, 1989.
13. Kosterlitz J. Taking care of Canada, Natl J 1989; 21(28):1792–7.
14. Iglehart JK. Canada's health care system: addressing the problem of physician supply. N Engl J Med 1986; 315:1623–8.
15. Canadian physician resources: report of the Canadian Medical Association committee on physician resources, August 21, 1989.
16. The 1989 survey of law firm economics. Ardmore, Pa.: Altman and Weil Management Consultants, 1989.
17. Lomas J, Fooks C, Rice T, Labella RJ. Paying physicians in Canada. Health Aff (Millwood) 1989; 8(1):80–102.
18. Iglehart JK. Canada's health care system. N Engl J Med 1986; 315:202–8.
19. Linton AI, Peachey DK. Utilization management: a medical responsibility. Can Med Assoc J 1989; 141:283–6.

POSTSCRIPT

Should the United States Adopt a National Health Insurance Program?

"An aura of inevitability is upon us," wrote George Lundberg, M.D., in *The Journal of the American Medical Association* (May 15, 1991). "It is no longer acceptable morally, ethically, or economically for so many of our people to be medically uninsured or seriously underinsured." Vicente Navarro expresses a similar opinion in "The Unhealth of Our Medical Sector," *Dissent* (Spring 1987). As millions of Americans remain uninsured, experts look to the Canadian program as a panacea for the problems facing the U.S. health care system. Would the Canadian system work in the United States?

Nearly one-third of U.S. states are currently investigating health insurance plans patterned to varying degrees after Canada's. In addition, labor unions and advocates for the poor continue to support moving to a Canadian-style system of health care. Those in favor of the Canadian system say Canadians have a valid claim: a successful, cost-efficient, working model with a long record of satisfying the majority of consumers and health providers. Opponents of the plan argue that although the United States and Canada have many fundamental similarities, Canada has a much smaller population that is considerably more racially and ethnically homogenous. Critics also argue that even if the United States adopted the Canadian system, costs would be significantly higher in the United States due to higher malpractice costs and the wasteful spending that results from defensive medicine.

What may surprise supporters of the current U.S. health care system is that some Canadian authorities doubt the wisdom of the United States trying to import a health care system from any other country. A major difference between Canadian and American patients is that Americans want health care on demand. Canadians accept and are more willing than Americans to wait for medical services. Physician J. Roy Rowland agrees that U.S. citizens are not used to waiting for health care, and he writes, "Countries with national health insurance invariably resort to rationing schemes which treat people in a discriminatory way and cause long waiting lines for treatment" ("Positive Cures Needed for Health Care Ills," *Private Practice*, February 1988).

ISSUE 2

Should Doctors Ever Help Terminally Ill Patients Commit Suicide?

YES: Timothy E. Quill, from "Death and Dignity: A Case of Individualized Decision Making," *The New England Journal of Medicine* (March 7, 1991)

NO: Leon R. Kass, from "Suicide Made Easy: The Evil of 'Rational' Humaneness," *Commentary* (December 1991)

ISSUE SUMMARY

YES: Timothy E. Quill, M.D., who describes a physician-assisted suicide, believes that doctors have roles other than healing and fighting against death.

NO: Physician Leon R. Kass argues that the weakening of the taboos against physician-assisted suicide is a bad idea whose time must never come.

Should doctors ever help their patients die? While doctors should provide every support possible to their dying patients, do they have the right or obligation to actually hasten the process if a patient requests it?

Some of the practices that were controversial a short time ago in the care of terminally ill patients have become accepted and routine. Many doctors now believe that it is ethical to use "do-not-resuscitate" orders on dying patients, while others feel that it is also acceptable to withhold food and water from patients who are hopelessly ill and dying. The word *euthanasia*, which comes from two Greek roots—the prefix *eu*, meaning good, fortunate, or easy, and the word *thanatos*, meaning death—describes a good or easy death. While withdrawing care or treatment (referred to as *passive euthanasia*) may be acceptable to many doctors, *active euthanasia*, or playing an active role in a patient's death, may not. One form of active euthanasia, physician-assisted suicide, has been the subject of numerous debates in recent years.

In early 1988, the *Journal of the American Medical Association* published a short article entitled "It's Over, Debbie" (January 8, 1988), which was written by an anonymous physician who described administering a lethal dose of morphine to a young woman with end-stage cancer. The doctor claimed her suffering was extreme and that there was absolutely no hope of recovery. The morphine was requested by the patient, who said, "Let's get this over

24

with." The patient died within minutes after receiving the drug, while the doctor looked on. This article generated a great deal of criticism because the doctor had only met the patient for the first time that evening and had not consulted with colleagues or family members before making his decision. The doctor did, however, believe he was correctly responding to the patient's request.

Soon after this incident, Dr. Jack Kevorkian assisted in the suicide of an Oregon woman who suffered from Alzheimer's disease. Dr. Kevorkian supplied the woman with a device that he developed—a "suicide machine"—which allowed her to give herself a lethal dose of drugs. Intense criticism followed regarding the ability of Dr. Kevorkian to diagnose the patient's illness (which was not immediately terminal) and whether or not the patient was able to make an informed decision to end her life.

In March 1991, Timothy E. Quill published an editorial in the *New England Journal of Medicine* that described an assisted suicide. A woman, Quill's patient for eight years, was dying of leukemia. She had decided not to undergo chemotherapy, which would have offered her only a 25 percent chance of long-term survival with considerable side effects. In addition to refusing treatment, the patient requested that Quill help her commit suicide.

In the following article, which is from that editorial, Quill discusses why he believes that an informed patient should have the right to choose or refuse treatment and to die with as much control and dignity as possible. Leon R. Kass, in opposition, argues against physician-assisted suicide and asserts that neither for love nor money should doctors ever kill.

YES

Timothy E. Quill

DEATH AND DIGNITY: A CASE OF INDIVIDUALIZED DECISION MAKING

Diane was feeling tired and had a rash. Her hematocrit was 22, and her white-cell count was 4.3 with some metamyelocytes and unusual white cells. I called Diane and told her it might be serious. When she pressed for the possibilities, I reluctantly opened the door to leukemia. Hearing the word seemed to make it exist. "Oh, shit!" she said. "Don't tell me that." I thought, I wish I didn't have to.

Diane was raised in an alcoholic family and had felt alone for much of her life. She had vaginal cancer as a young woman, and had struggled with depression and her own alcoholism for most of her adult life. I had come to know, respect, and admire her over the previous eight years as she confronted and gradually overcame these problems. During the previous three and a half years, she had abstained from alcohol and had established much deeper connections with her husband, her college-age son, and several friends. Her business and artistic work was blossoming. She felt she was living fully for the first time.

Unfortunately, a bone-marrow biopsy confirmed the worst: acute myelomonocytic leukemia. In the face of this tragedy, I looked for signs of hope. This is an area of medicine in which technological intervention has been successful, with long-term cures occurring 25 percent of the time. As I probed the costs of these cures, I learned about induction chemotherapy (three weeks in the hospital, probable infections, and hair loss; 75 percent of patients respond, 25 percent do not). Those who respond are then given consolidation chemotherapy (with similar side effects; another 25 percent die, thus a net of 50 percent survive). For those still alive to have a reasonable chance of long-term survival, they must undergo bone-marrow transplants (hospitalization for two months, a whole-body irradiation—with complete killing of the bone marrow—infectious complications; 50 percent of this group survive, or 25 percent of the original group). Though hematologists may argue over the exact percentage of people who will benefit from

From Timothy E. Quill, "Death and Dignity: A Case of Individualized Decision Making," *The New England Journal of Medicine*, vol. 324, no. 10 (March 7, 1991), pp. 691–694. Copyright © 1991 by The Massachusetts Medical Society. Reprinted by permission.

therapy, they don't argue about the outcome of not having any treatment—certain death in days, weeks, or months.

Believing that delay was dangerous, the hospital's oncologist broke the news to Diane and made plans to begin induction chemotherapy that afternoon. When I saw her soon after, she was enraged at his presumption that she would want treatment and devastated by the finality of the diagnosis. All she wanted to do was go home and be with her family. She had no further questions about treatment and, in fact, had decided that she wanted none. Together we lamented her tragedy. I felt the need to make sure that she and her husband understood that there was some risk in delaying, that the problem would not go away, and that we needed to keep considering the options over the next several days.

Two days later Diane, her husband, and her son came to see me. They had talked at length about the problem and the options. She remained very clear about her wish not to undergo chemotherapy and to live whatever time she had left outside of the hospital. Her family wished she would choose treatment but accepted her decision. She articulated very clearly that it was she who would be experiencing all the side effects of treatment and that one-in-four odds were not good enough for her to undergo so toxic a course of therapy. I had her repeat her understanding of the treatment, the odds, and the consequences of forgoing treatment. I clarified a few misunderstandings, but she had a remarkable grasp of the options and implications.

I HAVE LONG BEEN AN ADVOCATE OF THE idea that an informed patient should have the right to choose or refuse treatment, and to die with as much control and dignity as possible. Yet there was something that disturbed me about Diane's decision to give up a 25 percent chance of long-term survival in favor of almost certain death. Diane and I met several times that week to discuss her situation, and I gradually came to understand the decision from her perspective. We arranged for home hospice care, and left the door open for her to change her mind.

Just as I was adjusting to her decision, she opened up another area that further complicated my feelings. It was extraordinarily important to Diane to maintain her dignity during the time remaining to her. When this was no longer possible, she clearly wanted to die. She had known of people lingering in what was called "relative comfort," and she wanted no part of it. We spoke at length about her wish. Though I felt it was perfectly legitimate, I also knew that it was outside of the realm of currently accepted medical practice and that it was more than I could offer or promise. I told Diane that information that might be helpful was available from the Hemlock Society.

A week later she phoned me with a request for barbiturates for sleep. Since I knew that this was an essential ingredient in a Hemlock Society suicide, I asked her to come to the office to talk things over. She was more than willing to protect me by participating in a superficial conversation about her insomnia, but it was important to me to know how she planned to use the drugs and to be sure that she was not in despair or overwhelmed in a way that might color her judgment. In our discussion, it was apparent that she was having trouble sleeping, but it was also evident that the security of having enough barbiturates available to commit suicide, if and when the time came, would give her the peace of mind she needed to live fully in the present. She was not despondent and, in fact, was making deep, personal connections with her family and close friends. I made sure that she knew how to use the barbiturates for sleep, and how to use them to commit suicide. We agreed to meet regularly, and she promised to meet with me before taking her life. I wrote the prescriptions with an uneasy feeling about the boundaries I was exploring—spiritual, legal, professional, and personal. Yet I also felt strongly that I was making it possible for her to get the most out of the time she had left.

The next several months were very intense and important for Diane. Her son did not return to college, and the two were able to say much that had not been said earlier. Her husband worked at home so that he and Diane could spend more time together. Unfortunately, bone weakness, fatigue, and fevers began to dominate Diane's life. Although the hospice workers, family members, and I tried our best to minimize her suffering and promote comfort, it was clear that the end was approaching. Diane's immediate future held what she feared the most: increasing discomfort, dependence, and hard choices between pain and sedation. She called her closest friends and asked them to visit her to say good-bye, telling them that she was leaving soon. As we had agreed, she let me know as well. When we met, it was clear that she knew what she was doing, that she was sad and frightened to be leaving but that she would be even more terrified to stay and suffer.

Two days later her husband called to say that Diane had died. She had said her final good-byes to her husband and son that morning, and had asked them to leave her alone for an hour. After an hour, which must have seemed like an eternity, they found her on the couch, very still and covered by her favorite shawl. They called me for advice about how to proceed. When I arrived at their house we talked about what a remarkable person she had been. They seemed to have no doubts about the course she had chosen, or about their cooperation, although the unfairness of her illness and the finality of her death were overwhelming to us all.

I called the medical examiner to inform him that a hospice patient had died. When asked about the cause of death, I said acute leukemia. He said that was fine and that we should call a funeral director. Although acute leukemia was the truth, it was not the whole story. But any mention of suicide would probably have brought an ambulance, efforts at resuscitation, and a police investigation. Diane would have become a "coroner's case," and the decision to perform an autopsy would have been made at the discretion of the medical examiner. The family or I could have been subjected to criminal prosecution; I could have been subjected to a professional review. Although I truly believe that the family and I gave her the best care possible, allowing her to define her limits and directions, I am not sure the law, society, or the medical profession would agree.

Diane taught me about the range of help I can provide people if I know them well and if I allow them to express what they really want. She taught me about taking charge and facing tragedy squarely when it strikes. She taught me about life, death, and honesty, and that I can take small risks for people I really know and care about.

NO

Leon R. Kass

SUICIDE MADE EASY: THE EVIL OF "RATIONAL" HUMANENESS

Americans have always been a handy people. If know-how were virtue, we would be a nation of saints. Unfortunately, certain old-fashioned taboos— brought to you by the people who know the difference between virtue and dexterity—have prevented Americans from gaining the ultimate know-how, the know-how to die. Until now. Riding atop the best-seller lists, outdistancing other manuals of self-help like *The Seven Habits of Highly Effective People*, *The T-Factor Fat Gram Counter*, and *Wealth Without Risk*, is Derek Humphry's latest book, *Final Exit*,[1] subtitled "The Practicalities of Self-Deliverance and Assisted Suicide for the Dying." Know-how in spades.

What can one say about this new "book"? In one word: evil. I did not want to read it, I do not want you to read it. It should never have been written, and it does not deserve to be dignified with a review, let alone an article. Yet it stares out at us from nearly every bookstore window, beckoning us to learn how to achieve the final solution—for ourselves or for those we (allegedly) love so much that we will help them kill themselves. Says the Lord High Executioner, Derek Humphry, prophet of Hemlock: I have set before thee life and death: therefore choose death. "Courageous," bleat the media; "Timely." "Rational." "Humane." Is there no one who will call evil by its proper name?

This is not the usual and notorious evil of malicious intent or violent manner; this is humanitarian evil, evil with a smile: well-meaning, gentle, and rational, especially rational. For this reason it is both harder to recognize as evil and harder to combat. Yet, also for this reason, it deserves our most vigilant attention, for it is an exquisite model of modern rationalism gone wrong, while looking oh so right.

Duty requires a few words about the contents of the book. Following an introduction which tells us that the book is "aimed at helping the public and the health professional achieve death with dignity for those who desire to plan for it," the (longer) first of two parts is addressed to the public and especially those interested in "exiting." Here there are 22 chapters guiding the gentle reader ever so gently, step by step, into that gentle good night, from "The Most Difficult Decision" (a mere 3½ pages, ending with "Once these documents [Living Will and Durable Power of Attorney] are completed you are ready to tackle the other aspects of bringing your life to an end"), through (among others) "Shopping for the Right Doctor," "Beware of the Law," "Storing Drugs," "Who Shall Know?," "Insurance," "Letters to Be Written," and "Self-Deliverance Via the Plastic Bag," all leading up to "The Final Act," complete with detailed instructions for doing the deadly deed. Chapter 23 provides a check list of 16 items, after which drug-dosage tables are supplied for eighteen effective drugs. A shorter second part, addressed to doctors and nurses eager to assist, concludes with a short pharmacopoeia, rich in detail and editorial advice. A brief (and one-sidedly pro-death) bibliography, the text of the Hemlock Society's Model Death with Dignity Act, and brief notes about the author and the Hemlock Society conclude the book, save for a copious index from Abalgin to Zyklon-B gas.

DEREK HUMPHRY, WHO ASSISTED IN THE suicide of his first wife (though it was a felony), and who (along with his second wife, Ann Wickett) founded the Hemlock Society in 1980, has been the country's leading spokesman and protagonist for euthanasia in all its forms. A journalist by profession, a euthanist by conviction, a diligent student and publicist, he has researched far and wide in preparing this most handy guide. . . .

[T]he author is calm, cool, and collected, and marvelously matter-of-fact. His confident voice of experience guides us through every step of the process,

allaying anxieties, dispelling doubts, showing us exactly how-to-do-it. Adopting a tone and manner midway between the Frugal Gourmet and Mister Rogers, Humphry has written a book that reads like "A Salt-Free Guide to Longer Life" or "How to Conquer Fear in Twenty-two Easy Lessons." The reader, blinded by blandness, nearly loses sight of the big picture: this self-appointed messiah is indiscriminately and shamelessly teaching suicide (and worse) to countless strangers.

Humphry sanctimoniously insists that his book is not intended for everyone.[2] He intends, he avers, to be helpful *only* to those who are (or will be) *terminally* ill and who wish a quiet release from pain, suffering, or indignity. He even publishes a "Euthanizer-General's Warning"—but buries it in the footnotes to the drug-dosage table on the last page of Part 1, after all the lethal instructions have been given—telling us that "this information is meant for consideration only for a *mature adult who is dying* and wishes to know about self-deliverance." His concern for the others is touching, if brief:

ADVICE:
If you are considering taking your life because you are unhappy, cannot cope, or are confused please do not read this table but contact a Crisis Intervention Center or Suicide Prevention Center. (Look in the telephone book. It may be under "Hotlines.") *An unfinished life is a terrible thing to waste.* [Emphasis added.]

Whom are we kidding? Ever since Socrates' attack on writing, everyone knows that one cannot control who reads what is written or what is done with it. Only a fool could believe—and only a knave would pretend—that Humphry's instructions will be heeded only by the desperately dying or that his belated, brief, and saccharine advice to the depressed will lead them to re-embrace their precious unfinished lives.

The Centers for Disease Control have just reported that one in twelve American high-school students (grades 9–12)—or nearly 276,000 teenagers—tried to commit suicide in 1990, and more than one in four seriously contemplated it. Of those attempting, one in four—2 percent of the entire population—sustained serious injuries. (The rate of "successful" suicide attempts is roughly eleven deaths per 100,000 students, or 365 teenage suicides per year.) Thanks to Derek Humphry's book, our youth need no longer fail. Though the drugs he recommends require a doctor's prescription, they are, in fact, ubiquitous and easily available, as he surely knows ("Inspect your medicine cabinet for any barbiturates left over . . ."). And thanks to his instructions about sleeping pills, alcohol, and the proper way to use plastic bags, successful "self-deliverance" is available to anyone who can read—or who has a "loving friend" who can read. Even if only one teenager is now helped to suicide, Derek Humphry will have a lot to answer for.

Humphry has no intention of aiding poisoners, any more than he wishes to improve the suicide rate of the young. But he is, here too, equally naive, reprehensibly so. He is not so innocent as to be unaware of the danger, and in one (but only one) brief sentence—buried in the chapter on secrecy, "A Private Affair?"—makes a dashing display of his eagerness to prevent foul play: "I do not propose to name the drugs which are hard to trace because that information could possibly aid people with evil intent toward the lives of others." But such

people need not have evil intent; they could be merely compassionate toward senile Aunt Agatha—or just tired of visiting her or of paying the medical and nursing bills. Anyone with homicidal intent has been taught more lethal pharmacology than he ever needs to know—and also how to avoid detection. Just two pages before this pious refusal to help the wicked, Humphry has counseled the aiders-in-dying to refuse permission for autopsy, in order that death might pass as from "natural causes."

EVEN IGNORING THE INTENDERS-OF-EVIL, the teenagers, and the others whom Humphry excludes from his audience because they are "emotional," not "rational," it is perfectly clear that his intended readership is in fact much broader than the now or soon-to-be terminally ill. In a chapter on "The Dilemma of Quadriplegics," he embraces the principle of self-determination, terminal disease or not: "I respect the right of that small number of quadriplegics who want—either now or in the future—to have self-deliverance without being preached to and patronized by those on the religious Right." Not just terminal cancer but *any* sort of illness can qualify: "Nobody wants to die, yet life with *an incurable* or *degenerative illness* can be *unacceptable* for some people. Therefore, death is the preferred alternative" (emphasis added).

The elderly or the infirm or the demented or the blind—and, presumably, also the lonely or the humbled or the unwanted—are also on Humphry's compassionate and philanthropic mind: "I am not for one moment *advocating* that elderly people, or patients with degenerative diseases, *should* take their lives. It is *too personal* a decision" (emphasis added). Advocacy no, able assistance yes.

On the very same page, Humphry coins a new term to cover those who, alas, have no fatal disease to carry them off—"what I call 'terminal old age' "—a euphemism that can now justify death for the not-dying.

Nor is Humphry shy about facilitating euthanasia for people with Alzheimer's disease: "There is a trend in the euthanasia movement to legislate only for physician aid-in-dying for the terminal patient who is rational. . . . But I believe that to duck responsibility for the incompetent patient is a serious gap in our humanitarian cause." Today the rational and terminal, tomorrow the blind and the lame, the deaf and the dumb: let there be nothing but compassion (and "aid-in-dying") for those who choose death—and even for those poor "incompetents" whose debility or loss of dignity convinces us that they *would* choose death had they only mind enough to do so. Thus does the right to choose one's own death become quickly mixed up with the right to "choose" someone else's.

One cannot exaggerate the importance of this difficulty, for it is buried by sloppy reasoning and by the (yes) emotional appeal of the insistence on choice. If suicide (and its assistance) is to be justified by a right to choose the time and manner of one's death, if the right of life, liberty, and the pursuit of happiness or the so-called right of privacy encompasses also a "right to die," then (as Humphry argues) the whole matter is "too personal" and subjective; and the case for suicide need not rest on *any* objective or demonstrable criteria—such as certifiable terminal illness or truly intractable pain. For who is to say what makes life "unbearable," or death "electable," for another person? The autonomy argument kicks out all criteria for

evaluating the choice, save that it be uncoerced.

Of course no one, not even Humphry, wants to leave it at that. Instead, reasons are given to justify choosing death: too much pain, loss of dignity, lack of self-command, poor quality of life. These are supposed to add up to a plausible verdict: life is no longer worth living. Such "useless" or "degrading" or "dehumanized" lives now plead for active, "merciful" termination—*choice or no choice.*

THE LINE BETWEEN VOLUNTARY AND NON-voluntary (or involuntary) euthanasia cannot hold in practice, not least because it cannot be sustained in theory. Once suicide and assisting suicide are okay, for reasons of "mercy," then delivering the dehumanized is okay, whether chosen or not. Humphry and his crowd are well aware of the slippery slope. Yet pretending to want only a partial slide, they have both embraced the principle and started us on a decline that will take us all the way—to eliminating everyone deemed unfit.

This is already happening in Holland, as we are now beginning to discover. Humphry, like many other enthusiastic euthanists, touts the Dutch experience of physician-assisted suicide and treats it as a model, presenting a disingenuously rosy picture of the practice.[3] But the newly emerging truth should help restore sanity. In a recent book, *Regulating Death,*[4] Carlos S. Gomez reports that the practice in fact ignores virtually all the self-imposed guidelines and standards imposed by the Netherlands Medical Society: physicians sometimes do not seek a second opinion before administering death; they do not report the deed or even note it on the death certificate; where they do report euthanasia, no one investigates the facts; where someone does investigate, the physician controls all the evidence; and—quite clearly—they euthanize some patients who have *not* requested death. The practice is utterly unregulated—no big surprise to anyone who has given the matter any forethought.

Even more alarming is the newly released report of the government's Committee to Investigate the Practice of Euthanasia in Holland.[5] The report contains the most extensive and most reliable information to date on euthanasia in the Netherlands. Its reassuring conclusions are, to say the least, at great variance with the wealth of disturbing data it provides. Here are just a few of the findings: 25,300 cases of euthanasia (active and passive) occur in the Netherlands every year, 19.4 percent of all deaths in the country. These include 1,000 cases of *direct active involuntary* euthanasia. In addition, there are 8,100 cases in which morphine was overdosed with the intention to terminate life, 61 percent of the time without the patient's knowledge or consent. And there are another 8,750 cases in which life-preserving treatment was stopped or withheld without consent of the patient and with the intention to shorten life. "Low quality of life," "no prospect of improvement," and "the family could not take it anymore" were among the most frequently cited reasons to terminate patients' lives without their consent. In 45 percent of cases in which the lives of hospital patients were actively terminated without their consent, this was done without the knowledge of the families. Are you duly reassured? Hail to the Dutch, says Uncle Derek.

Hail also Dr. Jack Kevorkian, inventor of the suicide machine and self-appoint-ed father of "obitiatry," the doctoring of death. Humphry gives him ten pages, the longest chapter in the book, and praises him for "notable public service by forcing the medical profession to rethink its attitude on euthanasia." Having been present at Dr. Kevorkian's civil trial—I was a witness for the state on matters of medical ethics—and having read his testimony, watched his demeanor in court, read letters in which he promised to "help" a woman who later was found to be suffering merely from treatable migraine, and, above all, having seen the self-serving and manipulative videotape he made of his only conversation with the unfortunate Janet Adkins the day before he helped her to "self-deliver," I feel the deepest shame for my profession that he should be counted a member.

But what does Humphry know or care about medical ethics or the meaning of permission to kill for the doctor-patient relationship? He celebrates the new age in which "physicians are now more likely to be seen as 'friendly body technicians.'" Though he acknowledges the right of individual physicians to abstain for *personal* reasons from assistance-in-suicide, he has absolutely no idea of a *professional ethic* as such, or of why, for several thousand years, doctors have vowed neither to give nor suggest a deadly drug, not even if asked for it.[6]

True enough, many physicians fall far short of the professional ideal; many lack empathy or rely too heavily on technology. But will it really restore the ethical dimension constitutive of the profession if we permit doctors to become technical dispensers of death? What will happen to the doctor's unswerving allegiance to the patient's best interests once he is entitled to start thinking that death by injection is a possible "treatment option"? Drunk on what passes for compassionate caring, Humphry does not truly care.

Two further passages show his colors. In the first, Humphry helpfully drafts a model suicide note, to be written and signed as "your last letter." Here are the last letter's last words:

> If I am discovered before I have stopped breathing, I forbid anyone, including doctors or paramedics, to attempt to revive me. *If I am revived, I shall sue anyone who aided in this.* [Emphasis added.]

Compassionate words, intended to soften the blow when one finds one's loved one a suicide?

In the second vignette, concerning physician-and-nurse-assisted suicide, Humphry insists that the entire medical team must be informed about time and manner of the planned death. Why? Because "while everything must be done to reduce the stress on the medical team, a degree of emotional involvement in the dying of the patient is eminently worthwhile *to preserve an appreciation of the inherent sanctity of life*" (emphasis added). What kind of man would use "the inherent sanctity of life," no less, as a club to browbeat possibly reluctant nurses or doctors into participating in plans to kill?

No discussion of this book, especially in this magazine, could be complete without commenting on Humphry's respect for the fine work of his German counterparts, expressed at length in the chapter, "The Cyanide Enigma." After a (single) paragraph condemning the Nazi atrocities (but appreciating the swiftness of death by their Zyklon-B), Humphry rehabilitates the German euthanasia of the present day:

In the 1980's, the situation with regard to the suffering of terminally ill people was as tragic in Germany as elsewhere. Regardless of the terrible connotation given to the word "euthanasia" (which means help with a good death) by the Nazi atrocities, some people felt that compassionate action to help the dying was needed. In 1980, a pro-euthanasia society was formed, *Deutsche Gesellschaft Für Humanes Sterben* (German Society for Humane Dying), by a small group of brave people under the leadership of Hans Henning Atrott.

Unlike other countries, DGHS found it did not need to campaign for a change in the law on assisted suicide. There was no legal prohibition on helping another to die in justified circumstances so long as the request for help was clear and convincing.

The favorite method of DGHS is cyanide; Humphry, though he professes skepticism about peaceful death with cyanide, describes the German technique in minute detail, dosages included. He then goes on to praise "the simple cleverness of the DGHS method," which obviates the need for Zyklon-B gas by having the gas's active ingredient produced in the stomach following ingestion of potassium cyanide in water. Is not German science splendid? Does the high priest of euthanasia think that we have forgotten how to shudder?

LET ME NOT BE MISUNDERSTOOD. DYING IN our technological age, even in humanitarian institutions, often comes attended by horrors unknown to our ancestors, often as an unintentional consequence of medical success in the battle against death. Medicine or no medicine, mortality remains our lot. Yet our secular and utopian culture does not prepare us well to face this truth and its consequences. Both painful personal experience and serious study for over two decades have taught me to appreciate deeply the anguish and fear of patients and families in the myriad matters surrounding decay and death; I know and feel the horror of the way many of us now end our lives. There are many, many circumstances—too numerous, too particular, too nuanced to lay out in advance—that call for the cessation of medical intervention, even if death comes as a result. There is rarely a good reason for withholding proper doses of pain medication, even if providing effective analgesia runs an increased risk of earlier death. And there is much more that we can do—most of it a matter of human relations, not of technological devices—to support the morale and dignity of people faced with incurable or fatal illness.[7] But to cross the line and accept active euthanasia, mercy killing, "aid-in-dying," death from doctor's healing hand, "dignified autoeuthanasia," and "self-deliverance"—that way lies madness.

At the very least, we must now open our eyes to the situation before us. We must not allow ourselves to be gulled by euphemisms and by falsely calming images like "final exit." We must not accept Humphry's shallow notion that "dignity" can be delivered by a hypodermic needle filled with lethal medicine. We must not forget the cost-containers and the eugenicists who stand ready in the wings to exploit the "choice" for death, to make sure that the burdensome and incurable take advantage of the deadly option.[8] And, above all, we must not fall for the calm and matter-of-fact talk of "rational suicide."

Calmness and coolness are, by themselves, no proof of rationality. Neither is

deliberate planning, or the stockpiling of "magic pills." All human conduct is motivated—by desire or fear or some other appetite or emotion; thought alone moves nothing. However much Humphry talks of rationality—"It was not done out of cowardice or escapism but from long-held rational beliefs"; "Very, very few physicians will prescribe a lethal dose for a fit person. The stigma of being associated with a possible emotional suicide (as distinct from a rational suicide) is too risky"; etc.—the truth is that passions, sentiments, desires drive our every action. In the case of those explicitly addressed by this book, the dominant motives—the true movers of the soul—will be fear, resignation, and despair, or, in other words, the desire to escape. It is surely not pure reason that finds life unbearable.

Let's get serious about "rationality" and reason. Do we know what we are talking about when we claim that someone can *rationally* choose nonbeing or nothingness? How can poor reason even contemplate nothingness, much less accurately calculate its merits as compared with continued existence? What we have in so-called rational suicide is a mere rationality of means, rationality of technique, but utter *non*-rationality regarding the end and its putative goodness. An act of "rational suicide" may be psychologically understandable and (even, in some cases) morally pardonable, but it is utterly *un*reasonable.

Humphry and others contend that it is religious dogma alone, not human reason, which regards suicide as unethical. But this is patent nonsense. Immanuel Kant, whose claim to rationality is second to none, regarded the will to suicide as inherently self-contradictory, and thus, precisely, irrational:

It seems absurd that a man can injure himself (*volenti non fit injuria* [Injury cannot happen to one who is willing]). The Stoic therefore considered it a prerogative of his personality as a wise man to walk out of this life with an undisturbed mind whenever he liked (as out of a smoke-filled room), not because he was afflicted by actual or anticipated ills, but simply because he could make use of nothing more in this life. And yet this very courage, this strength of mind— of not fearing death and of knowing of something which man can prize more highly than his life—ought to have been an ever so much greater motive for him not to destroy himself, a being having such authoritative superiority over the strongest sensible incentives; consequently, it ought to have been a motive for him not to deprive himself of life.

Man cannot deprive himself of his personhood so long as one speaks of duties, thus so long as he lives. That man ought to have the authorization to withdraw himself from all obligation, i.e., to be free to act as if no authorization at all were required for this withdrawal, involves a contradiction. To destroy the subject of morality in his own person is tantamount to obliterating from the world, as far as he can, the very existence of morality itself; but morality is, nevertheless, an end in itself. Accordingly, to dispose of oneself as a mere means to some end of one's own liking is to degrade the humanity in one's person (*homo noumenon*), which, after all, was entrusted to man (*homo phaenomenon*) to preserve.

So-called "rational suicide" is finally a sophism. Those who preach it and abet it are teachers of evil.

MODERN RATIONALISM, WHOSE LEADING branch is modern natural science and whose purest fruit is medical technology, has certainly made human life less poor, brutish, and short. Yet because, being morally neutral, it knows only the means, never the end, it has left us lost at sea without a compass. Worst of all, blinded by pride in our technique, we do not even suspect that we are lost, that we have become, as Churchill put it, "the sport and presently the victim of tides and currents, whirlpools and tornadoes amid which [we are] far more helpless than [we have] been for a long time." We do not yet understand that the project for the mastery of nature and the conquest of death leads only to dehumanization; that any attempt to gain the tree of life by means of the tree of knowledge leads inevitably also to the hemlock; and that the utter rationalization of life under the banner of the will tragically produces a world in which we all get to become senile and in which our loved ones get to do us in.

The taboos against homicide, suicide, and euthanasia—like those against incest, adultery, and fornication, central insights of the receding wisdom from a more sensible age—are today weak and increasingly defenseless against the rising tide of gentle dehumanization. Yet they are all that stands between us and the flood. Everyone who cares truly for human dignity and decency—that is, everyone who would be truly rational— must now come to their defense, before it is too late.

NOTES

1. The Hemlock Society, 192 pp., $16.95.
2. Just after I wrote this sentence, in an eerie coincidence, a telephone call informed me of the suicide of Derek Humphry's (divorced) second wife, an act which he apparently deplored. In a display of despicable shamelessness, Humphry took out a quarter-page ad in the New York *Times* (October 14, 1991) distancing himself and the Hemlock Society from such "irrational suicides." He neglected to mention his earlier penchant for dis-

tance: two years ago, he abandoned and divorced this woman when she was diagnosed as having cancer.

3. Euthanasia and assisting suicide are still illegal in Holland, but the authorities have decided not to enforce the law. Here at home, happy reports about the Dutch practice played a large part in a campaign to make the state of Washington the first jurisdiction actively to legalize killing-on-request practiced by physicians.

4. The Free Press, 172 pp., $19.95.

5. Portions of the report have been translated for me by a Dutch acquaintance.

6. See my essay, "Neither For Love Nor Money: Why Doctors Must Not Kill," *Public Interest*, Winter 1989.

7. See my essay, "Death With Dignity & the Sanctity of Life," COMMENTARY, March 1990.

8. There is not a word in this book about the current economic crisis in health care and the pressures that already throw people with chronic illness prematurely out of the hospital. The partisans of "right to die" and the partisans of "cut the costs," strange bedfellows, are incubating a deadly outcome for the vulnerable, the elderly, and the powerless.

POSTSCRIPT

Should Doctors Ever Help Terminally Ill Patients Commit Suicide?

As our population ages and the incidence of certain diseases, such as cancer and AIDS, continues to increase, it appears that the ranks of the dying and suffering will grow. In the past, there were limited means of prolonging life; however, due to advances in modern medicine and technology, the dying can be kept alive sometimes lengthy time periods. As a result, some doctors are beginning to speak more often of euthanasia. Euthanasia is already being practiced in the Netherlands, but in the United States the American Medical Association has unequivocally reaffirmed its opposition to the practice. It refers to euthanasia as a euphemism for intentional killing and claims that "this is not part of the practice of medicine, with or without the consent of the patient."

The Dutch have taken a different viewpoint: In the past several years, thousands of Dutch have died by their own choice with the help of their doctors. While Dutch law still refers to euthanasia as a crime, the highest courts there have determined that doctors may practice it if they follow specific guidelines set up by the Royal Dutch Medical Association. Currently, it is estimated that 11 percent of Dutch AIDS patients die in this manner. An article in *Hippocrates*, "The Gentle Death" (September/October 1989), discusses this ability of the Dutch to have their wish to die granted by their physicians. "Is It Time for Mercy Killing?" the *Washington Post* (August 15, 1989) debates the euthanasia issue. Susan Wolf, an associate for law at the Hastings Center, argues that the consequences of easing the restrictions against euthanasia are unacceptable in "Holding the Line on Euthanasia," *Hastings Center Report* (January/February 1989).

Many doctors seem to be uncertain as to whether or not they should have a role in a patient's death. Articles that support euthanasia include "The Physician's Responsibility Toward Hopelessly Ill Patients," *The New England Journal of Medicine* (March 30, 1989); "Suicide: Should the Doctor Ever Help?" *Harvard Health Letter* (August 1991); "The Physician Can Play a Positive Role in Euthanasia," *Journal of the American Medical Association* (December 1, 1989); "Mercy Mission," *U.S. News & World Report* (March 18, 1991); "Physicians' Aid in Dying," *The New England Journal of Medicine* (October 31, 1991); "Intentional 'Death with Dignity' Raises Moral, Ethical, Legal Issues," *Des*

Moines Register (March 5, 1989); and "Assisted Suicide—Is It Acceptable?" the *Washington Post* (April 4, 1989).

Opponents of euthanasia and physician-assisted suicide argue that all life has value and that doctors do not have the right to end it. Leon R. Kass, in "Neither For Love Nor Money: Why Doctors Must Not Kill," *The Public Interest* (December 1989), maintains that under no circumstances should doctors take a life. Other articles that agree with this viewpoint include "Holding the Line on Euthanasia," *Hastings Center Report* (January/February 1989) and "They Shoot Horses, Don't They?" *New Scientist* (September 14, 1991).

ISSUE 3

Should Health Care for the Elderly Be Limited?

YES: Daniel Callahan, from "Aging and the Ends of Medicine," *Annals of the New York Academy of Sciences* (June 15, 1988)

NO: Nat Hentoff, from "The Pied Piper Returns for the Old Folks," *The Village Voice* (April 26, 1988)

ISSUE SUMMARY

YES: Hastings Center director Daniel Callahan believes that medical care for elderly people who have lived their natural life expectancy should consist only of pain relief rather than expensive health care services, which serve only to forestall death.

NO: Author Nat Hentoff argues that it is immoral to limit health care services to any one segment of the population and that, under Callahan's proposal, the elderly poor would die sooner than those with the means to buy medical services.

In 1980, 11 percent of the U.S. population was over age 65, but they utilized about 29 percent ($219 billion) of the total American health care expenditures. By the end of the decade, the percentage of the population over 65 had risen to 12 percent, which consumed 31 percent of total health care expenditures, or $450 billion. Medicare, the government insurance for the elderly, is expected to increase costs from $75 billion to $114 billion by the year 2000. By the year 2040, it has been projected that people over 65 will represent 21 percent of the population and consume 45 percent of all health care expenditures.

Can the United States afford to keep pace with this growing number of elderly people in providing even the present level of care, much less in adding expensive new technologies? And will taking care of the elderly be at the expense of the health of the young? Currently, the federal government spends about six times as much on health care for individuals over 65 as for those under 18, much of it during the last year of life. The elderly clearly receive a disproportionate share of health care expenditures. But is rationing health care for the elderly a possible answer?

In England, the emphasis of health care is on improving the quality of life through primary care medicine and well-subsidized home care and institutional programs for the elderly rather than through life-extending acute care medicine. As a result, it is difficult if not impossible for those over 55 to get kidney dialysis, open heart surgery, intensive care units, and other forms of expensive technology. The British seem to value basic medical care for all rather than expensive technology for the few who would benefit from it. As a result, the British spend a much smaller proportion of their gross national product (6.2 percent) on health services than Americans (10.8 percent) for a nearly identical health status and life expectancy.

Daniel Callahan, in the following selection, argues that using medical technologies to extend the lives of elderly individuals who have lived out their natural life spans is not an appropriate use of modern medicine. Technology, he feels, should be used to avoid premature death and to relieve suffering, not to prolong full and complete lives. He believes that most elderly people agree with these principles: They indicate a wish that their lives not be aggressively extended beyond a point at which they still possess a good level of physical and mental functioning and a certain degree of value and meaning. Callahan also states that the attempt to indefinitely extend life combined with an endless goal to improve the health of the elderly can be an economic disaster. These goals also fail to put health in its proper place as only one among many human values and discourage the acceptance of aging and death as part of life.

Nat Hentoff disagrees with Callahan. He feels that the elderly who lack financial resources in need of certain kinds of medical care will die sooner than the elderly who do not have to rely on the government for medical aid. He also wonders what society would become if the elderly were refused medical care that could prolong their lives. And what of the doctors who would refuse to treat elderly patients?

YES

Daniel Callahan

AGING AND THE ENDS OF MEDICINE

In October of 1986, Dr. Thomas Starzl of the Presbyterian-University Hospital in Pittsburgh successfully transplanted a liver into a 76-year-old woman. The typical cost of such an operation is over $200,000. He thereby accelerated the extension to the elderly of the most expensive and most demanding form of high-technology medicine. Not long after that, Congress brought organ transplantation under Medicare coverage, thus guaranteeing an even greater extension of this form of life-saving care to older age groups.

This is, on the face of it, the kind of medical progress we have long grown to hail, a triumph of medical technology and a new-found benefit to be provided by an established entitlement program. But now an oddity. At the same time those events were taking place, a parallel government campaign for cost containment was under way, with a special targeting of health care to the aged under the Medicare program.

It was not hard to understand why. In 1980, the 11% of the population over age 65 consumed some 29% of the total American health care expenditures of $219.4 billion. By 1986, the percentage of consumption by the elderly had increased to 31% and total expenditures to $450 billion. Medicare costs are projected to rise from $75 billion in 1986 to $114 billion in the year 2000, and in real not inflated dollars.

There is every incentive for politicians, for those who care for the aged, and for those of us on the way to becoming old to avert our eyes from figures of that kind. We have tried as a society to see if we can simply muddle our way through. That, however, is no longer sufficient. The time has come, I am convinced, for a full and open reconsideration of our future direction. We can not for much longer continue on our present course. Even if we could find a way to radically increase the proportion of our health care dollar going to the elderly, it is not clear that that would be a good social investment.

Is it sensible, in the face of a rapidly increasing burden of health care costs for the elderly, to press forward with new and expensive ways of extending their lives? Is it possible to even hope to control costs while, simultaneously, supporting the innovative research that generates ever-new ways to spend money? These are now unavoidable questions. Medicare costs rise at an extraordinary pace, fueled by an ever-increasing number and proportion of the elderly. The fastest-growing age group in the United States are those over the age of 85, increasing at a rate of about 10% every two years. By the year 2040, it has been projected that the elderly will represent 21% of the population and consume 45% of all health care expenditures. Could costs of that magnitude be borne?

Yet even as this intimidating trend reveals itself, anyone who works closely with the elderly recognizes that the present Medicare and Medicaid programs are grossly inadequate in meeting the real and full needs of the elderly. They fail, most notably, in providing decent long-term care and medical care that does not constitute a heavy out-of-pocket drain. Members of minority groups, and single or widowed women, are particularly disadvantaged. How will it be possible, then, to keep pace with the growing number of elderly in even providing present levels of care, much less in ridding the system of its present inadequacies and inequities—and, at the same time, furiously adding expensive new technologies?

The straight answer is that it will not be possible to do all of those things and that, worse still, it may be harmful to even try. It may be harmful because of the economic burdens it will impose on younger age groups, and because of the skewing of national social priorities too heavily toward health care that it is coming to require. But it may also be harmful because it suggests to both the young and the old that the key to a happy old

age is good health care. That may not be true.

It is not pleasant to raise possibilities of that kind. The struggle against what Dr. Robert Butler aptly and brilliantly called "ageism" in 1968 has been a difficult one. It has meant trying to persuade the public that not all the elderly are sick and senile. It has meant trying to convince Congress and state legislatures to provide more help for the old. It has meant trying to educate the elderly themselves to look upon their old age as a time of new, open possibilities. That campaign has met with only partial success. Despite great progress, the elderly are still subject to discrimination and stereotyping. The struggle against ageism is hardly over.

THREE MAJOR CONCERNS HAVE, NONETHEless, surfaced over the past few years. They are symptoms that a new era has arrived. The first is that an increasingly large share of health care is going to the elderly in comparison with benefits for children. The federal government, for instance, spends six times as much on health care for those over 65 as for those under 18. As the demographer Samuel Preston observed in a provocative 1984 presidential address to the Population Association of America:

There is surely something to be said for a system in which things get better as we pass through life rather than worse. The great leveling off of age curves of psychological distress, suicide and income in the past two decades might simply reflect the fact that we have decided in some fundamental sense that we don't want to face futures that become continually bleaker. But let's be clear that the transfers from the working-age population to the elderly are also transfers away from children, since the working ages bear far more responsibility for childrearing than do the elderly.[1]

Preston's address had an immediate impact. The mainline aging advocacy groups responded with pained indignation, accusing Preston of fomenting a war between the generations. But led by Dave Durenberger, Republican Senator from Minnesota, it also stimulated the formation of Americans for Generational Equity (AGE), an organization created to promote debate on the burden to future generations, but particularly the Baby Boom generation, of "our major social insurance programs."[2] These two developments signalled the outburst of a struggle over what has come to be called "Intergenerational equity" that is only now gaining momentum.

The second concern is that the elderly dying consume a disproportionate share of health care costs. Stanford economist Victor Fuchs has noted:

At present, the United States spends about 1 percent of the gross national product on health care for elderly persons who are in their last year of life. . . . One of the biggest challenges facing policy makers for the rest of this century will be how to strike an appropriate balance between care of the [elderly] dying and health services for the rest of the population.[3]

The third concern is summed up in an observation by Jerome L. Avorn, M.D., of the Harvard Medical School:

With the exception of the birth-control pill, each of the medical-technology interventions developed since the 1950s has its most widespread impact on people who are past their fifties—the further past their fifties, the greater the impact.[4]

Many of these interventions were not intended for the elderly. Kidney dialysis, for example, was originally developed for those between the age of 15 and 45. Now some 30% of its recipients are over 65.

THESE THREE CONCERNS HAVE NOT GONE unchallenged. They have, on the contrary, been strongly resisted, as has the more general assertion that some form of rationing of health care for the elderly might become necessary. To the charge that the elderly receive a disproportionate share of resources, the response has been that what helps the elderly helps every other age group. It both relieves the young of the burden of care for elderly parents they would otherwise have to bear and, since they too will eventually become old, promises them similar care when they come to need it. There is no guarantee, moreover, that any cutback in health care for the elderly would result in a transfer of the savings directly to the young. Our system is not that rational or that organized. And why, others ask, should we contemplate restricting care for the elderly when we wastefully spend hundreds of millions of dollars on an inflated defense budget?

The charge that the elderly dying receive a large share of funds hardly proves that it is an unjust or unreasonable amount. They are, after all, the most in need. As some important studies have shown, moreover, it is exceedingly difficult to know that someone is dying; the most expensive patients, it turns out, are those who are expected to live but who actually die. That most new technologies benefit the old more than the young is perfectly sensible: most of the killer diseases of the young have now been conquered.

These are reasonable responses. It would no doubt be possible to ignore the symptoms that the raising of such concerns represents, and to put off for at least a few more years any full confrontation with the overpowering tide of elderly now on the way. There is little incentive for politicians to think about, much less talk about, limits of any kind on health care for the aged; it is a politically hazardous topic. Perhaps also, as Dean Guido Calabresi of the Yale Law School and his colleague Philip Bobbitt observed in their thoughtful 1978 book *Tragic Choices*, when we are forced to make painful allocation choices, "Evasion, disguise, temporizing... [and] averting our eyes enables us to save some lives even when we will not save all."[5]

Yet however slight the incentives to take on this highly troubling issue, I believe it is inevitable that we must. Already rationing of health care under Medicare is a fact of life, though rarely labeled as such. The requirement that Medicare recipients pay the first $500 of the costs of hospital care, that there is a cutoff of reimbursement of care beyond 60 days, and a failure to cover long-term care, are nothing other than allocation and cost-saving devices. As sensitive as it is to the votes of the elderly, the Reagan administration only grudgingly agreed to support catastrophic health care costs of the elderly (a benefit that will not, in any event, help many of the aged). It is bound to be far more resistant to long-term care coverage, as will any administration.

But there are other reasons than economics to think about health care for the elderly. The coming economic crisis provides a much-needed opportunity to ask some deeper questions. Just what is it that we want medicine to do for us as we age? Earlier cultures believed that aging should be accepted, and that it should be in part a time of preparation for death. Our culture seems increasingly to reject that view, preferring instead, it often seems, to think of aging as hardly more than another disease, to be fought and rejected. Which view is correct? To ask that question is only to note that disturbing puzzles about the ends of medicine and the ends of aging lie behind the more immediate financing worries. Without some kind of answer to them, there is no hope of finding a reasonable, and possibly even a humane, solution to the growing problem of health care for the elderly.

Let me put my own view directly. The future goal of medicine in the care of the aged should be that of improving the quality of their life, not in seeking ways to extend that life. In its longstanding ambition to forestall death, medicine has in the care of the aged reached its last frontier. That is hardly because death is absent elsewhere—children and young adults obviously still die of maladies that are open to potential cure—but because the largest number of deaths (some 70%) now occur among those over the age of 65, with the highest proportion in those over 85. If death is ever to be humbled, that is where the essentially endless work remains to be done. But however tempting that challenge, medicine should now restrain its ambition at that frontier. To do otherwise will, I believe, be to court harm to the needs of other age groups and to the old themselves.

Yet to ask medicine to restrain itself in the face of aging and death is to ask more than it, or the public that sustains it, is likely to find agreeable. Only a fresh understanding of the ends and meaning of aging, encompassing two conditions, are likely to make that a plausible stance. The first is that we—both young and old—need to understand that it is possible to live out a meaningful old age that is limited in time, one that does not require a compulsive effort to turn to medicine for more life to make it bearable. The second condition is that, as a culture, we need a more supportive context for aging and death, one that cherishes and respects the elderly while at the same time recognizing that their primary orientation should be to the young and the generations to come, not to their own age group. It will be no less necessary to recognize that in the passing of the generations lies the constant reinvigoration of biological life.

Neither of these conditions will be easy to realize. Our culture has, for one thing, worked hard to redefine old age as a time of liberation, not decline. The terms "modern maturity" or "prime time" have, after all, come to connote a time of travel, new ventures in education and self-discovery, the ever-accessible tennis court or golf course, and delightfully periodic but gratefully brief visits from well-behaved grandchildren.

This is, to be sure, an idealized picture. Its attraction lies not in its literal truth but as a widely-accepted utopian reference point. It projects the vision of an old age to which more and more believe they can aspire and which its proponents think an affluent country can afford if it so chooses. That it requires a medicine that is singleminded in its aggressiveness against the infirmities of old age is of a piece with its hopes. But as we have come to discover, the costs of that kind of war are prohibitive. No matter how much is spent the ultimate problem will still remain: people age and die. Worse still, by pretending that old age can be turned into a kind of endless middle age, we rob it of meaning and significance for the elderly themselves. It is a way of saying that old age can be acceptable only to the extent that it can mimic the vitality of the younger years.

THERE IS A PLAUSIBLE ALTERNATIVE: THAT OF a fresh vision of what it means to live a decently long and adequate life, what might be called a natural life span. Earlier generations accepted the idea that there was a natural life span—the biblical norm of three score years and ten captures that notion (even though, in fact, that was a much longer life span than was then typically the case). It is an idea well worth reconsidering, and would provide us with a meaningful and realizable goal. Modern medicine and biology have done much, however, to wean us away from that kind of thinking. They have insinuated the belief that the average life span is not a natural fact at all, but instead one that is strictly dependent upon the state of medical knowledge and skill. And there is much to that belief as a statistical fact: the average life expectancy continues to increase, with no end in sight.

But that is not what I think we ought to mean by a natural life span. We need a notion of a full life that is based on some deeper understanding of human need and sensible possibility, not the latest state of medical technology or medical possibility. We should instead think of a natural life span as the achievement of a life long enough to accomplish for the most part those opportunities that life typically affords people and which we ordinarily take to be the prime benefits of enjoying a life at all—that of loving and living, of raising a family, of finding and carrying out work that is satisfying, of reading and thinking, and of cherishing our friends and families.

If we envisioned a natural life span that way, then we could begin to intensify the devising of ways to get people to that stage of life, and to work to make certain they do so in good health and social dignity. People will differ on what they might count as a natural life span; determining its appropriate range for social policy purposes would need extended thought and debate. My own view is that it can now be achieved by the late 70s or early 80s.

That many of the elderly discover new interests and new facets of themselves late in life—my mother took up painting in her seventies and was selling her paintings up until her death at 86—does not mean that we should necessarily encourage a kind of medicine that would make that the norm. Nor does it mean that we should base social and welfare policy on possibilities of that kind. A more reasonable approach is to ask how medicine can help most people live out a decently long life, and how that life can be enhanced along the way.

A longer life does not guarantee a better life—there is no inherent connection between the two. No matter how long medicine enabled people to live, death at any time—at age 90, or 100, or 110—would frustrate some possibility, some as-yet-unrealized goal. There is sadness in that realization, but not tragedy. An easily preventable death of a young child is an outrage. The death from an incurable disease of someone in the prime of young adulthood is a tragedy. But death at an old age, after a long and full life, is simply sad, a part of life itself.

AS IT CONFRONTS AGING, MEDICINE SHOULD have as its specific goal that of averting premature death, understood as death prior to a natural life span, and the relief of suffering thereafter. It should pursue those goals in order that the elderly can finish out their years with as little needless pain as possible, and with as much vigor as can be generated in contributing to the welfare of younger age groups and to the community of which they are a part. Above all, the elderly need to have a sense of the meaning and significance of their stage in life, one that is not dependent for its human value on economic productivity or physical vigor.

What would a medicine oriented toward the relief of suffering rather than the deliberate extension of life be like? We do not yet have a clear and ready answer to that question, so long-standing, central, and persistent has been the struggle against death as part of the self-conception of medicine. But the Hospice movement is providing us with much helpful evidence. It knows how to distinguish between the relief of suffering and the extension of life. A greater control by the elderly over their dying—and particularly a more readily respected and enforceable right to deny aggressive life-extending treatment—is a long-sought, minimally necessary goal.

What does this have to do with the rising cost of health care for the elderly? Everything. The indefinite extension of life combined with a never-satisfied improvement in the health of the elderly is a recipe for monomania and limitless spending. It fails to put health in its proper place as only one among many human goods. It fails to accept aging and death as part of the human condition. It fails to present to younger generations a model of wise stewardship.

How might we devise a plan to limit health care for the aged under public entitlement programs that is fair, humane, and sensitive to their special requirements and dignity? Let me suggest three principles to undergird a quest for limits. First, government has a duty, based on our collective social obligations to each other, to help people live out a natural life span, but not actively to help medically extend life beyond that point. Second, government is obliged to develop under its research subsidies, and pay for, under its entitlement programs, only that kind and degree of life-extending technology necessary for medicine to achieve and serve the end of a natural life span. The question is not whether a technology is available that can save the life of someone who has lived out a natural life span, but whether there is an obligation for society to provide them with that technology. I think not. Third, beyond the point of natural life span, government should provide only the means necessary for the relief of suffering, not life-extending technology. By proposing that we use age as a specific criterion for the limitation of life-extending health care, I am challenging one of the most revered norms of contemporary geriatrics: that medical need and not age should be the standard of care. Yet the use of age as a principle for the allocation of resources can be perfectly valid, both a necessary and legitimate basis for providing health care to the elderly. There is not likely to be any better or less arbitrary criterion for the limiting of resources in the face of the open-ended possibilities of medical advancement in therapy for the aged.

Medical "need," in particular, can no longer work as an allocation principle. It is too elastic a concept, too much a func-tion of the state of medical art. A person of 100 dying from congestive heart failure "needs" a heart transplant no less than someone who is 30. Are we to treat both needs as equal? That is not economically feasible or, I would argue, a sensible way to allocate scarce resources. But it would be required by a strict need-based standard.

Age is also a legitimate basis for allocation because it is a meaningful and universal category. It can be understood at the level of common sense. It is concrete enough to be employed for policy purposes. It can also, most importantly, be of value to the aged themselves if combined with an ideal of old age that focuses on its quality rather than its indefinite extension.

I HAVE BECOME IMPRESSED WITH THE PHILOS-ophy underlying the British health care system and the way it meets the needs of the old and the chronically ill. It has, to begin with, a tacit allocation policy. It emphasizes improving the quality of life through primary care medicine and well-subsidized home care and institutional programs for the elderly rather than through life-extending acute care medicine. The well-known difficulty in getting dialysis after 55 is matched by like restrictions on access to open heart surgery, intensive care units, and other forms of expensive technology. An undergirding skepticism toward technology makes that a viable option. That attitude, together with a powerful drive for equity, "explains," as two commentators have noted, "why most British put a higher value on primary care for the population as a whole than on an abundance of sophisticated technology for the few who may benefit from it."[6]

That the British spend a significantly smaller proportion of their GNP (6.2%) on health care than Americans (10.8%) for an almost identical outcome in health status is itself a good advertisement for its priorities. Life expectancies are, for men, 70.0 years in the U.S. and 70.4 years in Great Britain; and, for women, 77.8 in the U.S. and 76.7 in Great Britain. There is, of course, a great difference in the ethos of the U.S. and Britain, and our individualism and love of technology stand in the way of a quick shift of priorities.

Yet our present American expectations about aging and death, it turns out, may not be all that reassuring. How many of us are really so certain that high-technology American medicine promises us all that much better an aging and death, even if some features appear improved and the process begins later than in earlier times? Between the widespread fear of death in an impersonal ICU, cozened about machines and invaded by tubes, on the one hand, or wasting away in the back ward of a nursing home, on the other, not many of us seem comforted.

Once we have reflected on those fears, it is not impossible that most people could be persuaded that a different, more limited set of expectations for health care could be made tolerable. That would be all the more possible if there was a greater assurance than at present that one could live out a full life span, that one's chronic illnesses would be better supported, and that long-term care and home care would be given a more powerful societal backing than is now the case. Though they would face a denial of life-extending medical care beyond a certain age, the old would not necessarily fear their aging any more than they now do. They would, on the contrary, know that a better balance had been struck between making our later years as good as possible rather than simply trying to add more years.

This direction would not immediately bring down the costs of care of the elderly; it would add new costs. But it would set in place the beginning of a new understanding of old age, one that would admit of eventual stabilization and limits. The time has come to admit we can not go on much longer on the present course of open-ended health care for the elderly. Neither confident assertions about American affluence, nor tinkering with entitlement provisions and cost-containment strategies will work for more than a few more years. It is time for the dream that old age can be an infinite and open frontier to end, and for the unflagging, but self-deceptive, optimism that we can do anything we want with our economic system be put aside.

The elderly will not be served by a belief that only a lack of resources, or better financing mechanisms, or political power, stand between them and the limitations of their bodies. The good of younger age groups will not be served by inspiring in them a desire to live to an old age that will simply extend the vitality of youth indefinitely, as if old age is nothing but a sign that medicine has failed in its mission. The future of our society will not be served by allowing expenditures on health care for the elderly endlessly and uncontrollably to escalate, fueled by a false altruism that thinks anything less is to deny the elderly their dignity. Nor will it be served by that pervasive kind of self-serving that urges the young to support such a crusade because they will eventually benefit from it also.

We require instead an understanding of the process of aging and death that looks to our obligation to the young and to the future, that recognizes the necessity of limits and the acceptance of decline and death, and that values the old for their age and not for their continuing youthful vitality. In the name of accepting the elderly and repudiating discrimination against them, we have mainly succeeded in pretending that, with enough will and money, the unpleasant part of old age can be abolished. In the name of medical progress we have carried out a relentless war against death and decline, failing to ask in any probing way if that will give us a better society for all age groups.

THE PROPER QUESTION IS NOT WHETHER WE are succeeding in giving a longer life to the aged. It is whether we are making of old age a decent and honorable time of life. Neither a longer lifetime nor more life-extending technology are the way to that goal. The elderly themselves ask for greater financial security, for as much self-determination and independence as possible, for a decent quality of life and not just more life, and for a respected place in society.

The best way to achieve those goals is not simply to say more money and better programs are needed, however much they have their important place. We would do better to begin with a sense of limits, of the meaning of the human life cycle, and of the necessary coming and going of the generations. From that kind of a starting point, we could devise a new understanding of old age.

REFERENCES

1. PRESTON, S. H. 1984. Children and the elderly: divergent paths for America's dependents. Demography 21: 491–495.
2. Americans for Generational Equity. Case Statement. May 1986.
3. FUCHS, V. R. 1984. Though much is taken: reflections on aging, health, and medical care. Milbank Mem. Fund Q. 62: 464–465.
4. AVORN, J. L. 1986. Medicine, health, and the geriatric transformation. Daedalus 115: 211–225.
5. CALABRESI, G. & P. BOBBITT. 1978. Tragic Choices. W. W. Norton. New York, NY.
6. MILLER, F. H. & G. A. H. MILLER. 1986. The painful prescription: a procrustean perspective. N. Engl. J. Med. 314: 1385.

NO   Nat Hentoff

THE PIED PIPER RETURNS
FOR THE OLD FOLKS

In 1983, the [*New York*] *Times* ran an Op-Ed piece, "Our Elderly's Fate," by
Northeastern University sociology professors Jack Levin and Arnold Arluke. The lead paragraph was, to say the least, compelling:

> "American society may be heading toward a *de facto* 'final solution' to the
> problem of a growing elderly population. This trend raises the unthinkable
> prospect of the elderly one day being exterminated as a matter of law."

Having seized the elderly reader by the throat, the authors backed off a
little. The deliberate massing of the old to take their last showers was not
quite what they saw ahead. But already, "there is strong evidence that
increasing numbers of frail, disabled, and financially dependent elders, most
of whom are over 78, are even now, as a result of our social policies, being
isolated from society and dying prematurely."

You don't need to rebuild Auschwitz to send a message to the old that it is
time for them to enter eternity. The signals are everywhere. "Self-help
manuals," wrote Levin and Arluke, "are showing the elderly how to commit
suicide. Studies show that emergency room personnel tend to spend less
time and effort to resuscitate elderly heart attack victims than their younger
counterparts.

> "There is also a growing tendency in medical circles to *emphasize quality over
> quantity of life*. 'Death with dignity' may in some cases be a euphemism for
> extermination." (Emphasis added.)

The two professors were also astute enough to look at the auguries in the
popular culture. *Logan's Run*, a science fiction movie, starred Michael York as
a man in the future who, at 30, had reached the age at which he must be
executed by the state. The book *Triage* "conjectures that the Government
would solve the problems of old age by burning all nursing homes and their
inhabitants."

Not in America. It can't happen here. Not that way. But five years ago,
there was no way Jack Levin and Arnold Arluke could imagine that a

distinguished, widely respected bioethicist would come forth with what his admirers call a "humane" way, a "morally courageous" way, of solving the problems of old age.

The method: persuading the elderly that they can be socially responsible by having the government take away from them certain forms of costly, life-extending medical care.

After all, the kind of medical care he has in mind—heart bypass operations, for instance—would only make them live longer, vainly dreaming of immortality. But the Pied Piper would show old folks how to leave us with grace by being content with a "natural life span."

The Pied Piper, in his autumnal colors, has brought the news of his gentle proposal in magazines, on television, and in a widely praised book.

By having their medical care rationed, he says, the aged will learn to savor the meaning and significance of their final years, for they will *know* they are final. And since the rest of society will no longer be spending so much on the health care of the old, the money saved can be used for the vast numbers of the population who are not old but need more care than they can afford—single or widowed women, members of minority groups.

This benefactor of the elderly is Daniel Callahan, director of the Hastings Center—a pacesetter in medical ethics—in Briarcliff Manor, New York. His book is *Setting Limits* (Simon and Schuster), and it has been respectfully received in just about every important periodical in the nation. He has been asked to speak about his solution to all kinds of groups. Some disagree with him, but they all take him seriously.

I confess that when I first heard distant word of this notion of the elderly going gently into that good Callahan night, I thought he was putting us on. (I should have realized that the Hastings Center—where he and other bioethicists labor to tell us how to fit our lives and deaths into their designs—long ago found humor far too spontaneous and certainly too personal for its religion of utilitarianism.

Still, I expect that the sardonic Dean of Dublin's Saint Patrick's Cathedral, Jonathan Swift, would appreciate Daniel Callahan's *Setting Limits*—though not in the way he would be supposed to. Swift, you will recall, at a time of terrible poverty and hunger in Ireland, wrote *A Modest Proposal*. Rather than having the children of the poor continue to be such a burden to their parents and their nation, why not persuade the poor to raise their children to be slaughtered at the right, succulent time and sold to the rich as delicacies for dining?

What could be more humane? The children would be spared a life of poverty, their parents would be saved from starvation, and the overall economy of Ireland would be in better shape.

So, I thought, Callahan, wanting to dramatize the parlous and poignant state of America's elderly, as described by Jack Levin and Arnold Arluke, had created his modern version of *A Modest Proposal*.

I was wrong. He's not jiving.

So let us look at the Callahan way of ordering the future of America's elderly.

First, Callahan sees "a natural life span" as being ready to say good-bye in one's late seventies or early eighties. He hasn't fixed on an exact age yet. Don't lose your birth certificate.

If people persist in living beyond the time that Callahan, if not God, has allotted them, the government will move in. Congress will require that anybody past that age must be denied Medicare payments for such procedures as certain forms of open heart surgery, certain extended stays in an intensive care unit, and who knows what else.

Moreover, as an index of how humane the spirit of *Setting Limits* is, if an old person is diagnosed as being in a chronic vegetative state (some physicians screw up this diagnosis), the Callahan plan mandates that the feeding tube be denied or removed. (No one is certain whether someone actually in a persistent vegetative state can *feel* what's going on while being starved to death. If there is sensation, there is no more horrible way to die.)

What about the elderly who don't have to depend on Medicare? Millions of the poor and middle class have no other choice than to go to the government, but there are some old folks with money. They, of course, do not have to pay any attention to Daniel Callahan at all. Like the well-to-do from time immemorial, they will get any degree of medical care they want.

So, *Setting Limits* is class-biased in the most fundamental way. People without resources in need of certain kinds of care will die sooner than old folks who do not have to depend on the government and Daniel Callahan.

I am aware that there are more limits—in all respects—to the lives of the poor than to the lives of the comfortable. But there is something almost depraved about so brazenly discriminatory a plan coming from the director of a place that derives all its income and its considerable prestige from its reputation as a definer of ethical behavior—in the healing arts particularly.

Callahan reveals that once we start going down the slippery slope of utilitarianism, we slide by—faster and faster—a lot of old-timey ethical norms. Like the declaration of the Catholic bishops of America that medical care is "indispensable to the protection of human dignity." The bishops didn't say that dignity is only for people who can afford it. They know that if you're 84, and only Medicare can pay your bills but says it won't pay for treatment that will extend your life, then your "human dignity" is shot to hell.

What does Daniel Callahan say about this—uh—imbalance of justice? In the course of an appearance on the *MacNeil Lehrer News Hour*, Callahan said:

" . . . After the age of 80 or 85, wherever we might set it [the age of limiting medical care], then I agree injustice might set in. However, it seems to me in the nature of the case, it would not be for a very long time."

There's a logical man. It would indeed not be for a very long time, and all the shorter for the intervention of Mr. Callahan.

He noted on the same program that his is not an ideal proposal, "but I think the hard choice of that injustice at a later age is well worth the kinds of gains we would get in a more rounded, coherent health care system."

Again, this is naked utilitarianism—the greatest good for the greatest number. And individuals who are in the way—in this case, the elderly poor—have to be gotten out of the way. Not murdered, heaven forfend. Just made comfortable until they die with all deliberate speed.

It must be pointed out that Daniel Callahan does not expect or intend his design for natural dying to be implemented soon. First of all, the public will have to be brought around. But that shouldn't be too difficult in the long run. I am aware of few organized protests against the court decisions in a number of states that feeding tubes can be removed from patients—many of them elderly—who are not terminally ill and are not in intractable pain. And some of these people may not be in a persistently vegetative state.

So, the way the Zeitgeist [spirit of the times] is going, I think public opinion could eventually be won over to Callahan's modest proposal. But he has another reason to want to wait: He doesn't want his vision of "setting limits" to go into effect until society has assured the elderly access to decent long-term home care or nursing home care as well as better coverage for drugs, eyeglasses, and the like.

Even if all that were to happen, there still would be profound ethical and constitutional problems. What kind of a society will we have become if we tuck in the elderly in nursing homes and then refuse them medical treatment that could prolong their lives?

And what of the physicians who will find it abhorrent to limit the care they give solely on the basis of age? As a presumably penitent former Nazi doctor said, "Either one is a doctor or one is not."

On the other hand, if the Callahan plan is not to begin for a while, new kinds of doctors can be trained who will take a utilitarian rather than a Hippocratic oath. ("I will never forget that my dedication is to the society as a whole rather than to any individual patient.")

Already, I have been told by a physician who heads a large teaching institution that a growing number of doctors are spending less time and attention on the elderly. There are similar reports from other such places.

Meanwhile, nobody I've read or heard on the Callahan proposal has mentioned the Fourteenth Amendment and its insistence that all of us must have "equal protection of the laws." What Callahan aims to do is take an entire class of people—on the basis only of their age—and deny them medical care that might prolong their lives. This is not quite *Dred Scott*; but even though the elderly are not yet at the level of close constitutional scrutiny given by the Supreme Court to blacks, other minorities, and women, the old can't be pushed into the grave just like that, can they?

Or can they? Some of the more influential luminaries in the nation—Joe Califano, George Will, and a fleet of bioethicists, among them—have heralded *Setting Limits* as the way to go.

Will you be ready?

POSTSCRIPT

Should Health Care for the Elderly Be Limited?

In October 1986, Dr. Thomas Starzl of Pittsburgh, Pennsylvania, transplanted a liver into a 76-year-old woman at a cost of over $200,000. Soon after that, Congress ordered organ transplantation to be covered under Medicare, which ensured that more older persons would receive this benefit. At the same time these events were taking place, a government campaign to contain medical costs was under way, with health care for the elderly targeted. Sociologist Amitai Etzioni argues that rationing health care for the elderly would encourage conflict between generations and would invite restrictions on health care for other groups in "Spare the Old, Save the Young," *The Nation* (June 11, 1988). In agreement with Etzioni is James F. Childress, "Ensuring Care, Respect, and Fairness for the Elderly," *Hastings Center Report* (October 1984).

Currently, about 40 million Americans have no medical insurance and are at risk of being denied basic health care services. About 20 percent of all children have not had proper immunizations, and one-third of all pregnant women do not receive prenatal care during their first trimester. Richard Lamm, writing in the *New York Times* (February 19, 1987), claims that the federal government pays 50 percent of the health care costs of the elderly. While it may not meet the needs of all older people, the amount of medical aid that goes to the elderly is greater than any other demographic group, and the elderly have the highest disposable income. Daniel Callahan, in "Limiting Health Care for the Old?" *The Nation* (August 15/22, 1987), maintains that we must confront the realities of economics and limit health care. Callahan also writes on the allocation of health resources in "Allocating Health Resources," *Hastings Center Report* (April/May 1988).

Most Americans have access to the best and most expensive medical care in the world. As these costs rise, some difficult decisions may have to be made regarding the allocation of these resources, whether by age, income, or other criteria. As the population ages and more health care dollars are spent on this population group, medical services for the elderly may become a natural target for reduction in order to balance the health care budget. Additional readings on this subject are the following: "Setting Limits," by Daniel Callahan (Simon & Schuster, 1987); "Justice Between Generations and Health Care for the Elderly," by Norman Daniels, *Journal of Medicine and Philosophy* (1988); and Timothy M. Smeeding et al., eds., *Should Medical Care Be Rationed by Age?* (Rowman & Littlefield, 1987).

ISSUE 4

Is AIDS Getting More Than Its Share of Resources and Media Attention?

YES: Michael Fumento, from "Are We Spending Too Much on AIDS?" *Commentary* (October 1990)

NO: Timothy F. Murphy, from "No Time for an AIDS Backlash," *Hastings Center Report* (March/April 1991)

ISSUE SUMMARY

YES: Writer Michael Fumento points out that Congress continues to allocate substantial amounts of money for research and the treatment of AIDS, which he feels is disproportionate to the number of people who die annually from the disease.
NO: Medical professor Timothy F. Murphy argues that the AIDS epidemic is still fairly new and has an unknown future, and that AIDS is a lethal, contagious disease affecting thousands of Americans; thus, current funding is justified.

AIDS could be called the world's most serious health concern since the bubonic plague, which killed off one-third of the population of Europe in the fourteenth century. Unless there is a major breakthrough, every person with AIDS will ultimately die (unlike the plague, which some survived). Currently there is no vaccine or cure for the disease.

It is not clear if AIDS is a "new" disease or one that has been around and has only recently begun to spread. As early as 1977, medical journals in the United States were reporting on a pneumonia-like disease that affected mostly young, homosexual males and intravenous drug users. The disease was ultimately called "acquired immunodeficiency syndrome," or AIDS. In 1983, scientists isolated the virus responsible for the disease, which eventually became known as human immunodeficiency virus (HIV)—a virus that invades and destroys white blood cells (T-lymphocytes), which are the cells directly involved in controlling the body's immune response. Once HIV has crippled a person's immune system, certain bacteria, viruses, and parasites that the body might ordinarily be able to fight off are able to take over. Persons who are infected may not have symptoms but are capable of passing the virus on to others. Transmission of HIV occurs through sexual contact and through exposure to infected blood. Infected women who are pregnant can transmit the virus to their unborn child. Blood, semen, and vaginal secretions are known to be infectious. Anyone who has unprotected sex with an infected person is at risk of being infected.

In the early 1980s, about 150 cases of AIDS were reported in the United States. In mid-1992, about 218,000 cases and approximately 130,000 deaths from AIDS were identified by the Centers for Disease Control. AIDS is found throughout the world: In Africa, over 1 million persons are thought to be infected, and whole villages have fallen victim to the disease. Thousands of Europeans, South Americans, and Asians also are infected with AIDS.

In the United States, AIDS funding for research and treatment has been steadily rising. Except for cancer, AIDS now receives more research money than any other illness. For example, AIDS currently gets approximately $1.5 billion annually, as compared to heart disease, which receives about half as much. Heart disease is the leading cause of death in the United States and kills 20 times more people each year than does AIDS. Despite these disparities, most Americans favor increasing spending for AIDS.

In the following selections, Michael Fumento argues that the United States is spending too much money and effort on AIDS, which could result in less spent on research or treatment for other diseases. While he agrees that AIDS is contagious whereas heart disease and cancer are not, he maintains that AIDS is spread almost exclusively through controllable and preventable behavior and that some of the research money currently going toward AIDS could be better spent elsewhere. Timothy F. Murphy argues that those who believe that AIDS is getting more than its share of resources and attention should remember that HIV remains a highly lethal, communicable virus and that, despite better medical management, the number of HIV-related deaths continues to increase. In view of the people who are still sick, who are dying, and who bear the costs of this epidemic, it is too shameful and early to claim that enough has been done.

YES

Michael Fumento

ARE WE SPENDING TOO MUCH ON AIDS?

If there is one thing Americans seem to agree upon about AIDS, it is that we are not spending enough on the disease. "The government has blood on its hands," reads a bumper sticker that is ubiquitous in major cities, "one AIDS death every half hour." AIDS activists, who are fond of asserting that AIDS is "not a homosexual disease," tell us in the same breath that the failure to spend more on it constitutes genocide against homosexuals. A recent public-opinion poll shows, indeed, that most Americans favor increasing spending on AIDS.

But consider. This past year, reported cases of AIDS in the U.S. increased only 9 percent over the previous year's tally. The federal Centers for Disease Control (CDC) of the Public Health Service (PHS) has been forced to lower greatly both its estimate of current infections and its projections of future cases. The World Health Organization, similarly, has lowered its original estimate of as many as 100 million infections by 1990 to a current eight to ten million. New York City, AIDS capital of the nation, has lowered its estimate of current infections from 500,000 to about 150,000.

Nor has the long-expected "breakout" of AIDS into the heterosexual middle class shown any sign of occurring. Former Surgeon General C. Everett Koop, who probably coined the expression "heterosexual AIDS explosion," now claims he knew "from the very beginning" that such a thing would never happen; Gene Antonio, author of *The AIDS Cover-Up?* (300,000 copies in print), which predicted as many as 64 million infections by this year [1990], now denies having made such a prediction. At the recent international AIDS conference in San Francisco, Dr. Nancy Padian put another nail in the coffin of the "breakout" theory when she reported the results of her study of 41 couples among whom the woman was originally infected and the man was not: over a period of years, only one man became infected, and that only after both he and his partner had experienced penile and vaginal bleeding on over 100 occasions.

This year, AIDS dropped from being the 14th biggest killer of Americans to number 15. Heart disease this year will kill about 775,000 Americans, a figure perhaps 20 times as high as the number of Americans who will die of

From Michael Fumento, "Are We Spending Too Much on AIDS?" *Commentary* (October 1990). Copyright © 1990 by The American Jewish Committee. Reprinted by permission of *Commentary*. All rights reserved.

AIDS in the next twelve months. In the next two months cancer will kill almost as many people as have died of AIDS in the course of the entire epidemic.

Nevertheless, the *current* PHS allocation of about $1.6 billion for AIDS research and education is higher than that allocated for any other cause of death. In 1990, the CDC will spend $10,000 on prevention and education for each AIDS sufferer as opposed to $185 for each victim of cancer and a mere $3.50 for each cardiac patient. Total federal research expenditures on AIDS this year will be more than 100 percent of nationwide patient costs; in the case of cancer, the corresponding ratio of research-and-development spending to patient costs is about 4.5 percent, in the case of heart disease about 2.9 percent, and in the case of Alzheimer's disease, less than 1 percent.

AIDS ACTIVISTS HAVE ANSWERS TO THESE statistics. Since AIDS strikes most often in the prime of life, they urge us to consider the years of lost productivity as a cost that could be avoided by more spending now on AIDS research. Yet every year cancer and heart disease *each* kills more than 150,000 Americans below the age of sixty, while this year AIDS will kill around 30,000 persons of all ages. Nor do the calculations of years lost take account of the fact that intravenous drug abusers, who make up a growing portion of those affected by the disease, have a very low life expectancy and an even lower expectancy of productivity.

But, say AIDS activists, the disease is overwhelming the nation's health-care system, and this alone justifies increased spending on research. A figure repeated often in the media has been the Rand Corporation's estimate that by 1991, direct medical costs for AIDS (that is, med-

ical expenses only, with lost wages not included) could be as high as $133 billion, with up to $38 billion in 1991 alone. *U.S. News & World Report* flatly declared, "What is now becoming clear to an array of leaders—in medicine, business, government, and academia—is that AIDS not only threatens untold death and suffering but could bankrupt America's health system as well." In fact, however, a typical AIDS case costs approximately the same as a terminal cancer case, about $40,000 to $50,000, which means that the 35,000 reported AIDS cases last year will end up costing the nation something less than $2 billion, or considerably less than 1 percent of this year's total U.S. medical costs of approximately $650 billion.

Of course, localized emergencies can exist. New York City's hospital system, running poorly even before AIDS, is clearly in a state of crisis even though cases in that city have peaked. The reason New York, San Francisco, Los Angeles, and other such cities have been hit so hard by AIDS is that they are refuges for homosexuals and drug abusers. With that in mind, the House and Senate are seeking to authorize $2.9 billion and $4 billion, respectively, over the next six years, mostly for these hard-hit cities and states. (Ironically, the bill has been cast as emergency relief for *rural* areas, apparently in the belief that voters have more sympathy for the problems of Peoria than for those of San Francisco or New York.) This special allocation for AIDS, which comes on top of an earlier special allocation to subsidize the drug AZT, is almost without precedent. There is nothing similar for people with heart disease or cancer or diabetes or lupus or any number of other potentially fatal diseases (with the exception of end-stage renal disease).

WHAT ABOUT THE ASSERTION THAT AIDS deserves more funding because it is contagious, while heart disease and cancer are not? In fact, AIDS is contagious almost exclusively through behavior, and modification of that behavior could in theory reduce future AIDS cases virtually to zero without another penny spent on research and without a single medical breakthrough. An as-yet uninfected homosexual who avoids high-risk behavior will almost certainly never contract AIDS; but his chance of dying of cancer remains one in five. Indeed, male homosexuals outside of such high-incidence areas as San Francisco, Los Angeles, and New York, and whose HIV status is unknown, currently have less chance of getting AIDS than of dying of either heart disease or cancer.

It is said that even if research on AIDS does not yield a cure, spin-offs from that research could lead to cures and treatments for other diseases. In line with this idea, Congressman Ted Weiss (D.-NY) requested the Office of Technology Assessment (OTA) to prepare a report titled, "How Has Federal Research on AIDS/HIV Contributed to Other Fields?" The reviewer in the British medical journal *Lancet*, struck by the contrast between this tiny report and OTA's customary "behemoth, exhaustive" efforts, noted that it was comprised of nothing more than opinions from an "unspecified organization of 'distinguished biomedical and social scientists,'" and that "For policy or polemics, this OTA production is a bust."

Nevertheless, Dr. Anthony Fauci, the director of the National Institutes of Allergies and Infectious Diseases (NIAID), a branch of the National Institutes of Health (NIH), and long an advocate of increased spending on AIDS, declared that "There's positive spin-offs already and certainly in the next decade or two you'll see more," adding that these included cancer. In fact, no life has ever been saved, no disease ever ameliorated, by AIDS spin-offs. As former NIH director Donald Fredrickson has pointed out, most AIDS research is far too narrowly targeted to lead to significant spin-offs. Indeed, most of the money spent by the PHS on AIDS (including for advertisements on late-night television like the one featuring a man who resolves not to go out on the town and "bring back AIDS to my family") does not involve clinical research at all.

This is not to say that no spin-offs are ever possible. After all, no one knew that the space program would end up introducing the world to velcro. But we did not embark on the space program because we wanted a new kind of fastener. If it is a cure for cancer we seek, we should spend money on cancer research, not on another disease entirely. As it happens, increasing spending on cancer at the expense of spending on AIDS might do more for both diseases: of the first three drugs approved for treatment of AIDS or its conditions, two—AZT and alpha interferon—were spin-offs of cancer research.

Among the deleterious effects of disproportionate spending on AIDS have been inevitable boondoggles, as great a problem in medicine as in national defense. In December 1988, NIAID announced two grants totaling $22.8 million to study non-drug-using heterosexuals in order, as the Associated Press put it, to "prevent a huge new epidemic." Speaking on condition of anonymity, one prominent federal epidemiologist said of the study, "I think it's complete bullshit." He added, "My sense was that a huge amount of money got dumped on NIAID and that by the time they got around to awarding the money a lot of good institutions had already been funded and all that was left was schlock."

CONCENTRATION ON AIDS HAS IN GENERAL prompted a de-emphasis of other medical diseases like Alzheimer's, a cruel, debilitating malady that will continue to exact an ever-higher yearly toll unless medical intervention becomes possible. Nobody is more conscious of this than researchers themselves. It takes up to a decade to put a high-school graduate through medical school; thus, for now and for the immediate future AIDS researchers are being drawn from other research areas, primarily cancer, and the rumblings from traditionally nonpolitical laboratories are growing louder and louder. Some are calling it "AIDS Resentment Complex," a play on "AIDS Related Complex." Dr. Vincent T. DeVita, Jr., just before stepping down from his position as director of the National Cancer Institute (NCI), said that AIDS "has been an extraordinary drain on the energy of the scientific establishment." In fact, AIDS research has now weakened cancer research to the point where NCI's ability to fund promising new proposals is lower than at any time in the past two decades.

Two top doctors left NCI in late 1988, partly out of frustration over this state of affairs. According to one of them, Dr. Robert Young, now president of the American Society of Clinical Oncology, "the superstructure of cancer research is being dismantled." Indeed, for non-AIDS work, NIH lost almost 1,100 employees between 1984 and 1989. At the same time, according to *Science* magazine, the number of NIH employees en-

gaged in AIDS work increased by more than 400 to 580 workers or their full-time equivalents.

The most vocal opposition to spiraling federal AIDS expenditures has probably come from women concerned about breast cancer, which kills about 44,000 a year; every two years as many women die of breast cancer alone as the number of men and women who have died of AIDS over the course of the entire epidemic. True, Congress is now considering bills that would appropriate funds for cancer screening in women, but the total to be allocated for both breast cancer and cervical cancer—the latter kills 6,000 women a year and is virtually always preventable if caught early enough—is only $50 million, as contrasted with the $3 to $4 billion which Congress wants to spend for AIDS treatment programs over the next six years and which will probably not save a single life, from AIDS or anything else.

THE BLUNT FACT IS, THEN, THAT A GREAT many people will die of other diseases because of the overemphasis on AIDS. We will never know their names and those names will never be sewn into a giant quilt. We will never know their exact numbers. But they will die nonetheless.

Is this right? Should a compassionate society allocate funds and research on the basis of media attention, on the basis of whoever makes the loudest noise? Or should it, rather, put its appropriations where they can do the most good for the greatest number of people?

NO

Timothy F. Murphy

NO TIME FOR AN AIDS BACKLASH

Writing in *Time*, Charles Krauthammer described the May 1990 protests by AIDS activists at the National Institutes of Health as a most misdirected demonstration: "The idea that American government or American society has been inattentive or unresponsive to AIDS is quite simply absurd." On the contrary, "AIDS has become the most privileged disease in America," this since Congress continues to allocate an enormous amount of money for research and for the treatment of people with HIV-related conditions. Except cancer research, HIV-related disease now receives more research funding than any other illness in the United States, a priority Krauthammer maintains is all out of proportion to its significance since AIDS kills fewer people each year than many other diseases. The privilege of AIDS even extends to access to certain experimental drugs—access others do not share.

Chicago Tribune columnist Mike Royko has also challenged the view that there is government indifference regarding AIDS. "That might have been true at one time. But it no longer is. Vast sums are being spent on AIDS research. Far more per victim than on cancer, heart disease and other diseases that kill far more people." In his view, some AIDS education posters have far more to do with the "promotion" of homosexuality than with the prevention of disease. Views of this kind reflect a movement that would assign AIDS a lesser standing in the social and medical priorities of the nation.

This view is not new in the epidemic; the sentiment that homosexuals with AIDS were being treated as a privileged class had surfaced as early as 1983. What is new, though, is the increasing prominence of this view in public discourse and the extent to which the view is defended. In *The Myth of Heterosexual AIDS*, Michael Fumento mounts a full-scale defense of the proposition that the AIDS epidemic has achieved national and medical priority all out of proportion to its dangers, especially since the disease will make few inroads against white, middle-class heterosexuals. Fumento writes in self-conscious sound-bites: "Other than fairly spectacular rare occurrences, such as shark attacks and maulings by wild animals, it is difficult to name any broad category of death that will take fewer lives than heterosexually transmitted AIDS." He also says that the mass mailing of the Surgeon General's report on AIDS to every household "makes every bit as much sense as sending a booklet warning against the dangers of frostbite to every home in the nation, from Key West, Florida, to San Diego, California." Because there is no looming heterosexual epidemic and because the nation has neglected other medical priorities by siphoning off talent and money for AIDS research, Fumento concludes that "the ratio of AIDS research and development spending to federal patient costs is vastly out of proportion to other deadly diseases." Fumento also believes that the priority assigned to AIDS will endanger the lives of other people: "The blunt fact is that people will die of these other diseases because of the overemphasis on AIDS. We will never know their names, and those names will never be sewn into a giant quilt. We will never know their exact numbers. But they will die nonetheless."

Not only the priority of AIDS on the national agenda but also the tactics used to put it there and keep it there have found their critics. Krauthammer concedes that the gains made by AIDS activists are a tribute to their passion and commitment, but he believes that such gains have been won by ingenuous strategy. He charges that the "homosexual community," to advance its own interests, first claimed that AIDS was everyone's problem because everyone was at risk and its solution required universal social urgency. As it became clear that people would not fall at random to the disease, he says activists changed their tactics and began to prey on social guilt:

how dare a society let its gay men, needle-users, their partners and their children get sick and die? But this guilt is unwarranted, Krauthammer believes, since for the most part HIV-related disease is the consequence of individual choices that ignore clear warnings.

Also objecting to activist tactics, the *New York Times* criticized the ACT-UP [AIDS Coalition to Unleash Power] disruption that made it impossible for the Secretary for Health and Human Services to be heard during his remarks at the 1990 international AIDS conference in San Francisco. "It is hard," that paper of record wrote, "to think of a surer way for people with AIDS to alienate their best supporters." The action was characterized as a pointless breakdown in sense and civility. "ACT-UP's members had no justification for turning a research conference into a political circus," especially since, in the standard refrain, society has not only not turned its back but has committed extravagant effort and resources to the HIV epidemic. The disruption, moreover, was all out of proportion to the matters protested: immigration restrictions (since lifted) for people with HIV infection and President Bush's absence from the conference by reason of an event important to the re-election of North Carolina Senator Jesse Helms.

In a different vein, Bruce Fleming suggests in *The Nation* that Americans have come to hype AIDS because of a distorted sense of what it means to be sick and dying. Westerners, he says, assume that absence of disease is the normal state of human being, and that disease thereby becomes a divergence to be named, isolated, and eliminated. Thus can there be the fury and anger he found in a presentation at a Modern Language

Association convention, an AIDS address full of Susan Sontag, Harvey Fierstein, and laments about the lost golden age of free sex. Accepting sickness and death as an integral part of life, he thinks, would free us from the frenetic feeling that AIDS and all disease was unfair treatment amenable to moral and medical control—control it is in any case impossible to achieve.

For all the good intentions here, intentions to remember people sick and dying with other conditions, intentions to keep priorities and discourse rational, intentions to recall the inevitable mortality of human beings as an antidote to their hubris, there is little good reason to shift the priority now devoted to the HIV epidemic, to smear the tactics that have made that priority possible, or to alter the view that sickness and dying with HIV-related disease are evils to be resisted.

Fumento's book makes the most direct claim that people are dying from neglect because the nation has chosen to worry about people with HIV-related conditions. For this reason he thinks AIDS needs to be put into perspective, but he offers not a word about what priority an infectious, communicable lethal disease should receive as against, for example, diabetes or certain heart conditions, which are noncommunicable and can be successfully managed by medicine throughout life. There is not a word, indeed, on how priorities ought to be set at all. Surely an infectious, communicable, lethal disease ought to receive priority over diseases that can currently be medically managed in a way that permits people to live into old age, a prospect not enjoyed by people with HIV-related disease. It is not even clear that funding should be allocated according to the number of persons affected by a particular disease, since such allocation would effectively orphan certain diseases altogether. Moreover, many of the diseases that do now kill people in numbers greater than AIDS have a *long* history of funding, and the expenditures made on behalf of AIDS research and treatment should be measured against that history, not against current annual budget allocations. It may be that AIDS is only now catching up with comparable past expenditures.

Perhaps it is the seemingly voluntary nature of infection that invites the notion that enough has been done for HIV-related conditions. After all, if only people refrained from behavior known to be associated with HIV infection, they wouldn't be at any risk of sickness and death. But HIV-related disease is simply a matter of individual failure to heed clear warnings. Many cases of AIDS were contracted *before any public identification* of the syndrome. Even after the identification of the syndrome, there was no clear identification of its cause or how to avoid it altogether. Early on, there were no efforts to protect blood used in transfusions even when certain screening tests were available. Even after the discovery of the presumptive causal virus and development of blood-screening tests, educational efforts to reach persons most at risk were inadequate and in any case no one knew what forms of education were capable of effecting behavioral change. What educational programs there were failed, then and now, to reach drug-users, their sexual partners, and persons in rural areas. Some persons were infected by means altogether beyond their control: by rape, by transfusion, by Factor VIII used in control of hemophilia, through birth to an infected mother, by accidental needle infection while providing health care or using drugs, through artificial insemination. Because of ambiguities and delays (culpable or not) in biomedicine, education, and public policy, it is not evident for the majority of people with AIDS that there were "clear warnings" that went unheeded.

Even now, when HIV-related disease is well known, it does not follow automatically that those people who contract an HIV infection do so in any morally culpable sense. Over ten years will soon have passed since the CDC [Centers for Disease Control] first reported the occurrence of rare diseases in gay men and drug-using persons. Since that time, ten years of new gay men and drug-users have come along, persons who may not have been educated about the dangers of HIV, young persons who will not yet have maturity of judgment in sexual and drug matters, persons who may not have access to clean needles or drug rehabilitation programs, who may not have the personal and social skills necessary to avoid risk behavior altogether. In some cases there may be cultural and social barriers to protection from risk as well, such as resistance to condom use. It is important to remember, too, that as regards the enticements of sex and drugs, people are weak and not always capable of protecting themselves even from those risks they know and fear. It is not surprising then that a considerable portion of *all* human illness is self-incurred, brought about through one's life choices. This is to vary the principle of double effect: what is chosen is not illness but sex, food, alcohol, drugs, and so on. Their aftermath, unchosen if inevitable, may be illness. But it is telling in this society that those whose heart or lung disease, for example, is related to their life choices are not asked to wait for research and treatment while those whose disease is accidental or genetic are served first.

It is odd that critics see misplaced privilege in the priority and attention AIDS has won where they might instead see a paradigm for other successes. Should the priority accorded to AIDS research and care be seen as an indictment of the wiles of AIDS activists or should it be required study in schools of public health? AIDS activists are not trying to bleed the government dry, and neither are they blind to the nation's other needs. They are merely trying to insure that government and medicine work together to achieve important goals. If other disease research and care is being neglected, the question is not whether activists have rallied the Congress or the American Medical Association into questionable priorities. The relevant question is why other health care research services cannot be delivered with the urgency and high profile that the HIV epidemic has received. In this sense, the HIV epidemic is an opportunity for critical thinking about the nature of health care in the United States: is it the nature of the disease itself or the design of the health care system that makes the HIV epidemic so formidable? Is it the transmissibility of the disease or social attitudes toward sexuality and drug use that make prevention so difficult?

But all this talk of the priority given to the HIV epidemic is likely to be misleading. It is important to remember that AIDS is no privilege. A diagnosis of AIDS amounts to a virtually unlimited onslaught against an individual's physical, emotional, familial, and economic resources. In addition, there is the burden of stigmatization, given that the disease has sometimes been seen as a punishment or deserved consequence of immoral behavior. For example, a 1988 report showed that, depending on the social category of the respondent, some 8 to 60 percent of persons surveyed considered AIDS to be God's punishment for immoral sexual behavior. A minority of Americans is prepared to tolerate considerable discrimination against people with HIV-related conditions. Varying but significant numbers of persons surveyed report that they would refuse to work alongside people with AIDS, would take their children out of school if a child with AIDS were in attendance, would favor the right of landlords to evict people with AIDS, and so on. Perhaps most tellingly, the majority of people in one survey believed health professionals should be warned if patients have an HIV infection, and a third would allow physicians to decide whether to treat such patients.

This last observation would be benign by itself except that medical students and faculty express a great deal of apprehension in working with people with AIDS and there is some evidence that some of them are choosing specialties and geographies that will keep them at a distance from such patients. Some physicians have even taken to the pages of the New York Times to announce that they will refuse to treat any patients with an HIV infection. Nursing recruitment has become difficult for hospitals that care for large numbers of people with HIV-related disorders. There are still places in the United States where hospital food trays are left at the doors of people with AIDS because the nutrition staff will not go into the rooms.

All the money thus far spent in the HIV epidemic has not by itself insured adequate medical care for all people with HIV-related conditions. This is most especially true for the homeless who have HIV-related illness. Neither have the dollars spent on HIV research produced any medical panacea. Treatment with zidovudine (AZT) has proved important for some people but not for all, and there are still many unresolved questions about its long-term ability to extend the lives of all people with HIV infection or to guarantee the quality of life. Zidovudine notwithstanding, as Larry Kramer has pointed out, there continues to be one HIV-related death every twelve minutes in the United States. Is it therefore surprising that ACT-UP now chants, "One billion dollars . . . one drug . . . big deal"?

As Charles Perrow and Mauro F. Guillén point out in The AIDS Disaster, it is of course hard to "prove" that funding for AIDS research and care has been inadequate. But as they also point out, a broad array of highly credible reports have each drawn attention to government and philanthropic failures to respond to the epidemic. These reports have come from the Office of Technology Assessment, the Congressional Research Service, the General Accounting Office, the Institute of Medicine, and the Presidential Commission on the Human Immunodeficiency Virus Epidemic. Whatever funding has occurred, it is hard to see that one can object to the amounts per se that need yet to be spent. The money called for by, for example, the Presidential Commission on the Human Immunodeficiency Virus Epidemic or the Institute of Medicine and the National Academy of Sciences is not an invented figure pulled out of the air as a way of keeping scientists and bureaucrats in fat salaries. The figures represent estimates made in good faith about the extent of funding needed. It was clear early on that billions would be required, and that estimation has not changed merely because headlines have moved on to other subjects.

Perhaps the public is used to thinking in terms of billions only for military budgets, but the medical expenditures of the nation are measured in billions as well. The research carried out by the National Institutes of Health has always been enormously expensive, as has been the provision of medical benefits to veterans, the elderly, and the poor. The federal funding of dialysis for end-stage renal disease alone, for example, provides life-saving therapy for only some seventy thousand people, yet its costs have been measured in the billions since Congress decided to pick up the bill for such services. If this kind of funding is any precedent, neither high cost nor small number of affected persons serve as a convincing rationale for limiting the funding now accorded to AIDS research and treatment.

Budget requests based on what should be done are one thing, of course, and budgets actually produced in government legislatures are another. The question at issue in discussions about the "privilege" of AIDS is the question of what priority should be assigned to AIDS funding given all the other funding needs that face the nation. Richard D. Mohr has argued that AIDS funding exerts a moral claim insofar as the disease is associated with gay men; in many of its most significant aspects, the HIV epidemic is the consequence of prejudicial social choices and arrangements. Because its rituals, laws, educational sys-

tem, and prevailing opinion fail to offer gay men any clear or supportive pathway to self-esteem or any incentives to the rewards of durable relationships, society has effectively forced some gay men into promiscuous behavior. Neither does society permit gay men the opportunity to form families that could shoulder at least part of the care their sick need. Patricia Illingworth has fleshed out this argument and extended it to drug users as well. These are powerful arguments; it is hard to think, for example, of a single public ritual in family life, education, the media, religion, or the law that dignifies the love of one man for another, that supports any abiding union there. It is also hard to see that society has protected its needle-users where it cannot prevent drug use or offer successful drug rehabilitation programs. American society's enthusiasm for wars on drugs has not, after all, been translated into action capable of helping any but a fortunate few stop their drug use. Needle-exchange programs have been rejected out of fear that such action will appear to "condone" drug use—a fear that is odd given the de facto acceptance of drug use at every stratum of American culture from Supreme Court justice nominees on down.

It is not surprising then, that left to their own devices, many gay men, drug users, their sexual partners and children find themselves at the mercy of an indifferent virus as they try to lead what lives they can. Victims of disease rarely "just happen." More often than not society's choices permit them to happen, indeed make them inevitable. Robert M. Veatch has observed that it is fair to permit inequality of outcome where opportunities have been equal, but such a conclusion as regards health care would "not apply to persons who are truly not equal in their opportunity because of their social or psychological conditions. It would not apply to those who are forced into their health-risky behavior because of social oppression or stress in the mode of production." Because many of the persons who have contracted HIV-related conditions have done so under circumstances implicating prejudicial social arrangements, there is a substantial claim that priority for HIV research and care is required for reasons of compensation.

But it is not compensation alone that frames the moral imperative about how a society should act here. Moral philosophy also avails itself of the supererogatory, those burdens we undertake beyond the call of formal obligation. Seen from this perspective, the society worth praising, the society worth *having* is the one that will find ways to care and to research, even though there is no formal obligation to do so and for no other reason than that its citizens are ill and dying. The care of those who contracted HIV infection through blood transfusions would be relevant in this regard, as would be women whose HIV risk was a secretly sexually active husband. The morally admirable society would do what it could to protect such persons from infection and care for them when they are sick whether or not society specifically *owes* them this concern and care as a form of compensation.

Cost alone should not be any obstacle for keeping AIDS research and care a national priority. The research is as important as any other research being conducted in the United States today. Delaying this research will not only impede therapy and vaccine development, but it will also subject the eventual costs to inflation; AIDS research will only get

more expensive the longer it is delayed. Delays in researching treatments and vaccines will also increase the number of people who may be potentially at risk of HIV-related disease. It is worth remembering that only one disease (smallpox) has ever been entirely eliminated. HIV-related disease is a problem for our time, and it will be a problem for future generations. It is not something that one can throw a fixed sum of money at before moving on. Even when fully effective vaccines and treatment become available, there will be people who will fail to benefit from either by reason of social deprivation, geography, choice, and chance. HIV-related disease therefore needs to be treated as a disease that is here to stay and not one that has already had its share of the limelight and public coffers.

Objections to ACT-UP disruptions of traffic and speech seem to share the view that quiet discourse, argued in mannerly fashion by legislators consulting with medical boards is enough to insure that the nation will set appropriate medical goals. But this view of rationally framed public policy is not entirely true to history. There are few important social reforms that did not require the abandonment of polite discourse and the disruption of business as usual. It is important to remember that government and policy in this country are as much a product of protests, strikes, and civil disobedience as of reasoned debate. It is wrong to pretend that civil disobedience and social disruption are not part and parcel of this nation's political techniques, and it is wrong to blame AIDS activists for using these techniques as others have used them. Perhaps we have forgotten that the United States owes its very origin to acts of rebellion that the

New York Times might have found easy to condemn as breakdowns in sense and civility.

Without protests, moreover, it is hard to see how the battle against AIDS would ever have gotten off the ground. In the early years of the epidemic, the sickness and death of small numbers of gay men did not lend itself to the advocacy of important legislators and medical commissions. It was necessary then that impolite discourse be used in order to be heard. That need continues to this day. Most of the many recommendations of the 1988 Presidential Commission Report on the Human Immunodeficiency Virus Epidemic, for example, are already collecting dust. If an analysis with the stature of a Presidential Commission report cannot spur action on important goals, what other recourse is there than the tried and true methods of protest that are as much a part of American democracy as its parliamentary rules of order? It is odd that where people do not see conspiracy behind AIDS activism, they see irrationality and impropriety when what they might see is a standard of urgency and passion by which to evaluate and improve the entire health care system in the United States.

It is hard to see moreover that an acceptance of disease and dying, in the way Fleming has urged, is anything but an invitation to quietism. If disease and dying are inevitable, what incentive is there to resist their damages? Granted, some Americans may have lost the sense of their mortality, but it is hard to see that much is gained by restoring it. On the contrary, it may be the perception of disease as "excrescence" that is the very spur to its control and eradication. There is no point in glorifying disease and dying; the lessons they teach are easily learned and do not require advanced instruction. There is a point at which sickness and dying cease to offer insights into the human condition or opportunities for strength and become instead unbearable, unredeemable absurdity. This is most often how AIDS appears to those who know it. To his credit, Fleming does say that hesitation by the U.S. government to carry out necessary HIV research would be criminal. But if this is so, then it's unclear that the change in the perception of death he counsels would make any practical difference in regard to the responsibility of government and medicine to resist the epidemic as much as it can with all the resources it can muster.

The sentiment nevertheless grows that AIDS is getting more than its share of media attention, resources, and social indulgence. But there really hasn't been any change in the status of the epidemic to warrant a change in the scope of intensity of research and treatment programs. HIV remains a highly lethal, communicable virus. Despite better medical management, the number of HIV-related deaths continues to increase. More and more hospital resources have to be directed to the care of people with HIV-related conditions. What accounts for the sentiment, then, that AIDS has gotten more than its share? From the onset of the epidemic, there have been many dire prophesies about the toll of the epidemic, predictions that millions to billions would die. Is it possible that critics can say that AIDS has gotten more than its share because it has not yet killed *enough* people? Is the same epidemic at the margins of national attention now inspiring the claim that enough has been done? The sentiment that enough has been done for AIDS has primarily been argued in the press or journalistic accounts and not in professional journals of medicine, bioethics, or public policy. Could it be that this sentiment belongs to those who do not know the epidemic at first hand?

If HIV research and therapy are relegated to a lesser rank in the nation's priorities, it will be gay men, needle-users, their sexual partners and their children who will continue to pay the price of neglect, and the epidemic will become again the shadow killer that it was in the beginning. In view of the people who are still sick, who are dying, who bear the costs of this epidemic, it is too early and shameful to say that enough has been done. In an epidemic not yet ten years old, it is too early for a backlash.

POSTSCRIPT

Is AIDS Getting More Than Its Share of Resources and Media Attention?

In the spring of 1990, 1,000 demonstrators camped outside the National Institutes of Health near Washington, D.C., to protest governmental and scientific neglect of AIDS. This was not the first protest claiming that the government was not doing enough to help find a cure for the disease and that the government had not issued warnings about the disease soon enough.

AIDS was officially diagnosed in 1981. However, President Reagan did not mention AIDS until 1985, even though the number of cases and deaths were rising toward epidemic proportions. Finally, in 1986, then–surgeon general C. Everett Koop issued a report on the AIDS virus and sent educational materials about AIDS to every household in the United States. Critics claim that had the government begun AIDS education and research sooner, many lives would have been saved. Randy Shilts, in his 1987 book *And the Band Played On* (St. Martin's Press), argues that the government had known about the AIDS epidemic for several years before anything was done.

In *The AIDS Disaster: The Failure of Organizations in New York and the Nation* (Yale University Press, 1990), Charles Perrow and Mauro F. Guillen describe how the reaction, from both public and private organizations, was very limited and slow after the first AIDS cases were identified in 1981. They document their case that government and private groups failed to proivde the necessary education and care in response to this epidemic.

The entire October 1988 issue of *Scientific America* is devoted to AIDS and is a good resource on the biology of AIDS and on early research into the origins of the AIDS virus.

There are also those who share the sentiments expressed by Charles Krauthammer in his June 25, 1990, essay in *Time* magazine. In his essay, Krauthammer writes that people with AIDS deserve to be cared for and treated, but he questions why they should be first in line—ahead of those dying of leukemia, breast cancer, or stroke—for the resources and compassion of a nation.

The disease of AIDS has generated thousands of articles and books since the epidemic first began. The following articles offer several different viewpoints on the seriousness of the epidemic and the government's response to the crisis: "AIDS So Far," *Commentary* (December 1991); "AIDS Poses a Classic Dilemma," *The New York Times* (February 10, 1987); "AIDS: A Crisis Ignored," *U.S. News & World Report* (January 12, 1987); "AIDS and a Duty to Protect," *Hastings Center Report* (February 1987); "The AIDS Epidemic Has Hit Home," *Psychology Today* (April, 1987); and "The Judgment Mentality," *Christianity Today* (March 20, 1987).

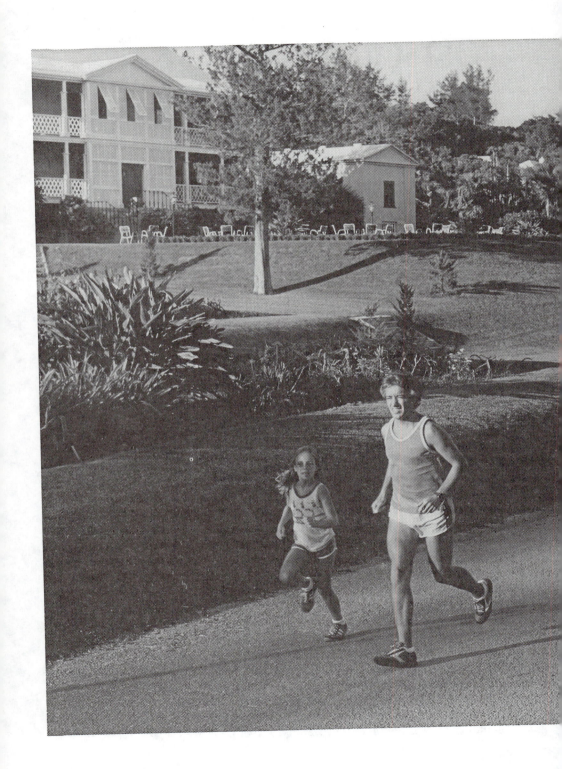

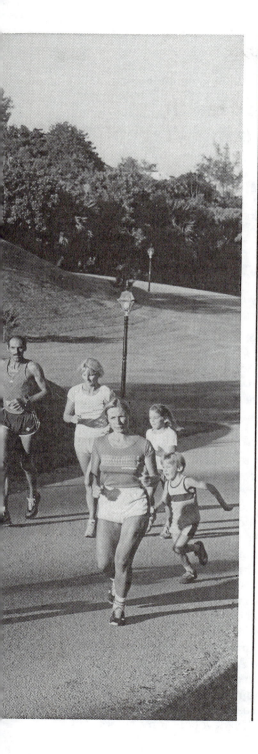

PART 2

Mind-Body Issues

Humans have long sought to extend life, eliminate disease, and prevent sickness. In modern times, people have depended on technology to develop creative and innovative ways to improve health. However, as cures for diseases such as cancer and heart disease continue to elude scientists and doctors, many people question whether or not modern medicine has reached a plateau in improving health. As a result, over the last decade emphasis has been placed on prevention as a way to improve health. Although millions of people have made changes in their life-styles in hopes of preventing the onset of disease, some scientists argue that people will always be plagued by illness and that overzealous emphasis on prevention and control is misplaced. The relationship between mind and body is the key to the issues debated in this section.

Will Practicing Positive Health Behaviors and Emphasizing Prevention Improve Health?

Can a Positive Mental Attitude Overcome Disease?

ISSUE 5

Will Practicing Positive Health Behaviors and Emphasizing Prevention Improve Health?

YES: Albert L. Huebner, from "The No-Win War on Cancer," *East West: The Journal of Natural Health and Living*

NO: Lenn E. Goodman and Madeleine J. Goodman, from "Prevention— How Misuse of a Concept Undercuts Its Worth," *Hastings Center Report* (April 1986)

ISSUE SUMMARY

YES: Professor of physics Albert L. Huebner believes that practicing healthy behaviors could both prevent and decrease the incidence of cancer.
NO: Professor of philosophy Lenn E. Goodman and professor of human biology Madeleine J. Goodman argue that the ability to prevent disease, especially cancer, is exaggerated and limited.

While it makes sense to try to prevent a disease rather than to place emphasis on treatment, prevention may not always be possible. To prevent disease, health behavior changes are often necessary, but such changes may be beyond the ability of some individuals, however motivated they may be. In addition, the beneficial effects of prevention on health are quite clear, but the risks and costs are not as obvious. These issues also need to be assessed.

During the past decade, there has been a movement toward self-care and prevention as a means to improve health. This movement has been based on several factors: Many diseases, such as cancer and heart disease, have no "magic bullet" cure; health care costs have been spiraling; and it is cheaper, more humane, and more sensible to try and prevent a disease rather than to attempt to cure it. If individuals could be encouraged to quit smoking and adopt low-fat diets, a significantly lower number of cancers would develop.

This viewpoint is of particular interest to Albert L. Huebner, who believes that the United States spends far too little on disease prevention. He presents research that relates cancer, the second leading cause of death in the United States, to specific life-style behaviors, such as smoking and eating a high-fat diet. Huebner argues that the government has devoted far more money and interest to treatment than to prevention. He cites examples of antismoking campaigns, the budgets of which equal a fraction of the money allocated to tobacco subsidies for farmers and agricultural research. He also claims that little interest or money has been spent promoting the anticancer diet.

Lenn E. Goodman and Madeleine J. Goodman argue that prevention campaigns are often based on limited scientific proof. They conclude that the ability of individuals to prevent cancer is somewhat restricted. The authors cite conflicting studies on the benefits of a low-fat diet in the prevention of cancer. They insist that cancer is caused by many factors and that merely changing one aspect (diet) will not necessarily prevent the disease. Goodman and Goodman also point out that all individuals respond differently to diet and other environmental substances. Making overall recommendations for populations, they argue, does not take into account individual differences within population groups.

YES

Albert L. Huebner

THE NO-WIN WAR ON CANCER

A fundamental principle of any rational approach to health is that it makes more sense to prevent a disease than to put the emphasis on treatment. This is especially important with cancer, for which strategies of prevention show enormous promise while the treatment hasn't gained much ground against major forms of the disease. Yet since passage of the National Cancer Act in 1971, repeated attempts to improve priorities in the "war on cancer" that was launched by this legislation have had little success.

During the mid-1970s, dispute raged over the small percentage of its budget the National Cancer Institute (NCI) allotted for prevention. It had been generally accepted by then that about 70 to 90 percent of human cancers have "environmental" causes, where environmental is used in a broad sense that includes food and tobacco smoke ("lifestyle" factors) as well as occupational chemicals and a wide range of industrial pollutants. The clear implication was that many of these cancers were preventable, yet the cancer establishment continued to concentrate its efforts on treatment. Criticism of priorities in the cancer war has continued, although frequently deflected by claims of remarkable new cures and rising survival rates.

Recently, however, cancer researchers John Bailar and Elaine Smith created new tremors with their well-documented claim, published in a May 1986 issue of the *New England Journal of Medicine*, that the war on cancer is being lost. They cited data from the National Center for Health Statistics indicating that, from 1962 to 1982, deaths from cancer, after adjustment for the increasing size and age of the population, increased by 8.7 percent. Perhaps equally important when focusing on causation, from 1973 to 1981 the age-adjusted *incidence* rate of the disease increased by 8.5 percent.

Bailar and Smith don't deny that there has been remarkable progress in treating some cancers. Childhood cancers and Hodgkin's disease, for example, provide remarkable success stories. But these forms of the disease are such a small proportion of the total that they are almost lost in the statistics. Vincent DeVita, director of NCI, acknowledges that "50 percent of all cures through chemotherapy occur in 10 percent of all cancer patients." That 10 percent consists mostly of children and patients with Hodgkin's disease.

It's the other 90 percent of patients that worry thoughtful analysts like Bailar, who insists that "the overall picture is pretty grim." His colleague at the

Harvard School of Public Health, cancer expert John Cairns, put it more forcefully. In *Science* magazine, the publication of the American Association for the Advancement of Science, Cairns said that "there have been no significant gains in survival from any of the major cancers since the 1950s" and that "the cancer data are so discouraging that it is difficult to discuss them in public." Lung cancer in particular, which has a major impact on cancer statistics, still has an extremely poor prognosis.

Given these trends, Bailar and Smith write, "The major conclusion we draw is that some thirty-five years of intense effort focused largely on improving treatments must be judged a qualified failure." And they renew a call for a "shift in emphasis, from research on treatment to research on prevention," essential "if substantial progress against cancer is to be forthcoming."

This recommendation is unlikely to find more tangible support now than it has in the past, however. A spokesperson for the NCI responded that, under the present program, steady progress is being made against the disease. He insisted that the institute's goal of cutting mortality in half by the year 2000 is realistic, although it isn't at all clear what might produce this dramatic drop in the cancer death rate in the next thirteen years.

THE NCI'S RESPONSE TO THE ARTICLE BY Bailar and Smith, like its response to earlier calls for greater emphasis on prevention, illustrates why the cancer war isn't being won. Soon after the Bailar and Smith study created a stir, the NCI announced, with great fanfare, that the cancer fatality rate decreased last year [1986] among Americans under age fifty-five. DeVita called this "one of the most encouraging cancer statistics we see," and attributed the decline to advances in treatment.

The realities are that the cancer death rate for people fifty-five and over, who account for more than three-fourths of all cancers, rose, so that the *total* death rate from cancer actually increased. The incidence rate for people under fifty-five also rose. And although NCI was elated over changes in the lung cancer rate among women, that rate didn't fall, it merely rose less rapidly than previously.

Bailar observed, "NCI is very selective in what figures it gives prominence," and he added, "I think it's unfair to the public and unfair to the news media and Congress to try to cover up the general failure [in the war on cancer] . . . by emphasizing the bright spots."

In the past, the NCI has acknowledged that a great deal is known about how to prevent cancer. When critics have voiced complaints about the low priority given to prevention, the NCI has drawn a distinction between trying to change lifestyle factors to curtail cancer, and trying to control industrial carcinogens. The NCI has argued in effect that smoking, diet, and other lifestyle factors, which account for about two-thirds of environmental cancers, are "voluntary" factors best left to the individuals for action. Only 10 to 15 percent of environmental cancers result from industrial pollution, so the institute claimed justification in directing roughly 10 percent of its budget to all environmental carcinogens, including those attributed to lifestyle. Even if NCI and other agencies had sharply reduced the threat from chemical pollutants—which they didn't—in ignoring most of the causes of cancer the institute was guaranteeing that cancer mortality would remain far higher than need be.

The NCI was also ignoring the problem inherent in viewing personal habits as completely voluntary, which suggests that the individual could easily eliminate these habits, and the cancer they cause, if he or she wanted to. This argument is the basis for the opinion that lung cancer, chiefly caused by cigarette smoking, shouldn't be included in cancer mortality statistics. And when proponents of this lifestyle doctrine push it to extremes, the implication is strong that if you get certain kinds of cancer, it's probably your own fault.

It can be argued, however, that this division into voluntary and involuntary exposures to cancer-causing substances is artificial, in view of the enormous advertising budgets used to push tobacco and processed food, and the influence advertising holds over the consuming public. Success against cancer will entail dealing broadly with these factors, as well as the toxic substances involved in many industrial and occupational cancers. The evidence indicates that the cancer establishment is marking time, or in many cases moving backwards, in confronting these issues. The problem is many-sided and complex, as we'll see, while attempts to solve it have been simplistic, fragmented, and frequently misguided.

THE CONTENTION THAT SMOKING IS A VOL-untary activity overlooks both the addictive properties of tobacco and the power advertising can have by instilling a product with an aura of glamor. Dr. William Polin, director of the National Institute of Drug Abuse, has correctly described cigarette smoking as "the most widespread drug dependence in our country." The statistics easily bear out the extent of use and the addictiveness.

Roughly one in three adult Americans smoke; national surveys indicate that 90 percent of smokers would like to quit, but 85 percent of those who try are unsuccessful.

Nicotine is believed to be the major reinforcer, or addictive component, in cigarette smoke, although there may be others. Pharmacologically, nicotine is similar to such central nervous system stimulants as the amphetamines, which are even more addictive than heroin and other opiates. Each inhaled puff of a cigarette delivers a dose of nicotine to the brain, resulting in 50,000 to 70,000 doses per person each year for an average smoker. No other form of drug use occurs with such frequency or regularity. It isn't surprising then that withdrawal from smoking can produce a wide range of physiological and psychological effects, or that many former drug addicts report that it's harder to give up tobacco than heroin.

With a drug this addictive, many smokers who start early stay hooked. Manufacturers know that 80 percent of regular smokers start by age eighteen and 90 percent by age twenty-one. This explains the special status of cigarettes as the most heavily advertised product in the U.S. It's well worth the investment—to the producer, if not the smoker.

Industry representatives insist that they advertise only to get existing smokers to switch brands, not to lure new smokers to the ranks and, in particular, never to influence young people. But a report prepared by Dr. Martin Fishbein for the Federal Trade Commission cites numerous U.S. and British studies showing that the level of cigarette advertising does influence smoking rates.

More importantly, these ads create images of smokers as sophisticated and socially secure people, images that have an enormous special appeal for youngsters. Consistent with this, a comprehensive survey conducted a few years ago among young Americans provided clear evidence, according to the investigators, that "cigarette advertising helps to reinforce and enhance the image of the teenage smoker as young, attractive, healthy, and sexy." What a cruel seduction!

The greatest recent tragedy in cancer mortality is that women have reached parity with men in making lung cancer their leading cause of cancer death. This isn't likely to change soon because women are giving up smoking even more slowly than men, and smoking among young women is actually increasing.

Here too, advertising plays a big role. The tobacco industry acknowledges that it directs much of its current advertising to the female market. A recent article in *Advertising Age*, headlined, "Women Top Cig Target," quoted the president of R. J. Reynolds describing the women's market as "probably the largest opportunity" for the company. Executives of other companies felt the same way, because during the 1970s cigarette ads increased tenfold in major women's magazines.

Despite this formidable combination of the addictive properties of tobacco and the youth-directed advertising, antismoking campaigns are not futile. On the contrary, they've been extremely successful on those rare occasions when they've been promoted seriously.

A program begun in 1967 provides a striking illustration both of the path toward conquest of cancer, and of the too-frequent turns away from that path. That year the Federal Communications Commission, in response to a petition from a young attorney, obligated radio and television broadcasters to give a "substantial" amount of time—although not equal time—to the "other side" of the cigarette controversy. For more than three years, creative ads urged smokers to quit and nonsmokers not to start. During that period, an unprecedented 10 million Americans quit smoking and, after years of virtually uninterrupted growth, per capita consumption of cigarettes plummeted.

The antismoking campaign was torpedoed when Congress passed legislation, privately supported by the manufacturers, that banned radio and television cigarette ads. The industry merely shifted its radio and television advertising to other media. But the ban on cigarette advertising over the electronic media eliminated the "Fairness Doctrine" obligation of stations that was at the heart of the effective antismoking campaign. Predictably, the sharp decline in cigarette consumption was reversed in 1971, the year the advertising ban went into effect.

This successful experiment in health education received scant financial support from the federal agencies publicly funded to conduct the war against cancer—never more than $1 million per year. Nearly twenty years later, a bill now before Congress would appropriate that same amount of money (actually much less when inflation is accounted for) to run some public service announcements informing women of tobacco's risks. Even during the highly publicized anticigarette campaign of former Health, Education, and Welfare Secretary Joseph Califano, however, total funding for this purpose was never more than a small fraction of what the government spends in *support* of tobacco use: federal price supports, tobacco agricultural research, market research, and most cynically, export to needy countries under the "Food for Peace" program.

A SECOND MAJOR LIFESTYLE FACTOR AFFECTing cancer is diet, which differs from smoking in that it plays both a positive and a negative role in influencing the disease. But as with smoking, the NCI has been ineffective in exploiting this opportunity to make progress against cancer.

As early as 1944 it was observed that the incidence of certain cancers changed dramatically when people moved from one country to another and adopted new eating habits. American blacks have much lower rates of liver cancer, but much higher rates of colon cancer, than African blacks. Similarly, there is a higher incidence of stomach cancer and a lower incidence of colon cancer in Japan compared with the U.S. But when Japanese migrate to the U.S. and adopt the diet of their new home, they acquire the U.S. stomach and colon cancer rates as well.

The implications that many cancer researchers drew from these epidemiological studies, and other early observations, is that compared to the current average American diet, a prudent anticancer diet would be lower in calories, lower in fat and higher in fiber, with more fruit, vegetables, and whole grains and less red meat, eggs, and fat-rich dairy products. Another implication is that additives such as nitrates and nitrites should be avoided, and intake of protective vitamins, notably A, C, and E, should be judiciously increased.

It's true that exactly *how* these dietary components prevent or promote cancer wasn't known when the cancer war was launched, and many of the details still aren't fully understood. A reasonable course for NCI would have been to vigorously publicize the prudent data (a healthful diet for reasons that go beyond cancer prevention) until every American got the message, while doing the research needed for a more precise understanding.

But despite its burgeoning budget, NCI did little. During the late 1970s, the agency was repeatedly chided by prominent members of Congress, in particular Senators Dole and McGovern, for neglecting the nutrition connection to cancer. It wasn't until quite recently that NCI finally took a firm stand on the low-fat, high-fiber diet, and the American Cancer Society, which does much of NCI's public relations, began promoting a few elements of the prudent diet in ad campaigns.

If advocacy of an anticancer diet has been at best lukewarm, research has also lagged behind. Dr. Ruth Shearer, an NCI-funded researcher with a passionate dedication to defeating cancer and an admirably independent mind, has pointed out that as late as 1977 only $3 million a year was going into nutritional research on cancer, while $57 million was being spent for the virus program. "There's more prestige in the virus theory," she has said, adding wryly, "Nutritional research conjures up the picture of a school lunch program."

IF SMOKING AND DIET, HOWEVER IMPORTANT as causes of cancer, are too humdrum to generate much enthusiasm among researchers, the toxicity of chemicals in the workplace and the environment ought to be more stimulating. Yet this aspect of cancer control has had no greater success.

In 1976, Congress passed the Toxic Substance Control Act (TSCA). Its stated goal was to provide a testing ground, other than "the nation's population and environment," for the potentially dangerous chemicals that pour into commerce in massive amounts each year. After several years of inaction by the Environmental Protection Agency (EPA), which administers TSCA, complaint was brought in federal court by an environmental group, the Natural Resource Defense Council (NRDC), along with the AFL-CIO. Significantly, the EPA was joined in defending itself by the Chemical Manufacturer's Association and the American Petroleum Institute.

Ruling on the case in 1984, a U.S. District Court judge found that "in the more than seven years since TSCA's enactment, though seventy-three chemicals have been designated by government scientists for priority rule-making consideration"—that is, formal testing procedures—"EPA has yet to finalize a single test rule. Congress could not have intended (or envisioned) this result."

Congress really had no right to expect much from the EPA, given its own performance. While a series of national scares took place around toxic substances ranging from DDT to vinyl chloride and from polychlorinated biphenyls to Tris, Congress delayed passage of TSCA. It was one thing to declare war on cancer, but quite another to crack down on the manufacturers of cancer-causing substances. Finally, after five years of debate, the bill passed was a thoroughly watered-down version of the original.

For obvious reasons, an especially critical group of environmental carcinogens are chemicals in food. In this case, rather than mere foot-dragging, the steps taken have been *backward*.

The Delaney clause, passed by Congress in 1958, bans the use of any substances that cause cancer in animals as additives to food, cosmetics, and drugs. The clause has been under increasing attack for more than a decade. In 1981, Secretary of Health and Human Services (HHS) Richard Schweiker officially took the position that it should be scrapped. He insisted, "We have to redefine the clause in terms of a risk-benefit ratio."

That redefinition has been eroding the clause ever since. For example, risk-benefit considerations were cited for the Food and Drug Administration in approving use of two drugs and cosmetic dyes recently, despite the language of the clause, which clearly imposes an absolute ban on cancer-causing additives. The FDA commissioner argued, "It makes no sense at all to brand as illegal, and by doing so to disrupt the marketing of a considerable number of products, additives that present a risk that is barely more than theoretical. . . ."

As a general principle, the risk-benefit approach might have some justification if the group taking the risk and the group reaping the benefits were the same, but usually they aren't. In the specific case of the dyes, the commissioner's own scientific staff argued against approval on grounds that the risk estimates used, based on industry calculations, may have significantly underestimated the true risk.

A variation of this risk-benefit gambit was recently supported by a ruling of the Supreme Court. The FDA can now substantially increase the "acceptable" levels of naturally occurring poisons in food without holding public hearings or publishing final regulations. Aflatoxins, a mold that grows on corn and peanuts, is one such substance. This mold is believed to be a major factor in the extremely high liver cancer rates in Africa, and the National Academy of Sciences has called it the "most potent carcinogen known in laboratory animals." Yet the allowed levels can now be increased fivefold if the FDA wants to.

IT'S CLEAR THAT MANY COMPONENTS OF what should be a coherent anticancer program are operating ineffectively. Individual agencies rarely pursue the war against cancer with the tactics and intensity required. The number of different agencies involved—NCI, EPA, FDA, OSHA, among others—has led to confusion about the causes of cancer, and how to prevent it. Commercial pressures add to the confusion.

The consequences of this fragmentation are illustrated by standard tabulations of the causes of cancer, where the numbers are made to add up to 100 percent. In a more realistic tabulation the totals would be greater than 100 percent, reflecting multiple, interactive causes.

The prevailing artificial tabulation obscures important preventative measures that need attention. For example, cancer epidemiologist Samuel Epstein believes that smoking, although certainly the most important single cause of lung cancer, nonetheless has been overestimated as a cause, and occupational carcinogens underestimated, because in many studies lung-cancer deaths of smoking workers were routinely attributed to smoking and not occupation. This underestimation of occupational cancers weakens attempts to regulate carcinogens in the workplace.

Similarly, Epstein and other prominent researchers think that one of the ways in which fat consumption increases cancer may be its ability to bring fat-soluble pesticides and industrial chemicals into the body. If so, then some cancers attributed to a high-fat diet should also be charged against pollution or occupational causes.

Insight into the artificiality in tabulating cancer causes, and of dividing cancer control among an alphabet soup of government agencies, reveals another artificiality: the division between regulating industrial and agricultural carcinogens to control cancer, and changing lifestyles to control cancer. As one researcher has observed, occupational hazards and toxic waste dumps are the production side of the cancer problem, while smoking, alcohol, improper diet, and polluting automobiles are the consumption side.

This holistic view shows clearly that cancer will not be stopped by government agencies alone, or by individuals acting alone. True, roads not taken by agencies are not necessarily barred to individuals, who can improve their odds by eating an anticancer diet, not smoking, and avoiding carcinogens as much as possible. But individuals need help that the agencies are well-qualified to supply, if their priorities are set straight. This reordering would free them to do needed research, to issue and enforce effective regulations against discharge of carcinogens into the environment, and to disseminate essential information to the public.

Needed, in short, are the responsible and harmonious efforts of both individuals and agencies, directed at the primary goal—prevention.

NO

Lenn E. Goodman and
Madeleine J. Goodman

PREVENTION—HOW MISUSE OF A CONCEPT UNDERCUTS ITS WORTH

Today the mounting costs of acute health care place an economic premium on preventive measures. The classic model is the mass vaccination campaign, but beyond that model lie notions and practices grafted to the image of prevention, sharing in its magic but lacking a sound conceptual basis for their claims. Misuse of the idea of prevention can occur in a variety of ways. The examples we have selected are not isolated incidents, nor are they limited to peripheral health promotion efforts.

As communicable diseases have gradually come under control in our society (with the exception of the newly discovered disease of AIDS), many public health workers are refocusing on chronic illnesses of complex or unknown etiology. They use statistical analysis to group associated "risk factors," which may be confounded either with one another or with their putative effects. Even as such a nexus is being identified, intervention efforts aimed at reducing risk are often undertaken. Since no biological model has been established, such efforts may yield unexpected results. . . .

In recent years claims that a specific dietary mode will decrease cancer risk have become more frequent and insistent. The Office of Technology Assessment, which undertook a study of cancer risk for the 97th Congress, concluded that the "overall association of cancer with diet exists, but there is no reliable indication of exactly what dietary changes would be of major importance in reducing cancer incidence and mortality." Nevertheless, in testimony before the Senate Subcommittee on Nutrition in October 1979, Arthur Upton, then director of the National Cancer Institute (NCI), forcefully laid a basis in policy for claims about the impact of diet on cancer risk: "Despite the . . . inability to pinpoint specific dietary carcinogens, scientists generally agree that factors in diet and nutrition—including drinking water contaminants—appear to be related to a large number of human cancers, perhaps 50 percent."

Reviewing a great body of pertinent studies Richard Doll and Richard Peto wrote in the *Journal of the National Cancer Institute,* "It may be possible to reduce U.S. cancer death rates by practicable dietary means by as much as 35% ('guestimated' as stomach and large bowel 90%; endometrium, gallbladder, pancreas, and breast 50%; lung, larynx, bladder, cervix, mouth, pharynx, and esophagus 20%; other types of cancer 10%)." The figures are impressive, and Doll and Peto explain in detail how they are derived: nations where meat and fat consumption are high are found to have high incidences and mortality rates of cancer.

But the inference that an altered diet can produce a corresponding change in incidence is problematic. [Researchers] have observed that in Greece the incidence of breast cancer is less than one-fourth that in Israel, but total dietary fat intake is essentially the same. Breast cancer mortality is three times higher in France and Italy than in Spain, although the total dietary fat intake is slightly higher in Spain. Puerto Rico has only 30 to 40 percent of the U.S. incidence of breast and colon cancers, despite substantially higher reliance on animal fat. Breast and colon cancer are twice as frequent in the Netherlands as in Finland, but animal fat consumption is estimated to be identical. Indians of the American Southwest have high intakes of animal fat but low breast cancer rates. [Researchers argue] that it is fallacious to attribute increased cancer rates in the United States to increased consumption of animal fat, since daily per capita consumption of animal fat decreased from 104 grams in 1909 to 97 grams in 1972.

A nineteen-year study of cancer in men suggests that milk, fatty fish, eggs, and butter—foods high in vitamin D but usually restricted in "anticancer" diets—may have a protective effect against colorectal cancer. The low rate of colon cancer found in Seventh Day Adventists is often attributed to vegetarianism, but Mormons have a similarly low rate. Their faith, like that of the Adventists, proscribes smoking, drinking, coffee, and stimulants. But they are not generally vegetarians. In a major international epidemiological study . . . GNP was as potent a correlate with cancer as any dietary factor.

Individual diets vary within nations geographically, culturally, ethnically, and with age, sex, and socioeconomic status. Familial and individual differences in food preparation, waste (for example, are cooking fats reused?), alcohol consumption, and other factors affect the impact of diet. Women of Japanese ancestry in the United States have a breast cancer rate closer to that of American women than to that of Japanese women living in Japan. But the changes in incidence have not been directly tied to diet. They are observed among the granddaughters of immigrants. There has not yet been a controlled study of the effects of diet over the lifespan of individuals. . . .

George Kerr of the Human Nutrition Center at the University of Texas School of Public Health cites the extremity of some recommendations as one factor justifying the promulgation of a cancer prevention diet before any dietary hypothesis is confirmed. The public, Kerr argues, demands information and will turn to the ill-founded, often dangerous diets of quacks and "health foodists" if reputable nutritionists do not provide responsible cancer preventive dietary guidelines. Recognizing that the causation of cancer must be multifactorial, Kerr does not simplistically equate reduction of a risk factor with reduction of risk: "Stating that diet is involved in the causation of 50% of cancers should not be interpreted to mean that dietary modification can prevent 50% of cancers," he points out. This important insight is lost sight of in the voluminous pages of Doll and Peto. . . . But Kerr himself does not believe that such reservations should inhibit efforts at dietary reform.

Kerr advocates dietary guidelines that are more moderate than those he seeks to preempt but they suffer nonetheless from some of the same weaknesses: the cancer prevention claims remain unproven, and the reasoning seems to be similar to that of the food culturists. The NRC [National Research Council] acknowledges that the contribution of diet to reducing cancer risk cannot be quantified presently; it even concedes that the crucial effects of diet may occur in childhood or adolescence and that dietary modifications later in life may have a negligible or negative effect. But proponents of the cancer prevention dietary guidelines argue that the recommended diet is a healthful one on general principles, even if it does not succeed in reducing cancer incidence and mortality.

OVERSELLING: THE ETHOS OF PROSPERO

A preventive health campaign is a marketing effort, subject to all the risks of motivational marketing—hyperbole, demagoguery, or playing upon fears and prejudices. Here ignorance is not the excuse for oversimplification: relevant data deemed contrary to the desired outcome, or not sufficiently productive of that outcome, are overlooked or under-

stated. But an oversold campaign can undercut its own authority, causing the audience to tune out or even respond adversely. . . .

In the case of swine flu, the use of a hard sell almost from the inception of contingency planning gave the program a momentum that inhibited deliberation. When swine flu was detected in February 1976 among recruits at Fort Dix, officials of the Centers for Disease Control in Atlanta rapidly recognized that the strain might represent a recurrence of the pandemic influenza of 1918, endangering perhaps a million American lives. Health planners proposed a voluntary immunization over three months of some 200 million Americans at a cost of $134 million.

The decision-making process throughout was characterized by concern about blame, eagerness to showcase preventive medicine, and a crisis mentality, all of which tended to eclipse clinical and epidemiological evidence. The rhetoric deployed at each level effectively forced the hand of those who would carry the decision to the next. External factors such as the attitude of the insurance industry, the outbreak of Legionnaires' disease, and the status of President Ford's anti-inflation campaign proved more decisive than the early production problems and the evidence from field trials concerning the difficulties of producing a vaccine both safe and effective for children between the ages of three and ten.

By mid-December 1976, over 45.6 million American civilians had received swine flu vaccine in what has been called the largest program of preventive medicine ever mounted. But the unexpected outbreak of 107 cases, six of them fatal, of Guillain-Barré Syndrome, a paralytic nerve disease, as an apparent complication of the immunization, and the failure of the feared flu epidemic to materialize led to discontinuation of the program, in an atmosphere as emotionally and rhetorically charged as that in which the program had begun. Earnestness and vigor proved insufficient guides to policy. Assigning greater weight to reified notions of prevention than to hard information about disease, vaccine modalities, and risks had seriously discredited the hitherto conservative and respected image of preventive medicine.

OVERKILL

It was not known in the 1940s that using X rays to prevent tissue regrowth after tonsillectomies might cause later thyroid cancers. But clearly such use of X rays exceeded the counsels of caution. A howitzer was being used not to swat a fly but to prevent flies from landing.

According to the tabloid, *Weekly World News* (February 28, 1984), Estelle Ramey, an endocrinologist, pronounced testosterone to be the reason men don't live as long as women: adrenalin, stimulated by testosterone in males, weakens the cardiovascular system. Castration appears to prolong life, a hypothesis that yellow journalism readily transformed into the headline "Castration Could Save Your Life." Ramey's actual prescription is small daily doses of aspirin. No one would seriously advocate castration as a prophylactic against cardiovascular disease, yet prophylactic hysterectomy and prophylactic mastectomy are seriously proposed.

As Diana Scully observes, only 15 percent of all hysterectomies in recent years have been performed for cancer. Thirty percent are prescribed for fibroid tumors, 35 percent for prolapsed uterus, and some 20 percent for sterilization, according to the American College of Obstetricians and Gynecologists. At one of its meetings reported in 1973, J. B. Skelton urged the College "to recognize and recommend prophylactic elective total hysterectomy and bilateral salpingo-oophorectomy after completion of childbearing as proper preventive medicine in obstetrics and gynecology." He argued that such complete removal of the female reproductive tract, placing women into immediate menopause, would preclude uterine and ovarian cancer, as well as pregnancy, forestall multiple gynecological operations, and eliminate "unpleasant and uncomfortable monthly bleeding" and "bothersome cyclic variations, tensions, and emotionally altered states which affect the woman's world." The procedure "decreases the frequency of unpleasant, humiliating pelvic exams and tests, and allows better utilization of available health personnel, facilities, and time." Follow-up "with feminizing hormones" could smooth mood variations. A Cornell study of 787,000 hysterectomies revealed 1,700 resultant deaths, at least 22 percent of them in cases where the surgery was judged unnecessary. Postoperative morbidity after vaginal hysterectomy was found to be 42.7 percent in another study, compared with 1.5 percent in laparotomy and 20.7 percent in abdominal tubal ligation.

Since 1937 Congress has mandated anticancer activities including cancer control, construed by the profession to include prevention. Lacking any effective preventive against breast cancer, health planners, researchers, and policy makers may present even outrageous proposals rather than admit that they are without alternative. Citing epidemiological studies from the 1950s to the 1970s, Robert Morgan and Damodar Vakil argue for surgical menopause as a means of reducing breast cancer risk. Admitting that preventive hysterectomy would be "a drastic step," they consider it "an available solution" for the high-risk woman. "Likewise, a case can be made for prophylactic bilateral mastectomy with silicone implantation for the person at very high risk and suffering from fibrocystic breast disease."

The authors write as though there were well-established criteria of breast-cancer risk. But such is far from the case. We do not have consistent, determinate correlations between benign breast disease and breast cancer. Further, the relative risk of breast cancer is only 1.6 to 2 times as high among women with all the known risk factors as that of the general population, and some 95 percent of all women have one or more risk factors. Ethically speaking, even if a discrete high-risk group could be identified, it would be questionable to propose a preventive measure as invasive as mastectomy. Logically it is problematic to speak of mastectomy as prevention, just as it is problematic to speak of amputation as prevention.

Morgan and Vakil are sanguine about cancer prevention: "One possible solution is the initiation of treatment with an oral contraceptive containing relatively large amount [sic] of estriol and low amounts of estrone or estradiol. This medication would provide the contraceptive effect desired by most women, while suppressing their natural ovarian function and supplanting it with a pattern of estrogens which is possibly less carcinogenic than their natural one." The word *possibly* here is a telling indication of the attitudes that influence preventive

health proposals affecting women's sexual and reproductive lives. It is unlikely that reliable indices of breast-cancer risk will ever simply be read from estrogen profiles. But if they could be, it is questionable whether a program as radically disruptive as Morgan and Vakil propose could be undertaken without systemic effects.

Estrogen replacement therapy (ERT) has been widely prescribed since the 1960s as treatment for menopause. In *Feminine Forever* Robert A. Wilson, a standard-bearer of ERT, describes menopause as a devastating disease for which ERT is both a therapy and a preventative of the worse ravages. ERT has brought "symptomatic relief" to many women. But there were also an estimated 7,500 excess cases of new endometrial cancer in women aged fifty to sixty-nine in the United States in 1975, a 171 percent increase over the 1970 figure. Publication in the *New England Journal of Medicine* of the finding that ERT had caused the increase led to substantial declines in incidence—down 27 percent from the 1975 peak within two years. But many physicians continue to prescribe ERT. Even after the FDA recommended a warning label concerning the risk of uterine cancer, Jane Brody, the *New York Times* health-science writer, found that all twelve physicians she checked around the country argued that ERT had not been proven guilty and that no major change was needed in its prescription.

A 1980 study based on national data gathered by the Commission on Professional and Hospital Activities in Ann Arbor, Michigan, indicates that "over 15,000 cases of endometrial cancer were caused by replacement estrogens during the five year period 1971–1975 alone." The authors write, "This represents one of the largest epidemics of serious iatrogenic disease that has ever occurred in this country." Women who have taken replacement estrogens for at least five years are now known to face a ten to thirty-five-fold increased incidence of endometrial cancer, an absolute risk of 1 to 3 percent per year. Where preventive health planners in the cancer field are considering widespread chemical blockage of estrogen activity as a preventative against breast cancer, an opposite set of would-be health engineers are urging the prevention or reduction of osteoporosis as a new justification for estrogen doses. But we have no neat bifurcation of women into those who would benefit from and those who would be harmed by ERT. . . .

TRANSFERENCE OF RESPONSIBILITY

A woman diagnosed at twenty-two with spina bifida reports, "My mother still to this day is asking herself what she ate or drank to cause this." The mother of a seven-year-old victim asks, "I'd like to know why it happened. I never drank, I never smoked, I never took drugs. . . ." When tragic accidents of birth or development occur, it is natural to seek a meaning, and in all human societies the terms of reference for that meaning may be moral. Something was wrongly done or left undone. Moralizing health concerns by treating them as foci of discipline and surrounding them with prudential counsels generates a context of expectations in which any tragic outcome may seem incomprehensible unless it can be ascribed to infraction of some hygienic rule. Adele Davis blamed her fatal stomach cancer on her failure to adopt a health-preserving diet early

enough in life. Followers of Jimm Fixx blamed his fatal heart attack at fifty-two on his late initiation into the running regimen. When disease strikes, solace and exoneration are found in assigning blame to doctors, patients, parents, genes. Explanation becomes a tug-of-war—your side of the family or mine, heredity or environment, society, economic conditions—in which something, preferably someone, must bear the blame. Doctors are professionals in this contest, having used the reproof "if only you had come sooner, something might have been done" at least since the days of Imperial China.

The obverse of blaming the victim is imparting a false sense of security. Even the most scrupulous observance of health warnings is clearly no guarantee of safety when the warnings themselves are derived from statistical trends. Studying the records of breast-cancer patients in Iowa (1980–81), Elaine Smith and Trudy Burns found no significant difference in tumor size, stage, or lymph node involvement between women who practiced breast self-examination monthly or more often and those who did not, and they found no evidence as yet of a decline in breast-cancer mortality to correspond with increased reliance on breast self-examination. Cancers detected by breast self-examination tend to be larger and more advanced tumors than those discovered by means such as mammography. Even massive educational programs on breast self-examination do not reduce tumor size or lymph-node involvement at detection, as the experience of the 1977–80 San Diego County Medical Society Breast Cancer Education Program has clearly shown. Mammographic screening does lead to earlier detection of tumors, but whether the lead time gained can be translated into a reduction in cancer mortality or whether it means only a prolongation of the interval between diagnosis and death remains to be determined.

The effects of shifting responsibility from the health care sector to the individual can be significant. Thomas Cole has shown skillfully how health reformers of the mid-nineteenth century preached a secular gospel: discipline and prophylaxis would preserve health and self-sufficiency to a vigorous old age. Hygiene and optimism were the works and faith of modern valetudinary salvation:

> Only the shiftless, faithless, and promiscuous were doomed to a premature death and old age . . . As late as 1901, Frederick L. Hoffman of Prudential Life Insurance, for whom the relationship between longevity and dividends was more than a metaphor, reiterated the increasingly unrealistic argument that temperance, frugality, and industry were the sole requirements for a comfortable, healthy old age.

Not surprisingly Hoffman became an ardent opponent of state pensions for elderly workers.

Today the attitude that individuals hold the power to preserve life and good health in relative unconcern for genetic frailties and environmental hazards might seem out of date and out of place. Yet in July 1979, at the climax of Jimmy Carter's administration, a Surgeon General's report titled *Healthy People* concluded that the foremost causes of illness lie in individual behavior and are to be met most effectively and economically through extensive changes in the lifestyles of almost everyone. The report was hailed as the manifesto of "a second public health revolution." Deane Neubauer and Rich-

ard Pratt have explained that assignment to the individual of the major responsibility for preventive health shifts the onus away from social agencies. Similarly, advocates of preventive health programs often present such programs as vehicles of social engineering, using the rhetoric and concern of prevention to redirect public attention and resources—a political act masquerading as a hygienic one.

An optimum mix of personal, familial, private, communal, social, and governmental responsibilities is probably best worked out in specific contexts. To address preventive health in moralistic terms—your diet, my exercise—diffuses the issue and directs attention away from the large and known area of world health needs such as pollution control, vector control, and vaccination to more nebulous areas like fiber in the diet. Rather than facing questions about social responsibility, it finesses them. Recognizing the effectiveness and relevance of individual human efforts and choices is a great step for professions that often see causation as completely divided between genetic and environmental "determinants." But recognizing the role of individual choice and discipline is no substitute for health insurance, research, therapy, or exercising responsibility for the environment.

MAGIC

In every society people project hopes and fears, using their own language and symbols. The amulets and incantations of shamans may seem primitive if they use alien language and exotic dyes and feathers. But the idea is universal that the wise, who know the workings of the cosmos, have the power to cure, prevent, or even cause disease. Only the symbols by which wisdom seeks outward recognition vary widely.

Since magic operates by the logic of association, its presence is readily identified. A practice, for example, may be deemed healthful because healthy people do it. (The commonplace confusion of the words *healthy* and *healthful* is indicative of the direction wishes take.) Running is perhaps the salient symbol of health in our society at the moment. The association is not arbitrary. Habitual exercise is associated empirically with reduction in the risk factors of cardiovascular disease. Enhanced energy and stress reduction are also associated with regular exercise. But the terms are difficult to define and quantify objectively. Many runners believe that exercise helps prevent colds and flu. Harvey Simon reviewed ten studies of 132 healthy volunteers ranging from the sedentary to marathoners; he found no evidence of such a relationship. Further studies may yet find one, perhaps masked by the contrary effects of overexertion. Orthopedic surgeons are growing increasingly alarmed at the bone damage associated with running, and a Rhode Island study estimates an annual fatality rate from running of one per 8,000 runners. But the belief among runners in the protective effects of exercise did not arise from scientific studies and will not disappear merely as a result of scientific counterevidence. The belief is partly a matter of projection and speaks more to the symbolic significance of exercise—and to the power of marketing—than to physiology.

Henry Solomon of Cornell Medical College, a cardiologist, points out that lack of exercise is among the least significant of the secondary risk factors for coronary artery disease. The primary factors are hypertension, high blood cholesterol, and cigarette smoking. The secondary include diabetes, socioeconomic status, stress, and abnormal EKGs. "Whatever benefits the human body derives from exertion are yours whenever you take a good brisk walk or enjoy yourself—without pushing yourself—at some other sport you enjoy," Solomon argues. Excessive exercise is a folly and a danger, a fad on which excessive hopes are lavished. The power of this fad derives in part from hope and fear, in part from the association of heroic exertion with virtue and of virtue with reward.

In the film *Fighting Back Cancer*, broadcast on BBC4's Broadside series in 1983, the Bristol Cancer Health Center is presented as a source of hope for cancer patients, especially those who reject or resent anticancer drugs. Controversial new research, we learn, suggests that a patient's determination and fighting spirit can be critical in facing cancer. A cancer patient must take charge of her own life, rather than "doctors having their will with me." The Bristol Center offers diet, counsel, and meditation. Absolutely pure raw foods containing "no chemicals" complement the spiritual purification, which "runs through your personality to find out what your defects are." The regimen is "enormously difficult." Some patients have trouble giving up meat. The vegetarian melange presented to the camera seems designed to appear unappetizing. But self-denial is the substance of catharsis: "We don't offer people a cure—[we say if you make certain changes in your lifestyle, you'll be] answering the questions the disease is asking."

While no medical claims are made about a cure, a patient can report "deep relaxation . . . visualizing my immune system getting rid of these malignant cells . . . a wildly exhilarating experience. . . . I just knew that I was actually getting rid of the cancer." As the film closes, a woman offers testimony that counseling "has prevented the disease."

Clearly morale effects the course of many diseases, but we lack evidence to sustain the suggestion that imagination, even aided by diet, has the power to "fight back" or exclude cancerous growths. Indeed Barrie Cassileth has found evidence that attitudinal factors among patients with advanced or inoperable cancers do not influence remission or survival. Marcia Angell argues in an accompanying editorial that medically encouraged "folklore" about the relation between cancer and mental outlook has led some patients to believe that they were to blame for their illnesses. Guilt, of course, along with fear, regret, and others of the emotions that Spinoza called passive are important factors in the pathology of superstition.

The purity of the Bristol diet and others like it is not merely hygienic but symbolic. "Chemicals" are a category only for the imagination. Meat is a symbolic issue in every culture, since animals' lives are involved. It has become even more a moral issue in recent years, through claims that eating meat appropriates an unfair share of the world's grain. But the idea that moral guilt can be expiated by vegetarianism or that moral guilt or innocence (however imputed) can be relevant to the incidence or course of cancer is a classic structural interchange: my guilt (symbolized through food) brings on my cancer; my purgation (through ascesis, symbolic rejection of sin) is my protection.

The dynamics of such symbolic exchanges are varied and complex. It is not a coincidence or even a paradox, we suspect, that a kind of moralistic vegetarianism, often linked with a narcissistic or excessive interest in exercise as fitness, should come into vogue simultaneously with the "sexual revolution" and, for that matter, with increased reliance on drugs for both mental and physical effects and the heightened prominence of new cults and old credos.

Our final point regarding magic has to do with the taboos of priestly language. The point can be made briefly, because the usages are familiar. Pap smears prevent cervical cancer deaths, but so does chastity:

> There is a striking association between cancer of the cervix and the number of sexual partners a woman has had. The death rate for this cancer among nuns is much lower than it is for the general population, suggesting the involvement of a venereally transmitted agent. A possible candidate is a virus (Herpes simplex type II) which has been found in association with both cervical cancer and other cervical cell abnormalities. . . .

If multiple sexual partners are a risk factor for cervical cancer, why is little said about this in the popular literature of disease prevention, or even in the massive output of sex education/birth control information? The answer, we suspect, is that the authors of such materials fear to weaken their authority and muddy their message by appearing in the eyes of their constituents to have taken open issue with the notion that sex as such and in all forms, with very rare and unmentionable exceptions, is (like "fitness" and unlike "stress") a Good Thing.

The appeal of the idea of prevention rests on a real but limited achievement. There is no great conspiracy to misuse the idea of prevention. But the fashionable tendency to rely too heavily on prevention is not confined to faddists or propagandists; it extends to the most respected and responsible health leaders and researchers. Most of the problems we have described arise in the over-enthusiastic promotional activities of well-meaning health practitioners. Yet taken together they constitute an abuse of the concept of prevention. Enthusiasts adulterate the value of this concept by conflating it with other ideas, hoping that its repute will carry over into projects of their own. But, like ancient alchemists, they are more likely to debase their own coinage than to transmute base metal into gold.

POSTSCRIPT

Will Practicing Positive Health Behaviors and Emphasizing Prevention Improve Health?

While Goodman and Goodman do not claim that smoking and high-fat diets are safe and unrelated to disease, they believe that arguments that emphasize disease prevention through individual health behaviors are misused and exaggerated. They feel that shifting the responsibility of health and well-being onto the individual relieves the government and health care industry of their responsibility to provide education, a clean environment, research into disease etiology (or causes), and adequate health care for everyone. Shifting responsibility for well-being and disease prevention onto individuals also ignores individual differences and genetics. Finally, the authors point out that individual responsibility for well-being comes at a high cost—the tendency to blame oneself when something goes wrong. A healthy life-style does not *guarantee* good health and longevity.

The view that a healthy life-style does not guarantee good health is shared by others. Cardiologist Henry A. Solomon argues that exercise will not necessarily improve longevity. Solomon believes that heredity is as much responsible for a long life as are health behaviors. Thomas Moore makes the same point for cholesterol reduction in *Heart Failure* (Random House, 1989). He claims that diet does not reduce serum cholesterol for many people and that heredity is as important as life-style in controlling cholesterol. In "The Cigarette Controversy," *Engage/Social Action* (September 1980), Horace Kornegay argues that even smoking may not be as harmful a practice as previously thought. He maintains that the case against tobacco is built on statistics that are not valid. All these writers argue that prevention via a healthy life-style may not be a valid way to maintain wellness.

Lawrence Green, in "When Health Policy Becomes Victim Blaming," *The New England Journal of Medicine* (December 17, 1981), also argues with the premise that individuals must always be responsible for their own health. He agrees with the Goodmans that government must not abandon its role in maintaining social conditions that support behavior conducive to health.

Donald B. Ardsell, writing in *High Level Wellness* (Ten Speed Press, 1986), maintains that individuals can join the ranks of those who look to themselves rather than their physicians for the maintenance of their health. He claims that what an individual can do for his or her own benefit is enormous; what medicine can do is quite limited. It is within our power to develop and maintain high levels of wellness and to avoid disease, doctors, and drugs.

ISSUE 6

Can a Positive Mental Attitude Overcome Disease?

YES: Bernard Dixon, from "Dangerous Thoughts," *Science86 Magazine,* a publication of the American Association for the Advancement of Science (April 1986)

NO: Marcia Angell, from "Disease as a Reflection of the Psyche," *The New England Journal of Medicine* (June 13, 1985)

ISSUE SUMMARY

YES: Writer and editor Bernard Dixon discusses studies indicating that stress negatively impacts the immune system and, conversely, that a positive mental attitude can prevent illness.

NO: Physician Marcia Angell argues that there is no proof that a positive mental attitude can slow or prevent disease.

Practitioners of holistic medicine believe that people must be responsible for their own health by practicing healthy behaviors and maintaining positive attitudes instead of relying on health providers. They also believe that physical disease has both behavioral and psychological components. These psychological components can be explained by the relationship between mental attitude and the immune system.

In 1979, the late journalist Norman Cousins published *Anatomy of an Illness.* In it, Cousins discusses how he cured himself of a serious illness that affected his collagen—*ankylosing spondylitis.* To battle the disease, he took massive doses of vitamin C (which aids in the synthesis of collagen) and kept a positive mental attitude by watching comedy movies. Since Cousins's book was published more articles and books have been devoted to the idea that people can control their immune systems, and therefore their health, with their minds. Sufferers of various illnesses have been told to have positive thoughts in order to assist their immune systems. Some studies have found that cancer patients with certain personality traits and those with a sense of helplessness are less likely to survive their disease.

Research over the past 20 years has shown that disease is not only an organic process but also a psychological one and that some personality types are more susceptible to disease than others. Research has also indicated that people are most at risk when exposed to certain types of stress, such as major life changes. It is as if our personalities determine what types of diseases we are most likely to suffer. Our health behaviors decide the levels of risk, and stress causes the outcome, which is disease.

In the following selections, Bernard Dixon asserts that the mind can have a significant influence over the body. In his article, Dixon presents research on how the immune system is influenced by mental attitude. He claims that the immune system can be negatively affected by depression, stress, and anxiety, as well as feeling of helplessness. These feelings prevent the immune system from responding to organisms and carcinogens that can bring on disease.

Marcia Angell disagrees with Dixon and claims that telling patients that they can change the courses of their diseases is harmful. For example, if a patient's cancer spreads, despite every attempt to think positively, is the patient at fault? Angell believes that individuals have responsibility for their health by practicing positive behaviors but that patients burdened by disease should not be further burdened by having to accept responsibility for its outcome. In addition, Angell maintains that viewing sickness as a personal failure is a form of blaming the victim.

YES

Bernard Dixon

DANGEROUS THOUGHTS

HOW WE THINK AND FEEL CAN MAKE US SICK

Until recently, Ellen hadn't seen a physician in years. When other people got a bug, she was the one who invariably stayed healthy. But then her luck seemed to change. First she caught a bad cold in January, then had a bout of flu in February, followed by a nasty cough that still lingers. What an infuriating coincidence that these ailments hit as her career was faltering—months of unemployment following companywide layoffs.

But is it a coincidence? Intuition may suggest that we have fewer colds when we are content with our lives, more when we are under stress. That the mind can influence the body's vulnerability to infection in an insidious but potent way is a perennial theme of folklore and literature. Now even scientists are beginning to take that idea seriously. An alliance of psychiatrists, immunologists, neuroscientists, and microbiologists, specialists who rarely look beyond their own disciplines, are beginning to work together in a field so new that it goes under a variety of names, including behavioral immunology, psychoimmunology, and neuroimmunomodulation. Behind these polysyllables lies the challenge of understanding the chemical and anatomical connections between mind and body and eventually, perhaps, even preventing psychosomatic illness.

Just 10 years ago, most specialists in communicable disease would have scoffed at any suggestion that the mind can influence the body in this way. Textbooks portrayed infection as the simple, predictable outcome whenever a disease causing microbe encountered a susceptible host. Various factors such as old age, malnutrition, and overwork could make a disease more severe. But there was no place for the fanciful notion that elation, depression, contentment, or stress could affect the course of disease.

Today, that once-conventional wisdom is being revised by scientists around the world. Playing a major role in these investigations are researchers at England's Medical Research Council Common Cold Unit near Salisbury. Their work shows that even this relatively trivial infection is affected by the psyche. And the lessons learned may apply to more serious diseases, including cancer.

For nearly four decades now, volunteers at the Common Cold Unit have helped test the efficacy of new antiviral drugs and have proven that colds are caused by rhinoviruses and a few related viruses. In 1975 psychologist Richard Totman at Nuffield College, Oxford, and Wallace Craig and Sylvia Reed of the Common Cold Unit conducted the first psychological experiments. The scientists infected 48 healthy volunteers by dribbling down their nostrils drops containing two common cold viruses. The researchers then offered 23 of their subjects the chance to take a new "drug," actually a placebo, that would presumably prevent colds. The investigators warned these subjects that if they accepted this treatment, they would have to have their gastric juices sampled with a stomach tube. The scientists had no intention of doing this; the warning was simply a ruse to put the volunteers under stress. The other half of the group was neither offered the drug nor cautioned about the stomach tube. Totman and his colleagues theorized that the 23 offered the placebo would experience either mild anxiety or regret, depending on the decision they made. This might cause them to allay their state of mind by justifying to themselves their decision—as a theory called cognitive dissonance predicts—which would result in greater bodily resistance and milder colds.

The experts were wrong. When an independent physician assessed the volunteers' symptoms, he found that the 23 offered the choice had cold symptoms that were significantly more severe than those given no option. Apparently anxiety generated by contemplating something unpleasant or refusing to help a worthy cause had a tangible influence on the course of the illness.

Totman's group also made some intriguing observations about the way stress affects people outside the laboratory. Volunteers were interviewed by a psychologist, received rhinoviruses, caught colds, and were monitored. Individuals who during the previous six months had experienced a stressful event, such as death of a loved one, divorce, or a layoff, developed worse colds than the others, and introverts had more severe colds than extroverts. Not only were the introverts' symptoms worse than those of their peers, their nasal secretions contained more rhinovirus, confirming that their illnesses were worse.

The Common Cold Unit is now trying to find out how stress affects people with strong social networks compared with their more introverted colleagues.

But how could an individual's mental state encourage or thwart the development of a cold? Research at several centers in the United States supports the most plausible explanation—that psychological stress impairs the effectiveness of the immune system, which has the dual role of recognizing and eliminating microbes from outside the body as well as cancer cells originating within.

The first line of defense of the immune system is the white blood cells called lymphocytes. These include B cells, which manufacture antibodies against microbes; helper T cells, which aid the B cells in making the right kind of antibodies; and killer T cells, which wipe out invading organisms if they have been exposed to them before. Another kind of lymphocyte, the natural killer cell, has received a lot of attention lately for its ability to detect and destroy harmful cells, including malignant ones, even if it hasn't encountered the invaders previously. Together with scavenging white blood cells that gobble up dead cells and debris, the various types of lymphocytes work in complex, coordinated ways to police the body's tissues.

Researchers can measure the efficiency of the immune system by measuring how well a patient's lymphocytes respond to foreign substances. For instance, they can grow the patient's lymphocytes in glassware and expose them to substances called mitogens, which mimic the behavior of microorganisms by stimulating the white cells to divide. Since a rapid increase in the number of white cells is a crucial early stage in the defense against invasion, patients whose white cells don't proliferate may have malfunctioning immune systems.

But most researchers are cautious about generalizing from the results obtained from a single technique of this sort, since the immune system has complicated backups to keep us healthy even when our lymphocytes aren't proliferating. Nevertheless, reports of stress reducing the efficiency of the immune system have been accumulating on such a scale—and with such variety—that it is becoming difficult to resist the conclusion that anxiety increases our vulnerability to disease.

In one landmark study, for example, Steven Schleifer and his colleagues at Mt. Sinai School of Medicine in New York sought help from spouses of women with advanced breast cancer. They persuaded 15 men to give blood samples every six to eight weeks during their wives' illnesses and for up to 14 months after the women died. While none of the men showed depressed lymphocyte response while their wives were ill, their white cell response was significantly lowered as early as two weeks after their wives died and for up to 14 months later. Schleifer believes he has shown, contrary to earlier studies, that it was bereavement, not the experience of the spouses' illness, that lowered immunity.

Prompted by his observations of the bereaved widowers, Schleifer wondered if serious, debilitating depression would also show up as weakened immunity. When he took blood samples from 18 depressed patients at Mt. Sinai and the Bronx Veterans Administration Hospital, he found their lymphocytes were significantly less responsive to mitogens than those of healthy individuals from the general population matched for age, sex, and race.

We sometimes think humans are uniquely vulnerable to anxiety, but stress seems to affect the immune defenses of lower animals too. In one experiment, for example, behavioral immunologist Mark Laudenslager and colleagues at the University of Denver gave mild electric shocks to 24 rats. Half the animals could switch off the current by turning a wheel in their enclosure, while the other half could not. The rats in the two groups were paired so that each time one rat turned the wheel it protected both itself and its helpless partner from the shock. Laudenslager found that the immune response was depressed below normal in the helpless rats but not in those that could turn off the electricity. What he has demonstrated, he believes, is that lack of control over an event, not the experience itself, is what weakens the immune system.

Other researchers agree. Jay Weiss, a psychologist at Duke University School of Medicine, has shown that animals who are allowed to control unpleasant stimuli don't develop sleep disturbances, ulcers, or changes in brain chemistry typical of stressed rats. But if the animals are confronted with situations they have no control over, they later behave passively when faced with experiences they can control. Such findings reinforce psychiatrists' suspicions that the experience or perception of helplessness is one of the most harmful factors in depression.

One of the most startling examples of how the mind can alter the immune response was discovered by chance. In 1975 psychologist Robert Ader at the University of Rochester School of Medicine and Dentistry conditioned mice to avoid saccharin by simultaneously feeding them the sweetener and injecting them with a drug that while suppressing their immune systems caused stomach upsets. Associating the saccharin with the stomach pains, the mice quickly learned to avoid the sweetener. In order to extinguish the taste aversion, Ader reexposed the animals to saccharin, this time without the drug, and was astonished to find that those rodents that had received the highest amounts of sweetener during their earlier conditioning died. He could only speculate that he had so successfully conditioned the rats that saccharin alone now served to weaken their immune systems enough to kill them.

If you can depress the immune system by conditioning, it stands to reason you can boost it in the same way. Novera Herbert Spector at the National Institute of Neurological and Communicative Disorders and Stroke in Bethesda, Maryland, recently directed a team at the University of Alabama, Birmingham, which confirmed that hypothesis. The researchers injected mice with a chemical that enhances natural killer cell activity while simultaneously exposing the rodents to the odor of camphor, which has no detectable effect on the immune system. After nine sessions, mice exposed to the camphor alone showed a large increase in natural killer cell activity.

What mechanism could account for these connections between the psyche and the immune system? One well-known link is the adrenal glands, which the brain alerts to produce adrenaline and other hormones that prepare the body to cope with danger or stress. But adrenal hormones cannot be the only link between mind and body. Research by a group under Neal Miller, professor emeritus of psychology at the Rockefeller University in New York City, has shown that even rats whose adrenal glands have been removed suffer depressed immunity after being exposed to electric shocks.

Anxiety, it seems, can trigger the release of many other hormones, including testosterone, insulin, and possibly even growth hormone. In addition, stress stimulates secretion of chemicals called neuropeptides, which influence mood and emotions. One class of neuropeptides known as endorphins kills pain and causes euphoria. Endorphins have another interesting characteristic: they fit snugly into receptors on lymphocytes, suggesting a direct route through which the mind could influence immunity.

This idea is borne out in the lab, where one of the natural pain-killers, beta-endorphin, can impair the response of lymphocytes in test tubes. Evidence from cancer studies shows that chemicals blocking the normal functions of endorphins can slow the growth of tumors. And other work suggests that tumor cells may be attracted to certain neuropeptides, providing a route for cancer to spread all over the body.

Neuropeptides are turning out to be extraordinarily versatile in their interaction with the immune system. At the National Institutes of Health in Bethesda, Maryland, Michael Ruff has found neuropeptides that attract scavenging white cells called macrophages to the site of injured or damaged tissue. There the macrophages regulate and activate other immune cells as well as gobble up bacteria and debris. What is even more surprising, however, is that the macrophages themselves actually release neuropeptides. This has led Ruff to speculate that these scavenging white cells may also serve as free-floating nerve cells able to communicate with the brain.

But why should that two-way communication sometimes have the effect of allowing stress to upset the body's defenses? One answer may lie in evolution. When early man was attacked by a sabertoothed tiger, for example, it may have been more important from a survival standpoint for his immune system to turn off briefly. In its zeal to get rid of foreign matter and damaged tissue, a revved-up immune system can also attack healthy tissue. Shutting down the immune system for a short time would avert any damage to the body's healthy tissues and would cause no harm, since it takes a while for infection to set in. As soon as the danger had passed, the immune system was able to rebound—perhaps stronger than before—and go about its main business of fighting invading organisms. But the kind of stress we modern humans suffer is of a different kind: it is rarely life threatening and often lasts a long time, weakening our immune defenses for long periods and making us vulnerable to infections and cancer.

The immune system is extraordinarily complex, and the mind is even more so. As Nicholas Hall of George Washington University School of Medicine says, "We're putting together two kinds of black boxes and trying to make sense of what happens."

In the process, researchers are wrestling with three issues of scientific and social import. First, what can be done to protect people at vulnerable times in their lives from a potentially catastrophic failure of their immune defenses? Second, should counseling and psychological support become as important as traditional therapeutic measures in the treatment of disease? And finally, what are the corresponding benefits to health of the positive emotions of hope, affection, love, mirth, and joy?

NO   Marcia Angell

DISEASE AS A REFLECTION
OF THE PSYCHE

Is cancer more likely in unhappy people? Can people who have cancer improve their chances of survival by learning to enjoy life and to think optimistically? What about heart attacks, peptic ulcers, asthma, rheumatoid arthritis, and inflammatory bowel disease? Are they caused by stress in certain personality types, and will changing the personality change the course of the disease? A stranger in this country would not have to be here very long to guess that most Americans think the answer to these questions is yes.

The popular media, stirred by occasional reports in the medical literature, remind us incessantly of the hazards of certain personality types. We are told that Type A people are vulnerable to heart attacks, repressed people (especially those who have suffered losses) are at risk of cancer, worry causes peptic ulcers, and so on. The connection between mental state and disease would seem to be direct and overriding. The hard-driving executive has a heart attack *because* he is pushing for promotion; the middle-aged housewife gets breast cancer *because* she is brooding about her empty nest.

Furthermore, we are told that just as mental state causes disease, so can changes in our outlook and approach to life restore health. Books, magazines, and talk shows abound in highly specific advice about achieving the necessary changes, as well as in explanations about how they work. Norman Cousins, for example, tells us how he managed to achieve a remission of his ankylosing spondylitis by means of laughter and vitamin C—the former, he assumes, operating through reversal of "adrenal exhaustion."[1] Carl and Stephanie Simonton prescribe certain techniques of relaxation and imagery as an adjunct to the conventional treatment of cancer.[2] The imagery includes picturing white cells (strong and purposeful) destroying cancer cells (weak and confused).

Clearly, this sort of postulated connection between mental state and disease is not limited to the effect of mood on our sense of physical well-being. Nor are we talking about relaxation as a worthy goal in itself.

From Marcia Angell, "Disease as a Reflection of the Psyche," *The New England Journal of Medicine*, vol. 312, no. 24 (June 13, 1985), pp. 1570–1572. Copyright © 1985 by The Massachusetts Medical Society. Reprinted by permission.

Cousins, the Simontons, and others of their persuasion advocate a way of thinking not as an end, but rather as a means for defeating disease. The assumption is that mental state is a major factor in causing and curing specific diseases. Is it, and what is the effect of believing that it is?

The notion that certain mental states bring on certain diseases is not new. In her book, *Illness as Metaphor*, Susan Sontag describes the myths surrounding two mysterious and terrifying diseases—tuberculosis in the 19th century and cancer in the 20th.[3] Tuberculosis was thought to be a disease of excessive feeling. Overly passionate artists "consumed" themselves, both emotionally and through the disease. In contrast, cancer is seen today as a disease of depletion. Emotionally spent people no longer have the energy to battle renegade cells. As Sontag points out, myths like these arise when a disease of unknown cause is particularly dreaded. The myth serves as a form of mastery—we can predict where the disease will strike and we can perhaps ward it off by modifying our inner life. Interestingly, when the cause of such a disease is discovered, it is usually relatively simple and does not involve psychological factors. For example, the elaborate construct of a tuberculosis-prone personality evaporated when tuberculosis was found to be caused by the tubercle bacillus.

The evidence for mental state as a cause and cure of today's scourges is not much better than it was for the afflictions of earlier centuries. Most reports of such a connection are anecdotal. They usually deal with patients whose disease remitted after some form of positive thinking, and there is no attempt to determine the frequency of this occurrence and compare it with the frequency of remission without positive thinking. Other, more ambitious studies suffer from such serious flaws in design or analysis that bias is nearly inevitable.[4] In some instances, the bias lies in the interpretation. One frequently cited study, for example, reports that the death rate among people who have recently lost their spouses is higher than that among married people.[5] Although the authors were cautious in their interpretation, others have been quick to ascribe the finding to grief rather than to, say, a change in diet or other habits. Similarly, the known physiologic effects of stress on the adrenal glands are often overinterpreted so that it is a short leap to a view of stress as a cause of one disease or another. In short, the literature contains very few scientifically sound studies of the relation, if there is one, between mental state and disease.

In this issue of the *Journal*, Cassileth et al. report the results of a careful prospective study of 359 cancer patients, showing no correlation between a number of psychosocial factors and progression of the disease.[6] In an earlier prospective study of another disease, Case et al. found no correlation between Type A personality and recurrence of acute myocardial infarction.[7] The fact that these well-designed studies were negative raises the possibility that we have been too ready to accept the venerable belief that mental state is an important factor in the cause and cure of disease.

Is there any harm in this belief, apart from its lack of scientific substantiation? It might be argued that it is not only harmless but beneficial, in that it allows patients some sense of control over their disease. If, for example, patients believe that imagery can help arrest cancer, then they feel less helpless; there is something they can do.

On the other hand, if cancer spreads, despite every attempt to think positively, is the patient at fault? It might seem so. According to Robert Mack, a surgeon who has cancer and is an adherent of the methods of the Simontons, "The patients who survive with cancer or with another catastrophic illness, perhaps even in the face of almost insurmountable odds, seem to be those who have developed a very strong will to live and who value each day, one at a time."[8] What about the patients who *don't* survive? Are they lacking the will to live, or perhaps self-discipline or some other personal attribute necessary to hold cancer at bay? After all, a view that attaches credit to patients for controlling their disease also implies blame for the progression of the disease. Katherine Mansfield described the resulting sense of personal inadequacy in an entry in her journal a year before her death from tuberculosis: "A bad day . . . horrible pains and so on, and weakness. I could do nothing. The weakness was not only physical. I must *heal my Self* before I will be well. . . . This must be done alone and at once. It is at the root of my not getting better. My mind is not *controlled*."[3] In addition to the anguish of personal failure, a further harm to such patients is that they may come to see medical care as largely irrelevant, as Cassileth et al. point out, and give themselves over completely to some method of thought control.

The medical profession also participates in the tendency to hold the patient responsible for his progress. In our desire to pay tribute to gallantry and grace in the face of hardship, we sometimes credit these qualities with cures, not realizing that we may also be implying

blame when there are reverses. William Schroeder, celebrated by the media and his doctors as though he were responsible for his own renascence after implantation of an artificial heart, was later gently scolded for slackening. Dr. Allan Lansing of Humana Heart Institute worried aloud about Schroeder's "ostrich-like" behavior after a stroke and emphasized the importance of "inner strength and determination."[9]

I do not wish to argue that people have no responsibility for their health. On the contrary, there is overwhelming evidence that certain personal habits, such as smoking cigarettes, drinking alcohol, and eating a diet rich in cholesterol and saturated fats, can have great impact on health, and changing our thinking affects these habits. However, it is time to acknowledge that our belief in disease as a direct reflection of mental state is largely folklore. Furthermore, the corollary view of sickness and death as a personal failure is a particularly unfortunate form of blaming the victim. At a time when patients are already burdened by disease, they should not be further burdened by having to accept responsibility for the outcome.

REFERENCES

1. Cousins N. Anatomy of an illness as perceived by the patient. New York: WW Norton, 1979.
2. Simonton OC, Matthews-Simonton S, Creighton J. Getting well again: a step-by-step, self-help guide to overcoming cancer for patients and their families. Los Angeles: JP Tarcher, 1978.
3. Sontag S. Illness as metaphor. New York: Farrar, Straus and Giroux, 1977.
4. Fox BH. Premorbid psychological factors as related to cancer incidence. J Behav Med 1978; 1:45–133.
5. Kraus AS, Lilienfeld AM. Some epidemiologic aspects of the high mortality rate in the young widowed group. J Chronic Dis 1959; 10:207–17.
6. Cassileth BR, Lusk EJ, Miller DS, Brown LL, Miller C. Psychosocial correlates of survival in

advanced malignant disease. N Engl J Med 1985; 312:1551–5.

7. Case RB, Heller SS, Case NB, et al. Type A behavior and survival after acute myocardial infarction. N Engl J Med 1985; 312:737–41.

8. Mack RM. Lessons from living with cancer. N Engl J Med 1985; 311:1640–4.

9. McLaughlin L. Schroeder kin, doctors try to lift his spirits. Boston Globe. December 17, 1984:1.

POSTSCRIPT

Can a Positive Mental Attitude Overcome Disease?

Physician Peter Ways, in his book *Take Charge of Your Health* (Stephen Greene Press, 1985), argues that illness is not a failure of the body, and he maintains that everyone should work to improve their attitude to overcome illness. Brian Inglis and Ruth West, in *The Alternative Health Guide* (Alfred A. Knopf, 1983), agree that personality is important to health maintenance.

Significant research into the relationship between stress and health indicates that the more stress one encounters, the sicker one will be. Physiologist Suzanne Kobasa has even found that executives exposed to high levels of stress are more likely to become ill if they possess certain personality traits. She claims that "hardy" workers who are challenged by new ideas, are committed to their work, believe they make a difference in the world, and are in control of their lives stay healthy in spite of leading stressful lives. See "How Much Stress Can You Survive?" *American Health* (September 1984). Yale psychologist Judith Rodin also believes that a sense of control is important for individuals who wish to lose weight or make their lives more productive. See "A Sense of Control," *Psychology Today* (December 1984). And Dr. Bernard Siegel, writing in his bestseller *Love, Medicine & Miracles* (Harper & Row, 1986), claims that there are no "incurable diseases, only incurable people" and that illness is a personality flaw.

Ellen Switzer disagrees with the view that the mind controls the body. She points out that the cure to our illnesses is not always in our heads, our personalities, or our attitudes (*Vogue*, September 1987). Research agrees with her assessment. B. R. Cassileth and associates, in "Psychosocial Correlates of Survival in Advanced Malignant Disease," *The New England Journal of Medicine* (vol. 312, 1985), report the results of a study of 359 cancer patients, which showed no correlation between psychosocial factors and the progression of the illness. Other research by R. B. Case et al., described in "Type A Behavior and Survival After Acute Myocardial Infarction," *The New England Journal of Medicine* (vol. 312, 1985), indicated no relationship between personality and heart attacks. Based on these studies, it is possible that personality may not be an important factor in the cause and cure of disease. While further research is needed, blaming the victims of disease for not "trying hard enough" to rid their body of disease may do them a great disservice.

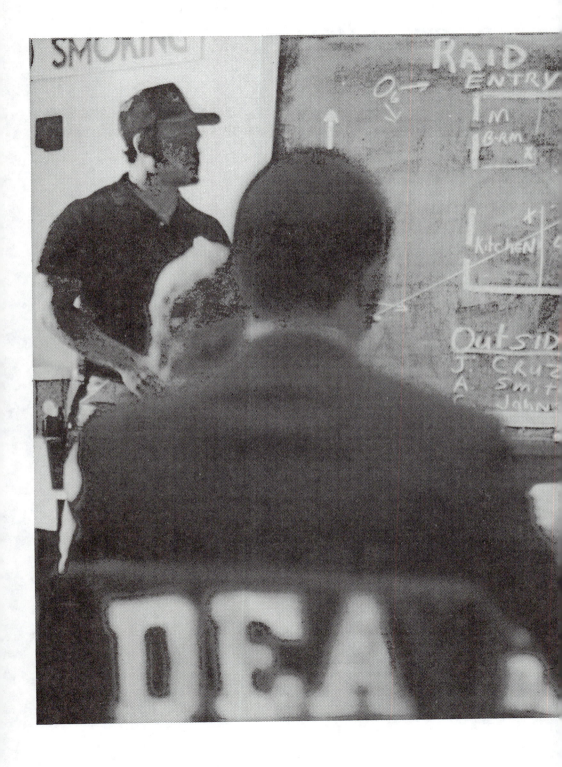

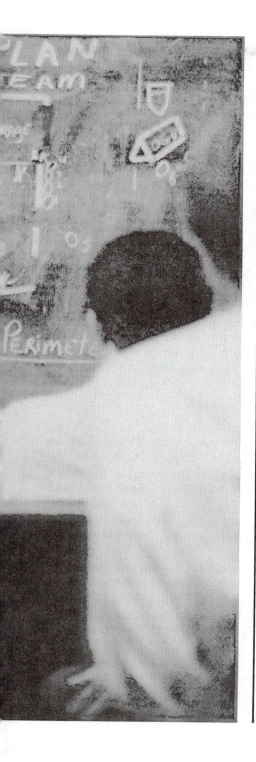

PART 3

Substance Use and Abuse

While millions of Americans use and abuse drugs ranging from cocaine to alcohol and tobacco, experts continue to seek solutions for the related problems. The use of illegal drugs often leads to crime, while drinking and smoking are clearly associated with sickness and death. Smoking also has become an issue of personal rights as well as health—nonsmokers claim that secondhand smoke is a hazard to their well-being. The issues in this section deal with the complex concerns about drugs in our society.

Do Smokers Have a Right to Smoke in Public Places?

Should Alcoholism Be Treated as a Disease?

Should Drugs Be Legalized?

ISSUE 7

Do Smokers Have a Right to Smoke in Public Places?

YES: B. Bruce-Briggs, from "The Health Police Are Blowing Smoke," *Fortune* (April 1988)

NO: Robert E. Goodin, from "The Ethics of Smoking," *Ethics* (April 1989)

ISSUE SUMMARY

YES: Policy analyst B. Bruce-Briggs believes that the war on passive smoking, which he argues is based on inaccurate data relating passive smoking with a myriad of health problems, is both a campaign against smokers and a trial run for a larger program of social manipulation.

NO: Professor of political and moral philosophy Robert E. Goodin argues that the health of nonsmokers suffers when they are forced to breathe tobacco smoke and that nonsmokers should have the right to a smoke-free environment.

Smoking has become an established part of our culture. When cigarette manufacturing became a major industry at the turn of the century, the typical smoker was a middle-class working man. Beginning in the 1920s, however, cigarettes began to seem sophisticated and even fashionable, and women, too, in increasing numbers, started to smoke. As advertising successfully penetrated the youth market and encouraged more and more young smokers, the number of smokers increased, and by 1964, 40 percent of the adult population smoked.

In 1964 the first major blow to smoking occurred: Then-surgeon general of the United States Luther L. Terry made his now-famous report positively linking smoking to lung cancer, heart disease, and other ailments. Other reports and stronger warnings on cigarette packs have contributed to the steady decline of smoking in the United States. Currently, only about one-third of adults continue to smoke.

While the health effects of cigarette smoking are well known, until 1981 the risks associated with breathing others' smoke, or *passive smoking,* were not as clear. A Japanese study completed during that year showed that nonsmoking women who were married to smokers had a higher risk of lung cancer than those who were married to nonsmokers. This study proved that breathing in the smoke from a family member's cigarettes on a daily basis is a significant risk factor for lung cancer. Since the publication of the Japanese study, passive smoking has been linked to numerous other diseases. Not only are nonsmokers who are exposed to passive smoke, also called *environmental tobacco smoke*, at risk for lung cancer, they are also more susceptible to heart disease, asthma, and other upper respiratory diseases. The children of smokers are particularly vulnerable.

In addition to the specific health risks associated with passive smoking, there are also vague health complaints made by nonsmokers who are forced to inhale someone else's smoke. These complaints include headaches, eye irritations, coughing, and nasal symptoms.

As a result of these health risks and complaints, 41 states now restrict smoking in public places, and smoking is banned on most domestic airplane flights and in many workplaces. With the proliferation of clean indoor air regulations, smokers' freedom to light up in public is becoming more and more curtailed.

In the following selections, B. Bruce-Briggs argues that the war against smoking is turning into a war against smokers. Smokers, he claims, are being exiled from public and are facing discrimination in the workplace. He believes that the liberty of smokers is now being threatened. He also dismisses the evidence linking passive smoking with health problems. Bruce-Briggs claims that "scam science," as generated by the government, is responsible for the so-called evidence against smoking. He points out that studies linking lung cancer among nonsmoking wives of smokers failed to take into account other factors, such as heredity, environment, and infection, and he discusses statistical exaggerations for other investigations that claim passive smoking is linked to disease. Finally, he voices his fear that other habits may make the "federal hit list," including alcohol and fatty diets.

Robert E. Goodin discusses the harms associated with passive smoking and argues that the nonsmoking majority (they outnumber smokers 3 to 1) have the right to breathe smoke-free air. He claims that nonsmokers cannot avoid places where there might be smoking, such as public buildings, shopping malls, public transportation, and the workplace. Gooding believes that however much smokers might want to smoke, the risks to nonsmokers are too great to continue allowing them to do so in public places.

YES

B. Bruce-Briggs

THE HEALTH POLICE ARE
BLOWING SMOKE

The war against smoking is turning into a jihad against people who smoke. Smokers are being exiled from public and private places and are facing discrimination in employment. The reason, we are told, is that tobacco is deadly not only to users but also to innocents exposed to its noxious fumes.

The truth is that America is suffering an epidemic of politically motivated hypochondria. Not only the liberty of smokers is threatened. Three decades ago the U.S. Public Health Service [PHS] had apparently defeated its statutory enemy, communicable diseases, and decided to preserve itself by policing our *private* health. Smoking was the first target—a trial run in social manipulation. Sniffing victory in this skirmish, the feds are now turning their weapons on drinking, eating, and sex.

But, you sputter, isn't the evidence conclusive that my smoke affects your health? Let me introduce you to the basics of scam science as generated for the feds. Smoking will be the example because it is the test case, but much of this mode of argumentation will be familiar to victims of the pollution, radiation, and toxic scams. All have their roots in the ambitions of the Public Health Service.

Note first the duplicitous use of words: *Toxic* means poisonous, but does not specify at what dose. Everything is toxic if ingested in sufficient quantity. This magazine is toxic—eat enough copies and you will get sick. Anyone who describes a substance as toxic without stating the dose level is engaging in flimflam; e.g., the Surgeon General informing us that cigarette smoke is "toxic."

Carcinogenic usually means that a group of rodents exposed to megadoses of a substance will have slightly higher cancer rates than a control group. Or it may mean merely that the unfortunate rodents had a few more tumors, or that slight genetic differences appeared in later generations. Too much oxygen, one scientist has determined, is carcinogenic. Anyone who says that something is carcinogenic without specifying the circumstances is a faker. And beware such labels as "linked," "associated with," "suspected," and "related"—these are pseudoscientific McCarthyscam.

Then there is the "no-threshold" scam: If megadoses kill rats, any dose, however tiny, must be assumed lethal to people, absent evidence to the contrary. A more elaborate version is the "linear no-threshold extrapolation." Take data purported to show adverse health at high dosages and draw a straight line to zero to invent ill effects of infinitesimal exposures.

This perversion of toxicology has a cozy symbiosis with "epidemiology." The curiously mislabeled study of health statistics, epidemiology was a benign academic backwater, infested by harmless drudges, until federal funding made it malignant. Most of the work is crude input-output analysis masquerading as precise statistical correlations, using data that are often appallingly inaccurate. The input is typically behavioral or environmental activity—smoking, for instance—established by survey questionnaires, which are notoriously unreliable. Output usually takes the form of death rates, as established by death certificates—documents quite unsuited for statistical research, since physicians often diagnose causes of death only roughly.

When no data exist, the health statisticians generate their own. A favored device is the "case control" method of comparing an affected group with a control group. The drawback here is that researchers have enormous latitude in picking control groups. Even studies using apparently similar groups can yield incredibly varied conclusions that cannot be replicated. For example, in studies cited by the Surgeon General using nonsmokers as control groups, putative lung cancer rates for smokers range from 20% to 3,500% higher.

Here's how the drill works: A toxie gets a government grant to terminate rats by all but drowning them in a suspect compound. He reports that whatzatapyrene is "carcinogenic." Because of the no-threshold principle, the feds can tell the public that "no safe dose level has been established." Next an epie gets a bigger grant to conduct a body count. He discovers that of 87,000 whatzat workers over 30 years, 46 succumbed to cancer. But the epie has calculated 22.7 "expected" deaths from the cancer in a comparable normal group, so the relative risk of whatzatapyrene exposure is 2.03. The feds tell the press that whatzateers are "twice as likely to get cancer."

EPIDEMIOLOGICAL RESULTS ARE CONVENtionally reported as "risk ratios." For example, contract researchers for the FAA might calculate that people who live near airports have a risk ratio of death from falling aircraft engines of 7.5 to 1 compared with the normal population, meaning their risk is $7\frac{1}{2}$ times higher, to hide the vital fact that falling engine fatalities are rather infrequent. Today all seriously untoward health events are rare. That's surely why the feds and their vendors are loath to inform us of the relevant risk data, which are the actual rates at which people suffer falling-engine trauma or contract lung cancer. Although the Public Health Service has been reticent about publicizing the fact, every study cited in support of the statement that "cigarette smoking causes cancer" reveals that a smoker is thoroughly unlikely to get cancer—only that he is statistically more likely to get it than a nonsmoker. No one can say precisely how much more likely. This is true of all supposed "carcinogens."

Perhaps this is why people continue to smoke despite the increasingly shrill scoldings they are subject to. So lately the feds have escalated the war. Their most ingenious weapon for converting private health into public health is the "determination" that secondhand smoke—or passive smoking, or in fed parlance, environmental tobacco smoke (ETS)—harms the public at large. In late 1986 two general surveys of the state of knowledge on ETS were published by the PHS and its contractors. Now follow closely and track scam science in action.

The heart of the health service report is a series of epidemiological studies comparing the lung cancer deaths of the spouses (mostly wives) of smokers with the spouses of nonsmokers, expressed as ratios, not rates. None of the studies took into account effects of common heredity, environment, and infection. Of the 13 studies, three showed that the smokers' wives had comparable or slightly better health—but these studies are worthless because they fail to meet conventional statistical standards. Eight more studies show that the smokers' wives are 3% to 103% more likely to get lung cancer—but these studies are also statistically suspect. That leaves a Greek case-control study and a Japanese study, both of which seem to show that having a smoking husband can be more dangerous than smoking. Both have been attacked in the medical press.

Yet the Surgeon General has announced that these 13 studies prove the evils of passive smoking.

The other survey of environmental tobacco smoke was conducted by the National Research Council of the National Academy of Sciences. The NRC used to be the premier source for fairly accurate and disinterested evaluations of current science, but lately has become a prestige vendor of sci-prop. An NRC panel, engaged by the PHS and the Environmental Protection Agency, averaged a group of studies that included most of the ones cited above and came up with a risk ratio for spouses of smokers of 1.34 to 1 (1.32 to 1 for women). They then concluded that the probable risk was about 1.25 to 1, though in the executive summary the risk was boosted to 1.3 to 1.

It is worth noting that the largest study of smoking conducted to date, by the American Cancer Society in the 1960s, found that women who smoked one to nine cigarettes a day had a lung cancer risk ratio of 1.3 to 1 compared with nonsmokers. Passive smoking is not only bad for women, it seems; it is just as bad as active smoking.

Alcohol is next on the feds' hit list. A study has already "determined" that alcohol "causes" cancer, and learned scientists have taken the next step. In a catalogue of cancer risks posed by various substances, British researchers Richard Doll and Richard Peto estimate that alcohol is responsible for 3% of American cancer deaths. Wine has been discovered to contain carcinogens. The Public Health Service, among other groups, is urging warning labels for alcoholic beverages. Can we doubt that ingenious researchers will ultimately calculate the toxic effects of passive drinking—errant molecules of alcohol from highballs in the box seats statistically killing innocents in the bleachers?

The authorities also complain that we eat too much, and that we don't eat what they think we should. Our heart attacks are a public health problem. Doll and Peto suspect that 35% of cancer deaths are caused by diet, even more than by smoking. Other epidemiologists are calculating how much cancer is caused by burning food. Watch out, restaurant operators and bachelor cooks. The new guardians of the public virtue have even begun collecting information on sexual conduct—when women lose their virginity, the proportion who marry when pregnant—under the rubric of health data. One researcher avers that sperm may be carcinogenic.

WHAT ARE THE IMPLICATIONS FOR BUSINESS? The entrepreneurial reader may already be slobbering to get his snout into the pork barrel. The federal government, after all, funds about 85% of basic health research. Alas, the business is a classic cartel, administered by a narrow trust, with strictly controlled entry. The big winners include the disease lobbies and such institutions as the Harvard School of Public Health.

More to the point, no industry is immune to the ravages of scam science. The feds are now trying to ban tobacco advertising in its surviving forms. As the Surgeon General has said, "There is no safe cigarette." And no such thing as a safe automobile, or a safe food, or a safe airline flight, or a safe ski, or a safe cosmetic, or a safe condom. Nothing is safe as long as the authorities define private health as public health.

NO
Robert E. Goodin

THE ETHICS OF SMOKING

Philosophically, smoking has long been regarded as a paradigmatically private-regarding vice, best treated as such. It is a vice, to be sure: a dirty, disgusting habit, in the view of nineteenth-century moralists, best confined to smoke rooms and male company. But it is a private vice harming only smokers themselves; and it is therefore best left to their personal discretion and moderation. Smoking has thus long been regarded as something best controlled through codes of etiquette and social pressure, and completey unsuited to any very much more serious social sanctions. . . .

In current controversies, the conventional wisdom is being questioned in both its parts. That smoking is a merely private-regarding vice, harming only smokers themselves, is challenged by evidence of the harmful effects of "passive smoking" (i.e., nonsmokers' inhalation of smoke given off by others smoking around them). That smoking is best treated as we would an ordinary private-regarding vice—by informal social pressure, rather than by formal legal sanctions—is also being challenged by evidence of the addictive nature of the habit, making it difficult for smokers to start and stop at will. . . .

HARM TO OTHERS

The Nature of the Risks

Broadly speaking, there are three classes of negative effects on others arising from a person's smoking. Two are clearly harms. The third is of only a slightly different character.

First, there is the well-established harm to the fetus inflicted by the mother's smoking. The extent of the effects, and the mechanism by which they are produced, is obvious. The only real question, perhaps, is whether mother and fetus really are two separate people yet, especially in the first trimester that is so crucial for the fetus's development.

Second, there is the harm to others arising from "passive smoking," that is, the inhalation of "sidestream" smoke from the burning tip of a lit

From Robert E. Goodin, "The Ethics of Smoking," *Ethics*, vol. 99 (April 1989). Copyright © 1989 by The University of Chicago. Reprinted by permission of University of Chicago Press. All rights reserved. Notes and references omitted.

cigarette and of smoke exhaled by a nearby smoker. The technical literature on this subject, though less overwhelming in sheer bulk weight than that on the direct effects of smoking on smokers, is nonetheless voluminous and increasingly compelling in its conclusions. Again, the best guides to the settled scientific view are official reports, dated 1986, from both the National Academy of Sciences and the U.S. surgeon general. They report that chemical analysis shows sidestream smoke to be richer in known carcinogens than the smoke actually inhaled by smokers themselves. Furthermore, evidence (from, e.g., studies of nonsmoking wives living with smoking husbands) shows that passive smokers run a 34 percent greater risk of lung cancer. That is a large increase in a tiny initial probability, of course, so the absolute number of people thus reckoned to die annually from passive smoking is rather small: anything from several hundred to a few thousand, depending upon how many nonsmokers actually are exposed regularly to smoke-filled environments. Those numbers are "small but not negligible." Even by that modest count, passive smoking would still constitute a greater risk to life than that posed by all airborne pollutants regulated by the Environmental Protection Agency, asbestos excepted. Passive smoking also aggravates a number of other conditions (among them bronchitis, asthma, emphysema, angina, and allergies), and it causes irritation of the eyes, nose and throat that can be especially severe in particularly sensitive individuals.

All of those are "real harms"—real health hazards imposed on one person by another's smoking nearby. Third, there are the mere disamenities that nonsmokers experience when breathing others' smoke.

As the Royal College of Physicians argues, whether or not passive smoking damages health, "there is already sufficient evidence as to the discomfort and annoyance, that breathing other people's smoke can cause. Non-smokers at work and play, in transport and in public places, should have the right not to be so exposed."

Emitting offensive odors, when done by a factory, is subject to public regulation. In Malaysia, it is illegal to carry the evil-smelling durian fruit on public transportation. Many nonsmokers (especially ex-smokers) find the smell of burning tobacco similarly offensive, and it might therefore be banned on similar grounds. . . .

"Offense," of course, is not quite harm, though it may be the first cousin to it. That makes it a notoriously tricky notion to fit into the essentially harm-based rationales central to standard moral and legal justifications for social regulation. In such schemes, "harmless immoralities" are ordinarily deemed permissible—especially when they touch upon values of free speech and expression— whether or not others are offended by them. Certainly we have grievous qualms about letting the notion of "offense" range so widely as to ban sexually explicit plays, politically pointed protest, or interracial marriage in the deep South. We are nonetheless comfortable in regulating, as "offensive nuisances," smelly or noisy factories. They may be "mere nuisances," posing no real harms to health, but showing that they are a nuisance is more than enough to justify us in restricting what they may do and where they may do it, according to some larger calculation of social utility.

So too, perhaps, with smoking. After all, nonsmokers are in an increasingly large majority among the population, outnumbering smokers three to one. Insofar as they find smoking similarly a public nuisance, we might appeal to similar standards to justify its regulation as we do to justify regulation of smelly factories. Showing "real harm" to health is always a stronger argument for regulation, of course; and there is evidence of that, too. . . . The point here is just that that might not be strictly necessary. The nuisance argument ought in itself suffice.

The Right to Smoke and the Right to Breathe

The argument for restricting smoking in enclosed public spaces is characteristically couched in deontological terms of the rights of nonsmokers to clean air (WHO 1986). The issue has been joined on this high deontological plane from the other side, too. The tobacco industry's UK pressure group, the Tobacco Advisory Council, maintains that smokers also enjoy a right to smoke, and that "neither group [smokers or nonsmokers] has any absolute right to dictate to the other."

I take it that the rights-based argument can be settled, presumptively at least, in favor of the nonsmoker. In the old adage, your freedom stops at the end of my nose; and in the case of environmental tobacco smoke, your smoke obviously transgresses the privacy of my nasal passages. "Just as my bodily integrity is violated by a punch in the nose, so too is it threatened by toxins and carcinogens others place in the environment. . . . Just as I have a rights claim against those who would punch me in the nose, so too I have one against those who would batter my lungs." The surgeon general has rightly concluded, "The right of smokers to smoke ends where their behavior affects the health and well-being of others; . . . the choice to smoke cannot interfere with the non-smoker's right to breathe air free of tobacco smoke."

In this way, we can break down the apparent symmetry between the loss that would be suffered by the smoker, denied the pleasures of tobacco to spare the nonsmoker, and those that would be suffered by the nonsmoker, denied the pleasures of clean air to indulge the smoker. "Each interferes with the other," it is true. But the nonsmoker "merely wishes to breathe unpolluted air and, in the pursuit thereof, and unlike the smoker, does not reduce the amenity of others" in so doing. "The conflict of interest does not arise from *reciprocal* effects and does not imply equal culpability. The conflict arises from the damage inflicted by one of the parties on the other." The symmetry suggested by the "right to smoke versus the right to clean air" formulation is thus illusory. The crucial asymmetry is that the smoker would be neither better nor worse off if the nonsmoker did not exist, whereas the nonsmoker would be better off if the smoker (qua smoker) did not exist.

At root, the grounds for assigning priority to the right to breathe clean air are simply that everyone—smoker and non-smoker alike—needs this right in order to flourish. The point is effectively evoked by a fanciful example offered by James Repace: "Suppose that individual non-smokers, in defense of their asserted right to breathe tobacco-smoke-free indoor air, were to release a gas into indoor spaces where they were forced to breathe tobacco smoke. Suppose further that when sucked through the burning cone of a cigarette, pipe, or cigar this gas decomposed into irritating byproducts which cause moderate to intense discomfort to the smoker, much the way ambient tobacco smoke affects the nonsmoker. Would smokers feel that they had the inalienable right to gas-free air?" If so, they must concede that nonsmokers have a right to smoke-free air, a right which takes priority over their right to smoke.

Some might say that the analogy is not a perfect one. For example, it might be argued that, unlike the antismoker gas bomber, the smoker is not intentionally harming anyone. The gas bomber actually intends to discomfort anyone who lights up a cigarette in the room. The discomfort caused to others by smokers smoking is regarded, even by smokers themselves, as an unfortunate by-product of their smoking; they would happily remove that side effect if they could do so, without undue cost or discomfort to themselves.

To this claim, the antismoker gas bomber might reply that he does not intend to harm anyone, either. Smokers will be discomforted by his gas only if they smoke. If they refrain from smoking, they will not be harmed in the slightest. Furthermore, the gas bomber might continue, if they do smoke then nonsmokers would have been analogously discomforted. The gas bomb can thus be construed as an act of self-defense which, though preemptive, has the endearing property of harming potential aggressors only if and when they turn into actual ones.

Some such argument might establish a presumptive priority of the right to clean air over the right to smoke. Like all presumptions, however, this one can always be overcome—in this case, in either of two ways. One is to show that nonsmokers have voluntarily consented to others' smoking. The other is to show, through a calculation of costs, and benefits, that the losses to smokers who are stopped from smoking would far exceed the losses to nonsmokers who are exposed to environmental tobacco smoke. Each of these possibilities will be considered, and rejected, in turn.

The Voluntariness of Passive Smoking

In the case of the smoker, it could (wrongly, as we have seen) be argued that the risks were somehow voluntarily incurred. In the case of the passive smoker, that argument would be far harder to sustain. Passive smokers do not themselves light up. They merely breathe. You can voluntarily choose to do something only if you can, realistically, choose not to do it; and no one can choose not to breathe. Since passive smoking—or, more technically, "exposure to environmental tobacco smoke"—"generally occurs as an unavoidable consequence of being in proximity to smokers, particularly in enclosed indoor environments," the surgeon general prefers simply to define passive smoking as "involuntary smoking."

Smokers might sometimes have sought and been granted the permission of all nonsmokers in the vicinity for them to light up. Assuming that that consent was given freely (i.e., that it was not a tyrannical boss 'asking' permission of a secretary and that it was based on full information about the hazards of passive smoking), nonsmokers' exposure to environmental tobacco smoke would indeed then be voluntary. Given the dangers of duress and of fraudulent claims that rights have been waived, we may prefer to treat the right to clean air as if it were as inalienable as the right to life itself. But in any case, this whole voluntary smoker scenario is plausible only among moderately small groups of people.

Among larger and more anonymous groups, the only sense in which passive smoking might be thought to be voluntary would be insofar as people voluntarily enter environments they knew were or would become smoky. Thus, it might be argued that if people do not want to breathe other people's smoke, they should not go into notoriously smoky places like English pubs.

There is, of course, the question of why nonsmokers should banish themselves rather than smokers controlling themselves. In any case, there is a range of places it is unreasonable to expect people to avoid going. One is to work. Another is onto public transportation. Another is into public buildings. Another, perhaps, is to public entertainments (restaurants, theaters, and such like). If people cannot reasonably be expected to avoid going to work, and getting there by public transportation, then the Humean doctrine ("no consent without the possibility of withholding consent") [David Hume, Scottish philosopher and historian] would imply that they have not voluntarily consented to the risks of passive smoking in those places either.

Costs and Benefits

Even if we supposed that the issue is properly couched in terms of rights—and especially if we do not—a calculation of the costs and benefits to all interested parties under all policy options is nonetheless relevant. Some rights violations matter more than others, after all. It would be a violation of bodily integrity for someone else to force smoke into

your lungs. It would equally be a violation of bodily integrity for someone else to brush against your arm, yet few courts would take cognizance of that invasion. Technically, it might count as a case of assault, but the law does not deal in trifles, as the saying goes. Neither should public policy.

When deciding which rights violations matter most, we tend to employ a rough-and-ready utilitarian calculus of a sort, taking into account both costs to the violated and benefits to the violator. In that calculus, the former weighs particularly heavily. If rights holders have suffered serious harm, then rights violators have wronged them, almost regardless of whatever benefits the rights violators themselves stood to gain (or losses to avert). Thus, insofar as the case against passive smoking can be made in terms of increased lung cancer and other potentially grave illnesses, the deontological case is once again quickly closed. But insofar as the stakes are more modest—offensive odors and watery eyes—we would have to take seriously into account costs and benefits to both parties on the model of nuisance law, for example (Feinberg 1985, chap. 8).

Dealing in straight utilitarian terms, the case against passive smoking is necessarily less strong than that against direct smoking. That is simply because the passive smoker gets only a small fraction of the dose of poisonous substances that is received by the active smoker. A smoker's chances of lung cancer are increased by 980 percent, a passive smoker's by only 34 percent; and so on. Since the costs of passive smoking are necessarily lower than those of active smoking, there is more of a chance that the benefits there might outweigh the costs, in a utilitarian calculus.

As before, one easy way to meet this challenge is to conceptualize "benefits" in terms of interests rather than of preferences. However much smokers might want to smoke, it is not in their interests to do so. We are doing them a favor—conferring upon them an objective health benefit—by stopping them from smoking, even for a little while. . . .

If dealing in preference-based terms, we must take account of the severity of the characteristic reactions involved: of smokers forced to suffer withdrawal for the period of time they would be constrained from smoking, on the one hand; of nonsmokers forced to suffer environmental tobacco smoke for the period of time they would be closeted with it, on the other. Of course, variable physiology on both sides means that some people will suffer more than others. Not all smokers would suffer withdrawal during a two-hour flight; not all nonsmokers would mind the smoke all that much. But most smokers would probably suffer some withdrawal symptoms over the course of a whole day at work, and surveys show that most nonsmokers suffer at least eye, nose and throat irritations from being subjected to day-long smoking in an enclosed office. Fine-grained interpersonal utility comparisons are notoriously difficult, but it would seem that those two are roughly on a par. Smokers might usually be bothered marginally more, but probably only marginally more, at least once they have had a chance to adjust as fully as they can to the new nonsmoking regime.

What is not on a par, and what decisively favors regulation of smoking in enclosed spaces, is the magnitude of the possible suffering by each party. At worst, the smoker prevented from smoking suffers discomfort. The nonsmoker exposed to environmental tobacco smoke for a prolonged period might, at worst, suffer lung cancer or other debilitating disease. This is not the most common outcome, by a long stretch. But in light of other less risky airborne contaminants that the Environmental Protection Agency does regulate, it certainly is a common enough outcome to take seriously in framing policies.

The second crucial element . . . is the number of people affected on both sides. Nonsmokers now outnumber smokers in the United States by a ratio of almost three to one. That is not a big enough differential to decide matters all by itself, perhaps. But conjoined with the above argument—that smokers will lose something less than three times what nonsmokers will gain from a ban—this fact does prove decisive. Numbers conspire with intensity in arguing for restricting passive smoking.

Policy Options

There are, again, several possible policy responses to the problem of passive smoking. Among them are these.

1. *Reduce smoking.*—First and foremost, notice that anything done to reduce smoking will also, simultaneously, reduce passive smoking. . . .

2. *Self-restraint/courtesy.*—Self-regulation, at the personal level, would amount to self-restraint among smokers to curb the passive smoking they inflict upon those around them. Ideally, "common sense and natural courtesy" should solve the problem; that has "long been the best approach to solving the occasional difference of opinion between smoking and non-smoking employees," as the tobacco industry's pamphlet on workplace smoking policies says. Ideally, smokers should ask others for permis-

sion before lighting up in confined quarters. Ideally, a polite request for them to cease should suffice. As Miss Manners instructs, "If you wish to smoke in the presence of clean people, you must ask their permission and be prepared to accept their refusal to grant it."

For those smokers who are considerate in such ways, self-restraint is indeed ideal. Not all are, however. Given the nature of addictions, internal sanctions of shame at discourtesy will often be overcome by internal compulsions of nicotine cravings; and, as an example of the theory of cognitive dissonance in action, surveys show that smokers when asked grossly underestimate the extent to which they think nonsmokers find their smoking behavior discourteous. In any case, the strategy of "polite requests" is more plausible to intimate company than in larger groups. No one presumes that one-to-one requests would be the appropriate way to regulate behavior in large, open-plan offices, on airplanes, or in restaurants.

Another form of self-restraint would be for smokers to shift over to using "smokeless" forms of tobacco: snuff, chewing tobacco, tobacco pouches, and so forth. (The recently announced "smokeless cigarette" may or may not be another example; there is some thought that it may just emit smaller particles of smoke that are harder to see, but contain much the same carcinogens [Helyar 1987]). There is no reason to suppose that any of these products pose fewer health hazards to smokers themselves, of course. But they do at least avoid inflicting similar hazards on others around them.

3. *Improved ventilation/air filters.*—Passive smoking is a problem arising principally in confined spaces. If windows can be opened without problems (of undue heat gain/loss, etc.), then that is one easy solution. But there are some places—airplanes, increasingly trains, and modern office blocks—where the windows do not open. In such places, we must rely instead upon technological fixes as filters, and such like. In practice, those presently available are both costly and inadequate. They are incapable of removing small particles and gases contained in cigarette smoke; typically, they serve merely to recirculate smoky air. Even air systems on aircraft—presumably the most controlled environments most of us regularly experience—fail to eliminate cigarette smoke from the air adequately, and increasing ventilation so that it is adequate to do so "is not technically feasible on existing aircraft." The next generation of aircraft is expected to be worse, if anything, in this respect. Of course, we should not rule out the possibility of some technological breakthrough that would clean the air of tobacco smoke perfectly. Neither, however, should we count on one.

4. *Market forces.*—To some extent, ordinary market forces might take care of the passive smoking problem. If people want nonsmoking provision, then they should be willing to pay for it; they should patronize establishments offering it, in preference to ones that do not; and so on. Airlines will win more flyers, restaurants more diners, and businesses more employees and customers if they cater to such demand. Insofar as this happens naturally, no government intervention would be required. . . .

5. *Bans/restrictions on smoking in public places.*—The best way to prevent people from being subjected to environmental tobacco smoke in confined public places is to ban (or, anyway, to restrict) smoking in those places, as a matter of public

policy backed, ultimately, by the force of law. On the basis of the evidence and arguments above, it seems that smoking should be curtailed especially in certain sorts of places: (*a*) Confined quarters generally. Enclosed spaces, if poorly ventilated, magnify the effects of tobacco smoke, both on the health and comfort of nonsmokers in the vicinity. (*b*) Places where a special "duty of care" is owed to others who might be harmed. Under common law, such duties traditionally fall upon: (i) public transport operators; (ii) inn keepers; (iii) employers, at least where it is impossible for workers to protect themselves from the hazards; (iv) jailers; and (v) heads of households. (*c*) Places where people cannot reasonably be expected to avoid going. If self-contained spaces are available, designating them as "smoking rooms" and restricting smoking to them might suffice to accomplish these goals. But "the simple separation of smokers and non-smokers within the same air space"—an open-plan office, for example—"does not eliminate the exposure of non-smokers to environmental tobacco smoke." So if no self-contained quarters are available for designation as smoking rooms, a total ban on smoking in the whole area might be required. Such bans or restrictions on smoking in public places are now in force in four-fifths of the American states and in forty-seven countries of the world. . . .

CONCLUSION

Forty-two states have now enacted restrictions—in at least nine cases extensive ones—on smoking in public places. Smoking is now banned or restricted in over a third of private-sector business establishments. Those responsible for governing our society have increasingly concluded that clean indoor air is a quality-of-life issue that is a fitting concern for socially enforced sanctions.

The evidence in this essay shows that there are more than adequate grounds for that conclusion. It also suggests that there are grounds, of an inoffensively weak paternalistic sort, for going even further—curbing the advertising, and perhaps even over-the-counter selling, of cigarettes. Smoking has long ago ceased to be a private-regarding vice best treated as such. It is high time that philosophers stopped talking as if it were.

POSTSCRIPT

Do Smokers Have a Right to Smoke in Public Places?

Because public smoking is an issue of both health and personal rights, it generates many arguments. Both nonsmokers and smokers claim that their rights are violated when one group's desires are allowed to prevail over the other's. In the battle over smoking, nonsmokers cite research showing that long-term exposure to passive smoke increases the risk of many illnesses, including heart disease and lung cancer. Researchers claim that passive tobacco smoke contains over 40 cancer-causing chemicals and is responsible for as many as 50,000 deaths each year. Lawrence Altman claims that passive smoke is a major risk factor in diseases such as lung cancer and heart disease in "The Evidence Mounts on Passive Smoking," the *New York Times* (May 29, 1990). Professor of pharmacology and toxicology K. H. Ginzel agrees in "What's In a Cigarette?" *Priorities* (Fall 1990).

Numerous research studies have confirmed that passive smoking is a health risk. The landmark investigation, which indicated that nonsmoking wives of smoking spouses have a higher risk of lung cancer, found that only a fraction of female lung cancer patients actually smoked cigarettes. It was concluded that the women who developed lung cancer were exposed to high levels of secondhand smoke from their husbands' cigarettes. See "Non-Smoking Wives of Heavy Smokers Have a Higher Risk of Lung Cancer: A Study from Japan," *British Medical Journal* (January 17, 1981). This classic study was followed by many others, all reaching the same conclusion: exposure to passive smoke is a risk for lung cancer and other smoking-related diseases. Further readings include "Passive Smoking and Lung Cancer," *The Lancet* (September 10, 1983); "Prevalence and Correlates of Passive Smoking," *American Journal of Public Health* (April 1983); "Cancer Risk in Adulthood from Early Life Exposure to Parents' Smoking," *American Journal of Public Health* (May 1985); "Passive Smoking May Cause Leukaemia," *New Scientist* (March 7, 1985); "Secondhand Smoke," *Newsweek* (June 11, 1990); "Passive Smoking, Active Risks," *American Health* (June 1990); and "Hazardous to Whose Health?" *Forbes* (December 11, 1989).

The groups that are in favor of smoking in public places believe that passive smoke is harmless and/or that smokers are entitled to the individual freedom to smoke wherever they please. To justify the claim that passive smoking is harmless to health, they argue that the research is inconclusive and lacking in valid data. Smokers believe that laws restricting smoking in public places violate their civil rights; after all, smokers are taxpayers too. Smokers believe that smoking is a personal choice and that the government has no right to restrict when and where they may light up. Articles supporting this view include "The Cigarette Controversy," by former Tobacco Institute president Horace Kornegay, *Engage/Social Action* (September 1980). Also see "Smoke and Mirrors," by Jacob Sullum, *Reason* (February 1991); "Zealots Against Science," *The American Spectator* (July 1990); and "Coping with Smoking," by Tibor Machan, *Freeman* (April 1989).

Since the classic Japanese study of 1981, it has been confirmed that smoking is harmful not only to the smoker but also to the persons surrounding the smoker. Yet, despite the overwhelming evidence against passive smoke, numerous writers continue to support the right to smoke in public. As the nonsmoking majority continue to vocally support a ban on public smoking, more and more work sites, public buildings, and retail establishments are restricting indoor smoking.

ISSUE 8

Should Alcoholism Be Treated as a Disease?

YES: George E. Vaillant, from "We Should Retain the Disease Concept of Alcoholism," *Harvard Medical School Mental Health Letter* (August 1990)

NO: Herbert Fingarette, from "We Should Reject the Disease Concept of Alcoholism," *Harvard Medical School Mental Health Letter* (September 1990)

ISSUE SUMMARY

YES: Physician George E. Vaillant maintains that since alcoholism is genetically transmitted, it should be treated as a disease and not as a character flaw.

NO: Philosophy professor Herbert Fingarette argues that alcoholism is voluntary behavior that is within the drinker's control and that the role of heredity and genes in alcoholism is limited.

According to the U.S. Department of Education, alcohol use and abuse is involved in 240,000 deaths per year from accidents, suicides, and alcohol-related diseases. Although the majority of adults drink alcohol, only a minority become problem drinkers or alcoholics. The National Council on Alcoholism defines *alcoholism* as a chronic, progressive, and potentially fatal disease characterized by physical dependency and harmful organ changes related directly or indirectly to the consumption of alcohol.

There are many different theories as to why some individuals become alcoholics. Historically, alcohol dependency was viewed as either a disease or a moral failing. In more recent years, other theories of alcohol addiction have been developed, including behavioral, genetic, sociocultural, and psychological theories.

The view that alcoholism is a moral failing maintains that overconsuming alcohol is voluntary behavior that the user chooses to do. Drinkers choose to overindulge in such a way that they create suffering for themselves and others. In order to control this abuse, American history is marked by repeated and failed government efforts to eliminate alcohol use with legal sanctions, such as the enactment of Prohibition in the late 1920s and the punishment of alcoholics via jail sentences and fines. However, there seem to be several contradictions to this model of alcoholism. Alcoholism appears to be a complex condition that is caused by multiple factors. It is also not totally clear that alcoholism is voluntary behavior. Finally, from a historical perspective, punishing alcoholics has been ineffective.

In the United States today, the primary theory for understanding the causes of alcoholism is the disease rather than the moral model. The disease model is especially strong among the medical and treatment communities as well as self-help groups such as Alcoholics Anonymous. The disease model implies that alcoholism is not the result of voluntary behavior, psychiatric problems, or lack of self-control; it is caused by biological factors. While there are somewhat different interpretations of the disease model, it generally refers to alcoholism as a disease with biological and genetic origins.

Many proponents of the disease model cite the claim that children of alcoholics are four times more likely to develop alcoholism than are children of nonalcholics. These figures, which support genetics as the cause of alcoholism, are largely based on a few studies that critics claim are flawed. George Vaillant is a proponent of the disease model of alcoholism. He believes that calling alcoholism a disease rather than a voluntary behavioral disorder is a useful device both to persuade the alcoholic to acknowledge the problem and to provide a ticket into the health care system.

Herbert Fingarette believes that it is a myth that certain people are genetically predisposed to becoming alcoholics and that once these people begin drinking, they cannot stop. He also claims that the scientific evidence for this model is flawed and that many people confuse the relationship of biological factors with drinking. Fingarette believes that biological factors are *correlated* with alcoholism but are not necessarily the *cause* of it.

YES
George E. Vaillant

WE SHOULD RETAIN THE DISEASE CONCEPT OF ALCOHOLISM

When I read expert discussions of why alcoholism is not a disease, I am reminded of the equally learned discussions by "the best and the brightest" of why the Viet Nam War was a good idea. These discussants had intelligence, advanced degrees, scholarship, prestige, literacy—every qualification but one. They lacked experience. None had spent much time in Viet Nam. Just so, the philosopher Herbert Fingarette, the psychoanalyst Thomas Szasz, the sociologist and theoretician Robin Room, and provocative, thoughtful psychologists like Stanton Peele and Nicholas Heather have every qualification but one for explaining why alcoholism is not a disease— they have never worked in an alcohol clinic. Why, I wonder, do experienced alcohol workers and recovering alcoholics, the thousands of competent common folk in the trenches, accept the view that alcoholism is a disease? Why is it mainly less competent people, the active alcoholics, who agree with Professor Fingarette that they are just "heavy drinkers"?

Let me summarize the evidence provided by the learned academics who have pointed out the folly of the medical model of alcoholism. First, alcohol abuse—unlike coughing from pneumonia, for example—is a habit under considerable volitional control. Second, there is compelling evidence that variations in alcohol consumption are distributed along a smooth continuum, although a medical model would suggest that in any individual, alcoholism is either present or absent. Third, when alcoholism is treated as a disease it can be used both by individuals and by society to explain away major underlying problems—poverty, mental deficiency, crime, and the like—which require our attention if efforts at prevention, treatment and understanding are to succeed. Fourth, to diagnose people as alcoholic is to label them in a way that can damage both self-esteem and public acceptance. Fifth, alcoholism should not be considered a disease if it is regarded as merely a symptom of underlying personality or depression.

From George E. Vaillant, "We Should Retain the Disease Concept of Alcoholism," *Harvard Medical School Mental Health Letter* (August 1990). Copyright © 1990 by the President and Fellows of Harvard College. Reprinted by permission of the *Harvard Medical School Mental Health Letter*, 164 Longwood Avenue, Boston, MA 02115.

REFUTATION OF OBJECTIONS

Let me try to refute these objections one by one. First, it may be true that there is no known underlying biological defect in alcoholism. Rather, alcohol abuse is a multidetermined continuum of drinking behaviors whose causes are differently weighted for different people and include culture, habits, and genes. But the same can be said of high blood pressure and coronary heart disease. The incidence of hypertension varies with measurement procedures and psychological circumstances. It lies on a physiological continuum which defies precise definition. It has no known specific cause. It is powerfully affected by social factors; for example, it has become epidemic among young urban black males. The point of using the term 'disease' for alcoholism is simply to underscore that once a person has lost the capacity to control consistently how much and how often he or she drinks, continued use of alcohol can be both a necessary and a sufficient cause of a syndrome that produces millions of invalids and causes millions of deaths.

The second objection to the medical model of alcoholism is that only opinion separates the alcoholic from the heavy drinker. Supposedly one either has a disease or does not have it; diagnosis should depend on signs and symptoms, not value judgments. But consider the example of coronary heart disease. We regard it as a medical illness, although its causes are diverse and often poorly understood and there is no fixed point at which we can decide that coronary arteries become abnormal. So it is with alcoholism. Normal drinking merges imperceptibly with pathological drinking. Culture and idiosyncratic viewpoints will always determine where the line is drawn.

The third objection is that alcoholism is affected by so many situational and psychological factors that the drinking must often be viewed as reactive. Some people drink uncontrollably only after a serious loss or in certain specific situations, and some alcoholics return to normal drinking by an act of will. But these observations are equally true of hypertension, which often has an extremely important psychological component. Nevertheless, prospective studies show that alcohol dependence causes depression, anxiety, and poverty far more often than the other way around. In citing psychological problems as a cause of alcoholism, Fingarette reverses the position of cart and horse.

The fourth objection to calling alcoholism a disease is that it involves both labeling and a disparagement of free will. But in this case both labeling and the denial of free will are therapeutic. Some people believe that the label 'alcoholic' transforms a person into an outcast, akin to a leper. Well, should a doctor who knows that a person has leprosy keep the fact secret lest the patient be labeled a leper? Some people believe that if alcoholics are taught to regard alcoholism as a disease they will use this label as an excuse to drink or a reason why they should not be held responsible for their own recovery. It does not work out that way. Like people with high blood pressure, alcoholics who understand that they have a disease become more rather than less willing to take responsibility for self-care. That is why the self-help group, Alcoholics Anonymous, places such single-minded emphasis on the idea that alcoholism is a disease.

DIAGNOSIS HELPS

Once patients accept the diagnosis, they can be shown how to assume responsibility for their own care. Physicians stress the value of diagnosing hypertension early because it can provide a rational explanation for headaches and other symptoms that were hitherto regarded as neurotic or irrational. For years alcoholics themselves have labeled themselves 'wicked,' 'weak,' and 'reprehensible.' The offer of a medical explanation does not lead to irresponsibility, only to hope and improved morale.

The fifth argument against calling alcoholism a disease is the most compelling; it is said that uncontrolled maladaptive ingestion of alcohol is not a biological disorder but a disorder of behavior. Like compulsive fingernail biting, gambling, or child molesting, this form of deviant behavior can often be better classified by sociologists than by physiologists, and better treated by psychologists skilled in behavior therapy than by physicians with their medical armamentarium.

But unlike giving up gambling or fingernail biting, giving up alcohol abuse often requires skilled medical attention during acute withdrawal. Unlike gamblers and fingernail biters, most alcoholics develop secondary symptoms that do require medical care. Unlike child molesters, but like people with high blood pressure, alcoholics have a mortality rate two to four times as high as the average. In order to receive the medical treatment they require, alcoholics need a label that will allow them unprejudiced access to emergency rooms, detoxification clinics, and medical insurance.

The final argument for regarding alcoholism as a disease rather than a behavior disorder is that it often causes alcoholics to mistreat persons they love. Very few sustained human experiences involve as much abuse as the average close family member of an alcoholic must tolerate. Fingarette's "heavy drinking" model (which conveys a concept of misbehavior) only generates more denial in the already profoundly guilt-ridden alcoholic. Calling alcoholism a disease rather than a behavior disorder is a useful device both to persuade the alcoholic to acknowledge the problem and to provide a ticket for admission to the health care system. In short, in our attempts to understand and study alcoholism, we should employ the models of the social scientist and the learning theorist. But in order to treat alcoholics effectively we need to invoke the medical model.

Let me close with an anecdote. My research associate, reviewing the lives of 100 patients who had been hospitalized eight years previously for detoxification from alcohol, wrote to me that she mistrusted the diagnosis of alcoholism. To illustrate, she described one man who drank heavily for seven years after his initial detoxification. Although the alcohol clinic's staff agreed that his drinking was alcoholic, neither he nor his wife acknowledged that it was a problem. Finally he required a second detoxification, and the clinic staff claimed that they had been right.

"How can you call such behavior a disease," my associate wrote, "when you cannot decide if it represents a social problem [that is, requires a value judgment] or alcohol-dependent drinking?" Then she shifted her attention to the ninety-nine other tortured lives she had been reviewing. Oblivious of the contradiction, she concluded: "I don't think I ever fully realized before I did this follow-up what an absolutely devastating disease alcoholism is." I respectfully submit that if Professor Fingarette were to work in an alcohol clinic for two years, he would agree with the last half of my research associate's letter rather than the first half.

NO
Herbert Fingarette

WE SHOULD REJECT THE DISEASE CONCEPT OF ALCOHOLISM

Why do heavy drinkers persist in their behavior even when prudence, common sense, and moral duty call for restraint? That is the central question in debates about alcohol abuse. In the United States (but not in other countries such as Great Britain) the standard answer is to call the behavior a disease, "alcoholism," whose key symptom is a pattern of uncontrollable drinking. This myth, now widely advertised and widely accepted, is neither helpfully compassionate nor scientifically valid. It promotes false beliefs and inappropriate attitudes, as well as harmful, wasteful, and ineffective social policies.

The myth is embodied in the following four scientifically baseless propositions: 1) Heavy problem drinkers show a single distinctive pattern of ever greater alcohol use leading to ever greater bodily, mental, and social deterioration. 2) The condition, once it appears, persists involuntarily: the craving is irresistible and the drinking is uncontrollable once it has begun. 3) Medical expertise is needed to understand and relieve the condition ("cure the disease") or at least ameliorate its symptoms. 4) Alcoholics are no more responsible legally or morally for their drinking and its consequences than epileptics are responsible for the consequences of their movements during seizures.

The idea that alcoholism is a disease has always been a political and moral notion with no scientific basis. It was first promoted in the United States around 1800 as a speculation based on erroneous physiological theory, and later became a theme of the temperance movement. It was revived in the 1930s by the founders of Alcoholics Anonymous (AA), who derived their views from an amalgam of religious ideas, personal experiences and observations, and the unsubstantiated theories of a contemporary physician.

The AA doctrine won decisive support in the 1940s when a reputable scientist, E. M. Jellinek, published an elaborate statistical study of the "phases of alcoholism." He portrayed an inevitable sequence of ever more uncontrollable drinking that led progressively to such symptoms as blackouts, tolerance, and withdrawal distress, until the drinker "hit bottom" as a derelict, became insane, or died. Jellinek's work seemed to put a scientific seal of confirmation on the AA portrait of the alcoholic. That was hardly surprising, since he had taken his data from questionnaires that were prepared and distributed by AA and answered by fewer than 100 self-selected members. Jellinek conscientiously acknowledged the source of his data and his reservations about its scientific adequacy. Nevertheless, his dramatic-tragic portrait of the alcoholic became widely accepted and is now part of American folk beliefs.

NO CONSISTENT PATTERN

Recent scientific literature shows that in reality the typical pattern of heavy drinking fluctuates. Some drinkers with numerous and severe problems deteriorate; others markedly improve, or develop different problems. Some claim loss of control; others do not. Many heavy drinkers report no serious social problems associated with their drinking and are not recognized as alcoholics by friends, colleagues, or even their families.

The idea that alcoholics are constantly drunk is quite false. One leading researcher points out that "in any given month, one half of alcoholics will be abstinent, with a mean of four months of being dry in any one-year to two-year period." During any ten- to twenty-year period, about a third of alcoholics "mature out" into various forms of moderate drinking or abstinence. The rate of maturing out is even higher among heavy problem drinkers not diagnosed as alcoholics. Undoubtedly there is a small group who follow a pattern resembling Jellinek's four phases; one objection to the disease concept of alcoholism is that it focuses attention mainly on this marginal group.

It is now widely believed that a biological cause of alcoholism has been discovered; some people are said to have a biochemistry or a genetic predisposition that dooms them to be alcoholics if they drink. The truth is less dramatic. There are certain so-called biological markers associated with heavy drinking, but these have not been shown to cause it. One supposed marker is the metabolism of alcohol into acetaldehyde, a brain toxin, in the bodies of people who are independently identifiable as being at higher risk of becoming alcoholics. Another proposed marker is the high level of morphine-like substances supposedly secreted by alcoholics when they metabolize alcohol. But almost all people with serious drinking problems have intermittent periods of sobriety during which all metabolic products of alcohol have been excreted. It is implausible that any residual effects, whether physical or psychological, could be so powerful as to override a sober person's rational, moral, and prudential inclination to abstain.

Recent studies have also been said to imply that alcoholism is a hereditary disease. But that is not what the genetic research shows. In the first place, these studies provide no evidence of a genetic factor in the largest group of heavy drinkers—those who have significant associated problems but are not diagnosable as alcoholics. Even among the minority who can be so diagnosed, the data suggest that only a minority have the pertinent genetic background. And even in this category, a minority of a minority, studies report that the majority do not become alcoholics.

It is not only misleading but dangerous to regard alcoholism as a genetic disorder. Heavy drinkers without alcoholism in their genetic backgrounds are led to feel immune to serious drinking problems, yet they have the greatest total number of problems. On the other hand, people who do have some hereditary disposition to alcoholism could easily become defeatist. Their risk is higher, and they should be aware of that, but their fate is still very much in their own hands.

NO SINGLE CAUSE

The idea of a single disease obscures the scientific consensus that no single cause has ever been established. Heavy drinking has many causes which vary from drinker to drinker, from one drinking pattern to another. Character, motivation, family environment, personal history, ethnic and cultural values, marital, occupational, and educational status all play a role. As these change, so do patterns of drinking, heavy drinking, and "alcoholism." For example, alcohol is used in many so-called "primitive" societies, but their drinking patterns are not ours, and what we call alcoholism does not exist among them before contact with Europeans. That would not be true if alcoholism were a disease caused by chemical and neurological effects of drinking in conjunction with individual genetic vulnerability. The crucial role of psychology in alcoholics' drinking is demonstrated by experiments in which they are deceived about whether the beverage they are drinking contains alcohol. Their drinking patterns then reflect their beliefs; the actual presence or absence of alcohol is irrelevant.

Alcoholics do not "lack control" in the ordinary sense of those words. Studies show that they can limit their drinking in response to appeals and arguments or rules and regulations. In experiments they will reduce or eliminate drinking in return for such rewards as money, social privileges, or exemption from boring tasks. To object that these experiments are invalid because they occur in protected settings is to miss the point, which is precisely that the drinking patterns of alcoholics can vary dramatically in different settings.

True, alcoholics often resist appeals to cease their alcohol abuse, and they ignore obvious prudential and moral considerations. The simplistic explanation that attributes this to an irresistible craving obscures a more complicated reality: they have developed a way of life in which they use drinking as a major strategy for coping with their problems. They have become accustomed to values, friends, settings, and beliefs that protect and encourage drinking. When they encounter drastically changed circumstances in a hospital, clinic, or communal group, they are capable of following different rules. Even some who "cheat" where abstention is expected nevertheless limit their drinking to avoid being found out. They do not automatically lose control because of a few drinks. Our focus of attention must shift from drinking per se to the meaning of drink for certain persons and the way of life in which its role has become central.

TERMS REDEFINED

Responsible scientists who are familiar with the research but want to preserve the disease concept of alcoholism have had to redefine their terms. What they now mean by "disease" and "loss of control" no longer coincides either with the customary meaning of those words or with what the public is encouraged to believe. Thus Mark Keller, one of the early leaders of the alcoholism movement, now reinterprets loss of control to mean that alcoholics who have decided to stop "cannot be sure they will stand by their resolution." This is said to be compatible with anything from constant heavy drinking to remission in the form of permanent moderation or total abstention. Although the medical term "remission" is used, this is not a medical or scientific explanation: we all know that someone who resolves to change a long-standing way of life cannot be sure whether the promise will be kept. Similarly, craving, still popularly understood as an overwhelming and irresistible desire, has now been extended by researchers to include mild inclinations, although this makes nonsense of the supposed compulsion to drink.

The disease concept is sometimes justified on the ground that although scientifically invalid, it is a practical way of encouraging alcoholics to enter treatment. This argument is based on false assumptions and has harmful consequences. The many heavy drinkers who see themselves (often correctly) as not fitting the criteria for alcoholism under some current diagnostic formula are likely to conclude that they have no cause for concern. Their inclination to deny their problems is thus encouraged. As for people who are diagnosable as alcoholics, the vast majority never become permanently abstinent, even after treatment or after they join AA. Yet the disease doctrine may cause them to develop a fatalistic conviction that even one slip is a disaster, since they have

been led to believe, falsely, that occasional or moderate drinking is never possible for them.

When behavior is labeled a disease, it becomes excusable because it is regarded as involuntary. This is an important result of the disease concept of alcoholism, and indeed an important reason for its promulgation. Thus special benefits are provided to alcoholics in employment, health, and civil rights law, provided they can prove that their drinking is persistent and very heavy. The effect is to reward people who continue to drink heavily. This policy is insidious precisely because it is well intended, and those who criticize it may seem to lack compassion.

SUPREME COURT VIEW

The United States Supreme Court, after reviewing detailed briefs pro and con, has consistently held in favor of those who say that alcoholics are responsible for their behavior, and has concluded that medical evidence does not demonstrate their drinking to be involuntary. Spokesmen for the National Council on Alcoholism (NCA) state publicly that they too believe alcoholics should be held responsible for their misdeeds, but they are being hypocritical. In the less visible forum of the federal courts, the NCA has repeatedly argued that alcoholics should be protected from criminal and civil liability for their acts and excused from the normal regulatory requirements.

But the greatest scandal of the argument for the disease concept as a useful lie is the claim that it helps alcoholics by inducing them to enter treatment. On the contrary, both independent and government research show expensive disease-oriented treatment programs to be largely a waste of money and human resources. Their apparent success proves illusory when they are compared in statistically rigorous studies with other programs, and with the rate of improvement in untreated alcohol abusers (which is much higher than the disease concept has led the public to believe). Very often, perhaps always, brief outpatient counseling works just as well as a long stay in a hospital or other residential clinic costing thousands of dollars. Some studies conclude that professional intervention is slightly better than no treatment, although the treatment method, duration, setting, or cost makes no difference. Other studies find no significant difference in results whether or not there is treatment.

We must refocus our compassion and redefine our policies on alcohol abuse. While continuing biological research, we should loosen the grip of physicians on the chief government agencies and research funding sources, and we should reject their deep bias in favor of the disease concept. Greater resources must be shifted to psychological and sociocultural research. We should consider promising new approaches to treatment that are being used in other countries. The public should be better informed about the scientific facts and above all about our scientific ignorance. Our policies should reflect the fact that heavy drinking is not primarily a biochemical or medical problem but a human and social one.

POSTSCRIPT

Should Alcoholism Be Treated as a Disease?

One of the most valuable aspects of the disease model is that it removes alcohol from the moral realm. It proposes that addiction sufferers should be treated and helped, rather than scorned and punished. Though the moral model of alcoholism has by no means disappeared in the United States, today more resources are directed toward rehabilitation than punishment. The disease model can be credited with this shift in attitude. Increasingly, it is being recognized and understood that fines and imprisonment do little to curb alcohol abuse in society.

Another strength of the disease model is its simplicity. It is straightforward and relatively easy to teach to recovering alcoholics. They, in turn, are often comfortable with the concept that what they have is a disease, rather than moral degeneration. And finally, the disease model provides the alcoholic with a mechanism for coping with any shame or guilt resulting from past misdeeds. The disease model teaches that problem behaviors are *symptoms*, not causes, of the disease process and that the alcoholic is not to blame. Further reading supporting the disease model include *Twelve Steps and Twelve Traditions* (Alcoholics Anonymous World Services, 1981); *The Story of How Many Thousands of Men and Women Have Recovered from Alcoholism (The Big Book)* (Alcoholics Anonymous World Services, 1977); *Alcoholism: The Genetic Inheritance*, by Kathleen W. FitzGerald (Doubleday, 1988); and "Thin Thinking About Heavy Drinking," by William Madsen, *The Public Interest* (Spring 1989).

The following selections discuss the role of genetics in alcoholism: "The Gene and the Bottle," *Newsweek* (April 30, 1990); "Drinking Habits May Be All In the Family," *Mademoiselle* (August 1990); "Roots of Addiction," *Newsweek* (February 20, 1989); "DNA and the Desire to Drink," *Time* (April 30, 1990); and "Genes With a Don't Drink Label," *U.S. News & World Report* (April 30, 1990).

While there are definite advantages of the disease model, it is not well supported by research. In fact, most of its major hypotheses are disputed by research findings. Critics argue that the model either underemphasizes or ignores the impact of environmental forces, learned behaviors, and many other factors of alcohol abuse. Furthermore, most treatment programs in the United States are based on the disease model, and most are considered to be generally ineffective when judged by their high relapse rates. A detailed, critical evaluation of the disease model can be found in Herbert Fingarette's *Heavy Drinking: The Myth of Alcoholism as a Disease* (University of California Press, 1988).

ISSUE 9

Should Drugs Be Legalized?

YES: Richard J. Dennis, from "The Economics of Legalizing Drugs," *The Atlantic* (November 1990)

NO: James A. Inciardi and Duane C. McBride, from "The Case *Against* Legalization," in James A. Inciardi, ed., *The Drug Legalization Debate* (Sage Publications, 1991)

ISSUE SUMMARY

YES: Richard J. Dennis, chairman of the Advisory Board of the Drug Policy Foundation, believes that the war on drugs has failed to reduce substance abuse or crime and argues that legalizing marijuana and cocaine would reduce the social and economic costs of drug abuse.

NO: Professors James A. Inciardi and Duane C. McBride maintain that the legalization of drugs would cause an increase in crime and produce an even greater number of addicts.

At one time there were no laws regulating the use or sale of drugs or alcohol. Rather than legislation, their use was regulated by religious teaching and social custom. As society grew more complex and more heterogenous, the need for more formal regulation of drug sales, production, and use developed.

Attempts at regulating patent medications through legislation began in the early 1900s. In 1920 Congress, under pressure from temperance organizations, passed an amendment prohibiting the manufacture and sale of all alcoholic beverages. From 1920 until 1933, the demand for alcohol was met by organized crime, who either manufactured it illicitly or smuggled it into the United States. The government's inability to enforce the law and increasing violence finally led to the repeal of Prohibition in 1933.

Many years later, in the 1960s, drug usage again began to worry many Americans. Heroin abuse had become epidemic in urban areas, while many middle-class young adults had begun to experiment with marijuana and LSD by the end of the decade. Cocaine also became popular—first among the middle class; later among inner-city residents. Today, crack houses, babies born with drug addictions, and drug-related crimes and shootings are the images of a new epidemic of drug abuse.

This new epidemic encouraged President Reagan to begin a drug education program in the 1980s, characterized by a "Just Say No" campaign. Later, President Bush declared a "war on drugs" and appointed former education secretary William J. Bennett—who resigned a year later—to the post of "drug czar." While Bennett declared a victory, drug usage continues to be of concern to most Americans. In a 1989 poll, a majority of Americans cited drugs as the nation's greatest threat.

The way to end these drug-related problems, some experts maintain, is to follow the example of the repeal of Prohibition—legalize drugs. Proponents of legalization believe that if laws prohibiting the sale, manufacture, and use of drugs were repealed, there would be a significant reduction in the enormous profits earned by major drug suppliers. This, in turn, would reduce the violent crimes related to drug dealing.

Opponents of drug legalization believe that repealing drug laws is not the answer to crime and other drug-related problems. Drug usage would probably rise, as did the use of alcohol following the repeal of Prohibition; alcohol consumption rose 350 percent after 1933. With more users, there would doubtlessly be an increase in crime, drug-addicted babies, and other social ills.

In the following articles, Richard J. Dennis argues that "safe" drugs, such as marijuana, should be legalized but that laws preventing children from using drugs should be maintained. Dennis believes that the legalization of drugs would reduce crime and corruption while saving society money. James A. Inciardi and Duane C. McBride are opposed to legalizing drugs. They argue that the high cost of illegal drugs restricts their usage and that making them legal would ultimately increase the number of users and, hence, the number of drug-related problems.

YES
Richard J. Dennis

THE ECONOMICS OF LEGALIZING DRUGS

Last year federal agents in southern California broke the six-dollar lock on a warehouse and discovered twenty tons of cocaine. The raid was reported to be the largest seizure of illegal narcotics ever. Politicians and law-enforcement officials heralded it as proof not only of the severity of our drug problem but also of the success of our interdiction efforts, and the need for more of the same. However, in reality the California raid was evidence of nothing but the futility and irrationality of our current approach to illegal drugs. It is questionable whether the raid prevented a single person from buying cocaine. Addicts were not driven to seek treatment. No drug lord or street dealer was put out of business. The event had no perceptible impact on the public's attitude toward drug use. People who wanted cocaine still wanted it—and got it.

If the raid had any effect at all, it was perverse. The street price of cocaine in southern California probably rose temporarily, further enriching the criminal network now terrorizing the nation's inner cities. William Bennett, the director of national drug-control policy, and his fellow moral authoritarians were offered another opportunity to alarm an already overwrought public with a fresh gust of rhetoric. New support was given to a Bush Administration plan that is meant to reduce supply but in fact guarantees more money to foreign drug lords, who will soon become the richest private individuals in history.

Indeed, Americans have grown so hysterical about the drug problem that few public figures dare appear soft on drugs or say anything dispassionate about the situation. In a 1989 poll 54 percent of Americans cited drugs as the nation's greatest threat. Four percent named unemployment. It is time, long past time, to take a clear-eyed look at illegal drugs and ask what government and law enforcement can really be expected to do.

Drug illegality has the same effect as a regressive tax: its chief aim is to save relatively wealthy potential users of drugs like marijuana and cocaine from self-destruction, at tremendous cost to the residents of inner cities. For this reason alone, people interested in policies that help America's poor should embrace drug legalization. It would dethrone drug dealers in the ghettos and release inner-city residents from their status as hostages.

Once the drug war is considered in rational terms, the solution becomes obvious: declare peace. Legalize the stuff. Tax it and regulate its distribution, as liquor is now taxed and regulated. Educate those who will listen. Help those who need help.

Arguments for the benefits of drug legalization have appeared frequently in the press, most of them making the point that crime and other social hazards might be reduced as a result. This article presents an economic analysis of the benefits of legalizing drugs.

SOME WRONG WAYS TO DISCUSS THE DRUG PROBLEM

In order to make any sort of sane argument about drugs, of course, we have to decide what the problem is. That isn't as simple as it might seem, Bennett's thirty-second sound bites notwithstanding. It's easier to say what the drug problem is not.

The drug problem is not a moral issue. There's a streak of puritanism in the national soul, true, but most Americans are not morally opposed to substances that alter one's mind and mood. That issue was resolved in 1933, with the repeal of Prohibition. There is no question that drugs used to excess are harmful; so is alcohol. Americans seem to have no moral difficulty with the notion that adults should be allowed to use alcohol as they see fit, as long as others are not harmed.

The drug problem is not the country's most important health issue. The use of

heroin and cocaine can result in addiction and death; so can the use of alcohol and tobacco. In fact, some researchers estimate the yearly per capita mortality rate of tobacco among smokers at more than a hundred times that of cocaine among cocaine users. If the drug-policy director is worried about the effect on public health of substance abuse, he should spend most of his time talking about cigarettes and whiskey.

The drug problem is not entirely a societal issue—at least not in the sense that it is portrayed as one by politicians and the media. Drug dealing is a chance for people without legitimate opportunity. The problem of the underclass will never be solved by attacking it with force of arms.

So what is the problem? The heart of it is money. What most Americans want is less crime and less profit for inner-city thugs and Colombian drug lords. Less self-destruction by drug users would be nice, but what people increasingly demand is an end to the foreign and domestic terrorism—financed by vast amounts of our own money—associated with the illegal drug trade.

This, as it happens, is a problem that can be solved in quick and pragmatic fashion, by legalizing the sale of most drugs to adults. Virtually overnight crime and corruption would be reduced. The drug cartels would be shattered. Public resources could be diverted to meaningful education and treatment programs.

The alternative—driving up drug prices and increasing public costs with an accelerated drug war—inevitably will fail to solve anything. Instead of making holy war on the drug barons, the President's plan subsidizes them.

Laws protecting children should obviously be retained. Some might question the effectiveness of combining legal drug use by adults with harsh penalties for the sale of drugs to minors. But effective statutory-rape laws demonstrate that society can maintain a distinction between the behavior of adults and that of minors when it truly believes such a distinction is warranted.

Legalization would require us to make some critical distinctions among drugs and drug users, of course. The Administration's plan approaches the drug problem as a seamless whole. But in fact crack and heroin are harmful in ways that marijuana is not. This failure to distinguish among different drugs and their consequences serves only to discredit the anti-drug effort, especially among young people. It also disperses law-enforcement efforts, rendering them hopelessly ineffective. Instead of investing immense resources in a vain attempt to control the behavior of adults, we should put our money where the crisis is. Why spend anything to prosecute marijuana users in a college dormitory when the focus should be on the crack pusher in the Bronx schoolyard?

The appropriate standard in deciding if a drug should be made legal for adults ought to be whether it is more likely than alcohol to cause harm to an innocent party. If not, banning it cannot be justified while alcohol remains legal. For example, a sensible legalization plan would allow users of marijuana to buy it legally. Small dealers could sell it legally but would be regulated, as beer dealers are now in states where beer is sold in grocery stores. Their suppliers would be licensed and regulated. Selling marijuana to minors would be criminal.

Users of cocaine should be able to buy it through centers akin to state liquor stores. It is critical to remove the black-market profit from cocaine in order to destabilize organized crime and impoverish pushers. Selling cocaine to minors would be criminal, as it is now, but infractions could be better policed if effort were concentrated on them. Any black market that might remain would be in sales of crack or sales to minors, transactions that are now estimated to account for 20 percent of drug sales.

Cocaine runs the spectrum from coca leaf to powder to smokable crack; it's the way people take it that makes the difference. Crack's effects on individual behavior and its addictive potential place it in a category apart from other forms of cocaine. The actual degree of harm it does to those who use it is still to be discovered, but for the sake of argument let's assume that it presents a clear danger to people who come in contact with the users. A crack user, therefore, should be subject to a civil fine, and mandatory treatment after multiple violations. Small dealers should have their supplies seized and be subject to moderate punishment for repeat offenses. Major dealers, however, should be subject to the kinds of sentences that are now given. And any adult convicted of selling crack to children should face the harshest prison sentence our criminal-justice system can mete out.

The same rules should apply to any drug that presents a substantial threat to others.

A serious objection to legalizing cocaine while crack remains illegal is that cocaine could be bought, turned into crack, and sold. But those who now buy powder cocaine could take it home and make it into crack, and very few do so. Moreover, legal cocaine would most likely be consumed in different settings and under different circumstances than still-illegal crack would be. Researchers believe that more-benign settings reduce the probability of addiction. Legalization could make it less likely that cocaine users will become crack users. In addition, an effective dose of crack is already so cheap that price is not much of a deterrent to those who want to try it. No price reduction as a result of the legalization of cocaine, then, should lead to a significant increase in the number of crack users.

As for heroin, the advent of methadone clinics shows that society has realized that addicts require maintenance. But there is little practical difference between methadone and heroin, and methadone clinics don't get people off methadone. Heroin addicts should receive what they require, so that they don't have to steal to support their habit. This would make heroin unprofitable for its pushers. And providing addicts with access to uninfected needles would help stop the spread of AIDS and help lure them into treatment programs. . . .

SOME OBJECTIONS CONSIDERED

The fear that legalization would lead to increased drug use and addiction is not, of course, the only basis on which legalization is opposed. We should address other frequently heard objections here.

Crack is our No. 1 drug problem. Legalizing other drugs while crack remains illegal won't solve the problem. Although crack has captured the lion's share of public attention, marijuana has always commanded the bulk of law-enforcement interest. Despite de facto urban decriminalization, more than a third of all drug arrests occur in connection with marijuana—mostly for mere possession. Three fourths of all violations of drug laws

relate to marijuana, and two thirds of all people charged with violation of federal marijuana laws are sentenced to prison (state figures are not available).

Crack appears to account for about 10 percent of the total dollar volume of the drug trade, according to National Institute on Drug Abuse estimates of the number of regular crack users. Legalizing other drugs would free up most of the law-enforcement resources currently focused on less dangerous substances and their users. It's true that as long as crack remains illegal, there will be a black market and associated crime. But we would still reap most of the benefits of legalization outlined above.

Legalization would result in a huge loss in productivity and in higher health-care costs. In truth, productivity lost to drugs is minor compared with productivity lost to alcohol and cigarettes, which remain legal. Hundreds of variables affect a person's job performance, ranging from the consumption of whiskey and cigarettes to obesity and family problems. On a purely statistical level it can be demonstrated that marital status affects productivity, yet we do not allow employers to dismiss workers on the basis of that factor.

If legal drug use resulted in higher social costs, the government could levy a tax on the sale of drugs in some rough proportion to the monetary value of those costs—as it does now for alcohol and cigarettes. This wouldn't provide the government with a financial stake in addiction. Rather, the government would be making sure that users of socially costly items paid those social costs. Funds from the tax on decriminalized drugs could be used for anti-drug advertising, which could be made more effective by a total ban on drug advertising. A government that licenses the sale of drugs must actively educate its citizens about their dangers, as Holland does in discouraging young people from using marijuana.

Drug legalization implies approval. One of the glories of American life is that many things that are not condoned by society at large, such as atheism, offensive speech, and heavy-metal music, are legal. The well-publicized death of Len Bias [a potential professional basketball star who died of a cocaine overdose] and other harrowing stories have carried the message far and wide that drugs are dangerous. In arguing that legalization would persuade people that drug use is safe, drug warriors underestimate our intelligence.

Any restriction on total legalization would lead to continuing, substantial corruption. Under the plan proposed here, restrictions would continue on the sale of crack and on the sale of all drugs to children. Even if black-market corruption continued in those areas, we would experience an immediate 80 percent reduction in corruption overall.

Legalization is too unpredictable and sweeping an action to be undertaken all at once. It would be better to establish several test areas first, and evaluate the results. The results of such a trial would probably not further the case of either side. If use went up in the test area, it could be argued that this was caused by an influx of people from areas where drugs were still illegal; if use went down, it could be argued that the area chosen was unrepresentative.

Even if current drugs are legalized, much more destructive drugs will be developed in the future. The most destructive current drug is crack, which would remain illegal. Many analysts believe that the development of crack was a marketing

strategy, since powder cocaine was too expensive for many users. If cocaine had been legal, crack might never have been marketed. In any case, if a drug presents a clear danger to bystanders, it should not be legal.

No matter how the government distributes drugs, users will continue to seek greater quantities and higher potency on the black market. If the government restricts the amount of a drug that can be distributed legally, legalization will fail. It must make drugs available at all levels of quantity and potency. The government should regulate the distributors but not the product itself. The model should be the distribution of alcohol through state-regulated liquor stores.

Legalizing drugs would ensure that America's inner cities remain places of hopelessness and despair. If drugs disappeared tomorrow from America's ghettos, the ghettos would remain places of hopelessness and despair. But legalization would put most drug dealers out of business and remove the main source of financing for violent gangs. At the least, legalization would spare the inner cities from drug-driven terrorism.

Marijuana in itself may be relatively harmless, but it is a "gateway drug." Legalization would lead its users to more harmful and addictive drugs. While government studies show some correlation between marijuana use and cocaine addiction, they also show that tobacco and alcohol use correlate with drug addiction. Moreover, keeping marijuana illegal forces buyers into an illegal market, where they are likely to be offered other drugs. Finally, 60 million Americans have tried marijuana, and there are one million cocaine addicts. If marijuana is a gateway drug, the gate is narrow.

Legalizing drugs would aggravate the growing problem of "crack babies." The sale of crack would remain illegal. Even so, it is difficult to believe that anyone ignorant or desperate enough to use crack while pregnant would be deterred by a law. Laws against drug use are more likely to deter users from seeking treatment. Crack babies probably would have a better chance in a less censorious environment, in which their mothers had less to fear from seeking treatment.

Drug use in the United States can be seen as a symptom of recent cultural changes that have led to an erosion of traditional values and an inability to replace them. There are those who are willing to pay the price to try to save people from themselves. But there are surely just as many who would pay to preserve a person's right to be wrong. To the pragmatist, the choice is clear: legalization is the best bet.

NO

James A. Inciardi and
Duane C. McBride

THE CASE *AGAINST* LEGALIZATION

Ever since the passage of the Harrison Act in 1914, American drug policy has had its critics. The basis of the negative assessments has been the restrictive laws designed to control the possession and distribution of narcotics and other "dangerous drugs," the mechanisms of drug law enforcement and the apparent lack of success in reducing both the *supply of* and the *demand for* illicit drugs.

. . . [C]oncerns over the perceived failure of American drug policy spirited a national debate over whether contemporary drug control approaches ought to be abandoned, and replaced with the decriminalization, if not the outright legalization, of most or all illicit drugs. . . .

The arguments posed by the supporters of legalization seem all too logical. *First*, they argue, the drug laws have created evils far worse than the drugs themselves—corruption, violence, street crime, and disrespect for the law. *Second*, legislation passed to control drugs has failed to reduce demand. *Third*, you cannot have illegal that which a significant segment of the population in any society is committed to doing. You simply cannot arrest, prosecute, and punish such large numbers of people, particularly in a democracy. And specifically in this behalf, in a liberal democracy, the government must not interfere with personal behavior if liberty is to be maintained. And *fourth*, they add, if marijuana, cocaine, heroin, and other drugs were legalized, a number of very positive things would happen:

1. drug prices would fall

2. users could obtain their drugs at low, government-regulated prices and would no longer be financially forced to engage in prostitution and street crime to support their habits

3. the fact that the levels of drug-related crime would significantly decline would result in less crowded courts, jails, and prisons, and would free law enforcement personnel to focus their energies on the "real criminals" in society

From James A. Inciardi and Duane C. McBride, "The Case *Against* Legalization," in James A. Inciardi, ed., *The Drug Legalization Debate* (Sage Publications, 1991). Copyright © 1991 by Sage Publications, Inc. Reprinted by permission. Notes and references omitted.

4. drug production, distribution, and sale would be removed from the criminal arena; no longer would it be within the province of organized crime, and therefore, such criminal syndicates as the Medellín Cartel and the Jamaican posses would be decapitalized, and the violence associated with drug distribution rivalries would be eliminated

5. government corruption and intimidation by traffickers as well as drug-based foreign policies would be effectively reduced, if not eliminated entirely

6. the often draconian measures undertaken by police to enforce the drug laws would be curtailed, thus restoring to the American public many of its hard-won liberties

To these contentions can be added the argument that legalization in any form or structure would have only a minimal impact on current drug-use levels. Apparently, there is the assumption that given the existing levels of access to most illegal drugs, current levels of use closely match demand. Thus there would be no additional health, safety, behavioral, and/or other problems accompanying legalization. And, finally, a few protagonists of legalization make one concluding point. Through government regulation of drugs, the billions of dollars spent annually on drug enforcement could be better utilized. Moreover, by taxing government-regulated drugs, revenues would be collected that could be used for preventing drug abuse and treating those harmed by drugs.

The argument for legalization seems to boil down to the basic belief that America's prohibitions against marijuana, cocaine, heroin, and other drugs impose far too large a cost in terms of tax dollars, crime, and infringements on civil rights and individual liberties. And while the overall argument may be well intended and appear quite logical, it is highly questionable in its historical, sociocultural, and empirical underpinnings and demonstrably naive in its understanding of the negative consequences of a legalized drug market.

Within the context of these opening remarks, what follows is an analysis of the content of legalization proposals combined with a discussion of the more likely consequences of such a drastic alteration in drug policy. . . .

Considerable evidence exists to suggest that the legalization of drugs would create behavioral and public health problems to a degree that would far outweigh the current consequences of the drug prohibition. There are some excellent reasons why marijuana, cocaine, heroin, and other drugs are now controlled, and why they ought to remain so. What follows is a brief look at a few of these drugs.

Marijuana. There is considerable misinformation about marijuana. To the millions of adolescents and young adults who were introduced to the drug during the social revolution of the 1960s and early 1970s, marijuana was a harmless herb of ecstasy. As the "new social drug" and a "natural organic product," it was deemed to be far less harmful than either alcohol or tobacco. More recent research suggests, however, that marijuana smoking is a practice that combines the hazardous features of both tobacco and alcohol with a number of pitfalls of its own. Moreover, there are many disturbing questions about marijuana's effect on the vital systems of the body, on the brain and mind, on immunity and resistance, and on sex and reproduction.

One of the more serious difficulties with marijuana use relates to lung damage. The most recent findings in this behalf should put to rest the rather tiresome argument by marijuana devotees that smoking just a few "joints" daily is less harmful than regularly smoking several times as many cigarettes. Researchers at the University of California at Los Angeles reported early in 1988 that the respiratory burden in smoke particulates and absorption of carbon monoxide from smoking just one marijuana joint is some four times greater than from smoking a single tobacco cigarette. Specifically, it was found that one "toke" of marijuana delivers three times more tar to the mouth and lungs than one puff of a filter-tipped cigarette; that marijuana deposits four times more tar in the throat and lungs and increases carbon monoxide levels in the blood fourfold to fivefold. . . .

Cocaine. Lured by the Lorelei of orgasmic pleasure, millions of Americans use cocaine each year—a snort in each nostril and the user is up and away for 20 minutes or so. Alert, witty, and with it, the user has no hangover, no lung cancer, and no holes in the arms or burned-out cells in the brain. The cocaine high is an immediate, intensively vivid, and sensation-enhancing experience. Moreover, it has the reputation for being a spectacular aphrodisiac: It is believed to create sexual desire, to heighten it, to increase sexual endurance, and to cure frigidity and impotence.

Given all these positives, it is no wonder that cocaine has become an "all-American drug" and a multibillion-dollar-a-year industry. It permeates all levels of society, from Park Avenue to the ghetto: Lawyers and executives use cocaine; baby boomers and yuppies use cocaine; college students and high school drop-outs use cocaine; police officers, prosecutors, and prisoners use cocaine; politicians use cocaine; housewives and pensioners use cocaine; Democrats, Republicans, Independents, and Socialists use cocaine; barmaids and stockbrokers and children and athletes use cocaine; even some priests and members of Congress use cocaine.

Yet the pleasure and feelings of power that cocaine engenders make its use a rather unwise recreational pursuit. In very small and occasional doses it is no more harmful than equally moderate doses of alcohol, but there is a side to cocaine that can be very destructive. That euphoric lift, with its feelings of pleasure, confidence, and being on top of things, that comes from but a few brief snorts is short-lived and invariably followed by a letdown. More specifically, when the elation and grandiose feelings begin to wane, a corresponding deep depression is often felt, which is in such marked contrast to users' previous states that they are strongly motivated to repeat the dose and restore the euphoria. This leads to chronic, compulsive use. And when chronic users try to stop using cocaine, they are typically plunged into a severe depression from which only more cocaine can arouse them. Most clinicians estimate that approximately 10% of those who begin to use cocaine "recreationally" will go on to serious, heavy, chronic, compulsive use. To this can be added what is known as the "cocaine psychosis." As dose and duration of cocaine use increase, the development of cocaine-related psychopathology is not uncommon. Cocaine psychosis is generally preceded by a transitional period characterized by increased suspiciousness, compulsive behavior, fault finding, and eventually paranoia. When the psychotic state is reached, individuals may experience visual and/or auditory hallucinations, with persecutory voices commonly heard. Many believe that they are being followed by police, or that family, friends, and others are plotting against them. Moreover, everyday events tend to be misinterpreted in ways that support delusional beliefs. When coupled with the irritability and hyperactivity that the stimulant nature of cocaine tends to generate in almost all of its users, the cocaine-induced paranoia may lead to violent behavior as a means of "self-defense" against imagined persecutors.

Not to be forgotten are the physiological consequences of cocaine use. Since the drug is an extremely potent central nervous system stimulant, its physical effects include increased temperature, heart rate, and blood pressure. In addition to the many thousands of cocaine-related hospital emergency visits that occur each year, there has been a steady increase in the annual number of cocaine-induced deaths in the United States, from only 53 in 1976 to almost 1,000 a decade later. And while these numbers may seem infinitesimal when compared with the magnitude of alcohol- and tobacco-related deaths, it should be remembered that at present only a small segment of the American population uses cocaine.

Crack. Given the considerable media attention that crack has received since the summer of 1986, it would appear that only a minimal description of the drug is warranted here. Briefly, *crack*-cocaine is likely best described as a "fast-food" variety of cocaine. It is a pebble-sized crystalline form of cocaine base, and has become extremely popular because it is inexpensive and easy to produce. Moreover, since crack is smoked rather than snorted, it is more rapidly absorbed than cocaine—reportedly crossing the blood-brain barrier within six seconds—creating an almost instantaneous high.

Crack's low price (as little as $3 per rock in some locales) has made it an attractive drug of abuse for those with limited funds, particularly adolescents. Its rapid absorption initiates a faster onset of dependence than is typical with cocaine, resulting in higher rates of addiction, binge use, and psychoses. The consequences include higher levels of cocaine-related violence and all the same manifestations of personal, familial, and occupational neglect that are associated with other forms of drug dependence.

Heroin. A derivative of morphine, heroin is a highly addictive narcotic, and the drug historically most associated with both addiction and street crime. Although heroin overdose is not uncommon, unlike alcohol, cocaine, tobacco, and many prescription drugs, the direct physiological damage caused by heroin use tends to be minimal. And it is for this reason that the protagonists of drug legalization include heroin in their arguments. By making heroin readily available to users, they argue, many problems could be sharply reduced if not totally eliminated, including the crime associated with supporting a heroin habit; the overdoses resulting from problematic levels of heroin purity and potency; the HIV (human immunodeficiency virus) and hepatitis infections brought about by needle-sharing; and the personal, social, and occupational dislocations resulting from the drug-induced criminal life-style.

The belief that the legalization of heroin would eliminate crime, overdose, infections, and life dislocations is for the most part delusional, for it is likely that the heroin use life-style would change little for most American addicts, regardless of the legal status of the drug. And there is ample evidence to support this argument—in the biographies and autobiographies of narcotics addicts and in the treatment literature. And to this can be added the many thousands of conversations conducted by the authors with heroin users during the past two decades.

The point is this: Heroin is a highly addicting drug. For the addict, it becomes life consuming: It becomes mother, father, spouse, lover, counselor, confidant, and confessor. Because heroin is a short-acting drug, with its effects lasting at best four to six hours, it must be taken regularly and repeatedly. Because there is a more rapid onset when taken intravenously, most heroin users inject the drug. Because heroin has a depressant effect, a portion of the user's day is spent in a semistupefied state. Collectively, these attributes result in a user more concerned with drug-taking than health, family, work, or anything else. . . .

For the better part of the current century there has been a concerted belief in what has become known as the "enslavement theory of addiction"—the conviction that because of the high prices of heroin and cocaine on the drug black market, users are forced to commit crimes in order to support their drug habits. In this regard, supporters of drug legalization argue that if the criminal penalties attached to heroin and cocaine possession and sale were removed, three things would occur: The black market would disappear, the prices of heroin and cocaine would decline significantly, and users would no longer have to engage in street crime in order to support their desired levels of drug intake. Yet there has never been any solid empirical

evidence to support the contentions of this enslavement theory.

From the 1920s through the close of the 1960s, hundreds of studies of the relationship between crime and addiction were conducted. Invariably, when one analysis would support enslavement theory the next would affirm the view that addicts were criminals first, and that their drug use was but one more manifestation of their deviant life-styles. In retrospect, the difficulty lay in the way the studies had been conducted, with biases and deficiencies in research designs that rendered their findings to be of little value.

Research since the middle of the 1970s with active drug users in the streets of New York, Miami, Baltimore, and elsewhere, on the other hand, has demonstrated that enslavement theory has little basis in reality, and that the contentions of the legalization proponents in this behalf are mistaken. All of these studies of the criminal careers of heroin and other drug users have convincingly documented that while drug use tends to intensify and perpetuate criminal behavior, it usually does not initiate criminal careers. In fact, the evidence suggests that among the majority of street drug users who are involved in crime, their criminal careers were well established prior to the onset of either narcotics or cocaine use. . . .

There seem to be three models of drug-related violence—the psychopharmacologic, the economically compulsive, and the systemic. The *psychopharmacological model of violence* suggests that some individuals, as the result of short-term or long-term ingestion of specific substances, may become excitable, irrational, and exhibit violent behavior. The paranoia and aggression associated with the cocaine psychosis fit into the psychopharmacological model, as does most alcohol-related violence.

The *economically compulsive model of violence* holds that some drug users engage in economically oriented violent crime to support drug use. This model is illustrated in the many studies of drug use and criminal behavior that have demonstrated that while drug sales, property crimes, and prostitution are the primary economic offenses committed by users, armed robberies and muggings do indeed occur. The *systemic model of violence* maintains that violent crime is intrinsic to the very involvement with illicit substances. As such, systemic violence refers to the traditionally aggressive patterns of interaction within systems of illegal drug trafficking and distribution.

It is the systemic violence associated with trafficking in crack in the inner cities that has brought the most attention to drug-related violence in recent years. Moreover, it is concerns with this same violence that focused the recent interest on the possibility of legalizing drugs. And it is certainly logical to assume that if heroin, cocaine, and marijuana were *legal* substances, systemic drug-related violence would indeed decline significantly. But, too, there are some very troubling considerations. *First*, to achieve the desired declines in systemic violence, it would require that crack be legalized as well. For after all, it is in the crack distribution system that much of the drug-related violence is occurring. *Second*, it is already clear that there is considerable psychopharmacologic violence associated with the cocaine psychosis. Moreover, research has demonstrated that there is far more psychopharmacologic violence connected with heroin use than is generally believed. Given that drug use would

certainly increase with legalization, in all likelihood *any declines in systemic violence would be accompanied by corresponding increases in psychopharmacologic violence.* The United States already pays a high price for alcohol-related violence, a phenomenon well documented by recent research. Why compound the problem with the legalization of additional violence-producing substances? . . .

A timeless feature of cities has been concentrated poverty. Concentrations of poverty appear in all metropolitan areas and are greatest in inner cities. Moreover, poverty in American cities tends to be more concentrated among the members of minority groups than among whites. As such, minority group membership and living in the ghetto tend to go hand-in-hand across the American urban landscape. Numerous explanations for this situation have been offered: that cities tend to attract the poor, many of whom cannot or will not help themselves and, therefore, create and sustain the conditions of their own degradation; that in great part many of the poor adapt to their impoverished conditions by creating a set of attitudes and behaviors that tend to perpetuate poverty—the so-called "culture of poverty" thesis; that the cause of poverty is not with the poor but with the systemic limitation of opportunity imposed by the wider society; that attempts by the urban poor to improve their economic power are hindered by "ghetto colonialization"—the ownership of ghetto businesses by persons from outside the ghetto; and that the wider society encourages the persistence of poverty because it has positive functions, providing (a) an underclass to do the "dirty work" of society, (b) a pool of low-wage laborers, (c) a place where less qualified members of the professions can practice, (d) a population that can be exploited by businesses and served by social agencies, and (e) a reference point to justify the norms and behavior patterns of the wider society. And there are other reasons for urban poverty and its persistence that have been put forth. Whatever the reasons, it seems to be generally agreed that part of the problem lies in the wider society—that the American social structure has economically disenfranchised significant portions of its urban inner cities.

Urban ghettos are not particularly pleasant places in which to live. There are vice, crime, and littered streets. There is the desolation of people separated culturally, socially, and politically from the mainstream. There are the disadvantages of a tangle of economic, family, and other problems—delinquency, teenage pregnancy, unemployment, child neglect, poor housing, substandard schools, inadequate health care, and limited opportunities. There are many modes of adaptation to ghetto life. A common one is drug use, perhaps the main cause of the higher drug use rates in inner cities. And it is for this reason that the legalization of drugs would be a nightmare.

The social fabric of the ghetto is already tattered, and drugs are further shredding what is left of the fragile ghetto family. A great number of inner-city families are headed by women, and for reasons that are not all that clear, women seem to be more disposed to become dependent on crack than men. In New York City since 1986, this led to a 225% increase in child neglect and abuse cases involving drugs, and a dramatic rise in the number of infants abandoned in city hospitals and those born addicted or with syphilis, as well as a surge in children beaten or killed by drug-addicted parents.

Within this context, the legalization of drugs would be an elitist and racist policy supporting the neocolonialist views of underclass population control. In a large sense, since legalization would increase the levels of drug dependence in the ghetto, it represents a program of social management and control that would serve to legitimate the chemical destruction of an urban generation and culture. . . .

If not legalization in the light of a problematic "war" on drugs, what then?

It is eminently sensible to strengthen the supply-side programs aimed at keeping heroin, cocaine, marijuana, and other illegal drugs out of the country. However, the emphasis of federal policy has been a bit lopsided. Between 1981 and the passage of the Anti-Drug Abuse Act of 1986, federal funding for drug treatment was cut by 40%. The results included sharp reductions in the available number of treatment slots, overcrowded treatment centers, and the turning away of tens of thousands of drug abusers seeking help. Then, of the $1.7 billion authorized by the 1986 legislation, almost 80% was earmarked for enforcement efforts. Moreover, much of the $363 million Congress targeted for state education and treatment programs became bogged down by the red tape of an entrenched bureaucratic process.

The difficulty lies in the fact that allocating resources for warring on drugs is always more of a political rather than a commonsense process. Arrests and seizures are easy to count, making for attractive press releases and useful political fodder. And in recent years the figures were indeed dramatic. Reporting on the number of persons in treatment is far less impressive to a constituency. But the tragedy of it all is that the waiting time for treatment entry in some cities is up to a year.

In the final analysis, drug abuse is a complicated and intractable problem that cannot be solved with quick-fix approaches tended to by politically appointed boards. Deploying more patrol boats in the Caribbean or diverting additional high-technology military hardware will not guarantee an end to or even a slowing of the war. Intercepting drugs at the borders or cutting off illegal drugs at their sources are praiseworthy goals, but they are likely impossible ones. And pressuring source countries into compliance with U.S. objectives is also an elusive task, even when there is willingness.

Thus, if total elimination of the supply of drugs is impossible, then more attention must be focused on the demand side of the equation. For after all, without drug users there would be no drug problem. The weapons here are treatment and education, initiatives that seem to be both working and failing—working for some but failing for others.

On the treatment side, many drug users seeking help are unable to find it, for . . . treatment resources fail to match the demand. This problem is easily solved by a financial restructuring of the war on drugs. For the many thousands of users in need of help but unwilling to enter treatment programs, compulsory treatment may be in order.

On the education side, it is already clear that American youths are beginning to turn away from drugs. Moreover, surveys by the University of Michigan's Institute for Social Research suggest that this trend will continue. But all of these positive indicators relate only to mainstream American teenagers. Crack-cocaine is now tragically abundant in inner-city neighborhoods throughout the country.

The antidrug messages from government, schools, parent groups, sports figures, and the entertainment media are either not reaching, or have little meaning to, ghetto youth. Like the situation with treatment, the bottom line involves a restructuring of ideas, resources, and goals.

POSTSCRIPT

Should Drugs Be Legalized?

Prohibition is generally considered to have been a failure in curbing alcohol use, and today, many see the current drug laws as being similarly ineffective in halting the work of drug dealers or diminishing the number of drug users. But the debate continues over whether or not drugs should be legalized: If drugs were legal, dealers would be out of business, thus reducing drug-related crime. Legalization would not, however, necessarily reduce the usage or abuse of drugs. An overview of the debate can be found in *The Drug Legalization Debate*, by James A. Inciardi (Sage Publications, 1991).

A third route, decriminalization, is another option. Certain less dangerous drugs, such as marijuana, would be neither strictly legal nor illegal. There would be no penalty for personal use or possession, although there would continue to be criminal penalties for sale for profit and distribution to minors.

This third category appeals to journalist Robert Hough, who argues that marijuana should be decriminalized in "Reefer Sadness," *Toronto Globe and Mail* (November 9, 1991). This view is shared by D. Keith Mano who, in *National Review* (May 14, 1990), describes how he illegally supplied his dying mother with marijuana in order for her to overcome the side effects of cancer therapy. Mano argues that marijuana has genuine medicinal purposes and is, as a recreational drug, considerably less harmful than alcohol. Brian Hecht, in "Out of Joint," *The New Republic* (July 15, 1991), asserts that marijuana should be legalized for medicinal purposes. Hecht, responding to the announcement that the Public Health Service was phasing out its program of allowing seriously ill patients to smoke marijuana, claims that the reason has little to do with the effectiveness of marijuana; rather, the health service was responding to the mania surrounding illegal drugs.

In early 1992, the Drug Enforcement Administration published a document claiming that the government was justified in its continued prohibition of marijuana for medicinal purposes. The report indicated that too many questions surrounded the effectiveness of medicinal marijuana. See "Agency Says Marijuana Is Not Proven Medicine," *The New York Times* (March 19, 1992).

While the effectiveness of marijuana as therapy for cancer and AIDS patients continues to be debated, Brad Miner maintains that recent research on marijuana indicates that the drug is addictive and can wreck the lives of users, particularly teenagers. Miner argues that legalizing marijuana would undermine the forces of drug education and increase usage in "How Sweet Is Mary Jane?" *National Review* (July 7, 1991).

Additional views of the drug legalization issue can be found among the following selections: "Drug Laws Are Immoral," *U.S. Catholic* (May 1990); "How to Win the War on Drugs," *The New Republic* (May 21, 1990); "Has the Time Come to Legalize Drugs?" *USA Today* (July 1990); "Biting the Bullet: The Case for Legalizing Drugs," *The Christian Century* (August 8/15, 1990); and "Off the Pot," *The New Republic* (December 3, 1990).

There appear to be many different sides to the drug legalization debate. In many ways, the drug issues of the 1990s are similar to the alcohol problems of the 1920s. It remains to be seen if legalizing illegal drugs can eliminate drug-related violence and crime as well as reduce the number of users.

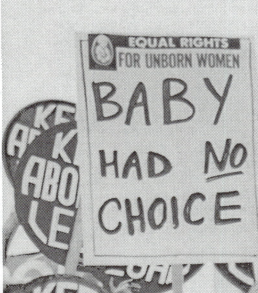

EQUAL RIGHTS
FOR UNBORN WOMEN
BABY
HAD NO
CHOICE

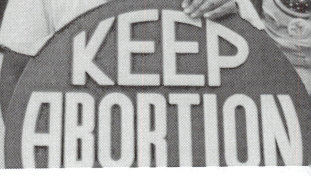

KEEP
ABORTION

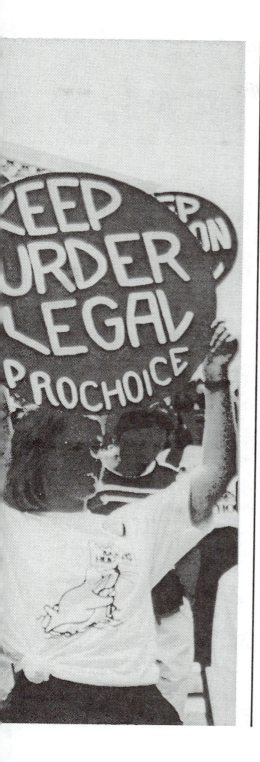

PART 4

Sexuality and Reproductive Issues

Few issues could promote greater controversy than those concerning sexuality and reproduction. Recent generations of Americans have thrown out "traditional" sexual values, which has resulted in a significant increase in the number of babies born out of wedlock, the spread of sexually transmitted diseases, and the decriminalization and proliferation of abortion. This section debates the role of sex education in the classroom and the morality of abortion.

Does Sex Education Prevent Teen Pregnancy?

Can Abortion Be a Morally Acceptable Choice?

ISSUE 10

Does Sex Education Prevent Teen Pregnancy?

YES: Michael A. Carrera and Patricia Dempsey, from "Restructuring Public Policy Priorities on Teen Pregnancy: A Holistic Approach to Teen Development and Teen Services," *SIECUS Report* (January/February 1988)

NO: Sarah Glazer, from "Sex Education: How Well Does It Work?" *Editorial Research Reports* (June 1989)

ISSUE SUMMARY

YES: Professors Michael A. Carrera and Patricia Dempsey discuss the success of sex education programs characterized by multiple intervention strategies, which they feel have decreased teenage pregnancy rates.
NO: Author Sarah Glazer argues that in the United States, sex education does not prevent teenage pregnancy, reduce teenage sexual activity, or increase the use of contraceptives.

Although many American schools teach sex education, controversy about it continues. Some parents and educators believe that in the age of AIDS and spiraling teenage pregnancy rates, there should be more, not less, sex education in the schools, taught at an earlier age. This view, however, is not shared by everyone. Opponents believe that sex education is harmful, not beneficial, to teenagers and that it actually encourages sexual experimentation, which leads to pregnancy.

Abstinence is an important goal of most sex education programs in the United States. Abstinence, it is felt, is the most effective way to prevent pregnancy and sexually transmitted diseases. Many teachers say they try to help students avoid sexual relations by providing techniques on how to resist peer pressure and how to say no to boyfriends and girlfriends. Although abstinence may be stressed, students are taught about contraception, which comes across as a mixed message. Does sex education actually work? Does it prevent teenage pregnancies and reduce sexual activity among teenagers?

While sex education, as currently taught, may not show proven results, Michael A. Carrera and Patricia Dempsey believe that a comprehensive program that includes sex education as well as well as health services and job counseling can significantly reduce teenage pregnancy in the United States. Schools can play an important role in giving adolescents the needed capacity to delay pregnancy through a combination of services. Sex education, taught along with family life, can be a part of these services. Examples of other countries have shown that those with the most extensive sex education and most accessible contraceptive services have the lowest rates of teenage pregnancy, abortion, and childbearing.

Sarah Glazer, in opposition, asserts that the available evidence indicates that school-based sex education has little or no effect on contraceptive usage, teenage pregnancy rates, or sexual activity. Part of the reason, she writes, is that sex education in many schools is based on a curriculum that attempts to offend no one and results in a stripped-down version of what should be taught. Glazer makes an example of educator Mary Lee Tatum, whose philosophy is that sex education should focus on the view that sexuality is part of who we are rather than merely an act we do. While there is considerable disagreement over what should be taught—abstinence, values, contraceptive usage, or morality—almost everyone seems to agree that the risks of AIDS and the high rate of teenage pregnancy (the United States has the highest teenage pregnancy rate of any developed nation) indicate that there is a problem that requires attention.

YES

Michael A. Carrera and Patricia Dempsey

RESTRUCTURING PUBLIC POLICY PRIORITIES ON TEEN PREGNANCY: A HOLISTIC APPROACH TO TEEN DEVELOPMENT AND TEEN SERVICES

THE FACTS

Each year, more than one million American teenagers become pregnant, the overwhelming majority unintentionally; 44% of these pregnancies result in births. Half of these births are to young women who have dropped out of school and have not yet reached their eighteenth birthdays; 50% are to young women who are not married. Young mothers are at an enormous risk of pregnancy complications and poor birth outcomes, and their infants face greater health and development risks. Teen males, even those who want to be involved, are often forgotten, excused, or written off, and teen marriages, which often compound the problem, are characterized by long-term welfare dependency and family instability.[1] Teenage parents are more likely than those who delay childbearing to experience chronic unemployment, inadequate income, and reduced educational experiences.

Teen pregnancy is a major factor in, and a contributor to, family poverty. One out of every five children are poor; one out of two children is in a female-headed household.[2] The emotional toll on teen parents is staggering, as is society's economic burden in sustaining them.[3]

SOME OF THE PROBLEMS WITH PRESENT APPROACHES TO TEEN PREGNANCY PREVENTION

In the face of such a daunting social problem, and with the knowledge that help must be given to our next generation of adults if they are to get off to a stable and healthy start, a number of individuals, agencies, and institutions have accepted the challenge to get involved with enthusiasm and resolve. However, it is our belief that the programs they have established, thus far, have promised too much, too quickly— and have spoken too prematurely about results. Although there have been *some* successful single intervention issue efforts that have addressed *some* of the problems of teen pregnancy, we have not yet begun to win the real war. There are no quick fix solutions, no single intervention programs, no slick "button" phrases which *by themselves* can reduce the haunting, unacceptable statistics and their impact—in human terms—on the lives of so many young people.

Because of this, we have repeatedly emphasized, in working with school family life and sex education. teachers and administrators, how important it is for them to understand the limits as well as the potential of their educational enterprises: *by themselves, programs of family life and sex education, in the schools and in agencies, also will not reduce unintended pregnancies among teens.* Family life and sex education programs are intrinsically worthwhile because of what they can offer young people in the cognitive and affective learning domains. Their educational desirability should be based on this. Family life and sex education programs should not, however, be seen as a panacea for the teen pregnancy problem.

It is also important to point out that it is only recently that government, program developers, and academics have begun to acknowledge that teen pregnancy is neither a moral problem nor a minority female problem. This acknowledgement should prove helpful in expediting future policymaking and program development that might have a realistic impact on present problems.

THE HOLISTIC APPROACH

It is our belief that the teen pregnancy problem is largely a symptomatic response to greater social ills and, because of this, it must concurrently be attacked on several levels. For example, unintended pregnancies among poor, urban teens can be more effectively curtailed if we reduce the impact of the institutional racism that is systemic in our society; if we provide quality education for everyone; and if we create more employment opportunities for young people and adults. If we could accomplish this, we would probably impact, in a more meaningful way, on the lives of teens than can any school or agency sexuality program.

We must also face another reality. In addition to educating young people, we must try to produce within them a desire to avoid unintended pregnancy and the ability to make responsible sexual decisions. At the same time, we must offer them the resources and opportunities that will provide them with a sense of the future and reasons not to become pregnant *at this time in their development.*

It is possible to convince teens to forego early pregnancy and childbearing if they have a more hopeful sense of their future. When more hopeful, they, in general, value and have a more positive sense of themselves. They develop appropriate coping skills; become more active and less passive; have more opportunities open up for them; and are more willing to communicate with a concerned adult about their sexuality.

Unfortunately however, many urban teen males and females today do not see any future for themselves: they live in poor communities; they see little employment opportunities; and have little, if any, reason to believe that they will fare as well as, let alone better than, their parents. Facing these conditions coupled with family problems, fragmentation, and inadequate opportunities for meaningful education, it is completely understandable that some young people become sexually intimate and fatalistic instead of industrious and hopeful. In New York state, Governor [Mario M.] Cuomo's adolescent pregnancy prevention initiative has shown some recognition of the complexities of these issues. (Our Teen Pregnancy Primary Prevention Program is funded under Governor Cuomo's Adolescent Pregnancy Prevention Program, through private funds, and by The Children's Aid Society [CAS].) He—and other state leaders—have stated that the rates of teen pregnancy and childbearing should be reduced through programmatic intervention that reflects an integrated, holistic approach. We have suggested, and they also agree, *that adolescence is not the best time to deal with adolescent sexuality, pregnancy, and childbearing. These should be addressed during the formative and development stages prior to the second decade of life.*

We would again like to emphasize, here, that as we begin to move in the direction of a more holistic approach we must make sure that our comprehensive programs are not short term attempts to contain the numbers of teen pregnancies. Rather, they should genuinely seek to address the root causes—political, social, and economic inequities—that contribute to our present problems.

In addressing these root causes, we must also fully address the issue of *quality of life* prevention and service programs. Primary prevention, that is, programs for young people who have not had a child in their early years, should be recognized as a separate strategy for

delaying unintended pregnancies. At the same time, while we rework service, health, and educational programs, we must work to increase the level of quality of life supports for young people and families, who continue to need services. This requires local and national commitments to overall restructuring of public policy priorities, and not simply grant allocations which reflect political expediency or value judgments about the client population. As fashionable as it is these days, political rhetoric is not a substitute for real problem-solving.

ONE SOLUTION: THE TEEN PREGNANCY PRIMARY PREVENTION PROGRAM OF THE CHILDREN'S AID SOCIETY

The Children's Aid Society's Teen Pregnancy Primary Prevention Program has been developed to create a holistic climate in which positive change can occur. To the best of our knowledge, taken altogether, a holistic program such as this—which has been established to serve the west, central, and east Harlem areas of the city of New York—has thus far not been replicated anywhere else in the country.

Our programmatic philosophy is based on the belief that, in order to create a climate where positive change can occur and where direction can be given to young people, it is necessary to influence multiple facets of their lives over a continuous period of time. This holistic type of approach represents a very complex intervention strategy.

Believing that such a comprehensive, quality of life, holistic approach can affect the life options that we seek for young people—even those who live within family systems which have experienced generations of economic deprivation—we have designed our program components to operate concurrently and sometimes simultaneously. These program components center on working with, and affecting, a young person individually, as well as within his or her family and community systems.

The programmatic vision of our Teen Primary Prevention Program is based on several organizing principles. We believe that young people are capable of more than simply avoiding problems and situations which will complicate their lives. We believe that they are capable of "doing good" for themselves, their family, and their community. Our staff's attitudes and behavior sustain this notion and encourage young people to realize their potential for such achievements. This belief affects our entire program.

We believe that parents, grandparents, foster parents, and other adults in the community are significant influences on the sexual development of young people. Their roles, therefore, should be respected and should be included in holistic, quality-of-life programs—and in meaningful ways.

We believe that people should delay having intercourse, for as long as possible, because intercourse is the kind of special intimacy that best fits a relationship later in life. However, we are mindful that intercourse for some teens is a way of coping with their feelings of poor self-image, fatalism, and unhappiness. Therefore, we are prepared to replace this coping mechanism with options, possibilities, and experiences which are meaningful, which will make sense, and which will also be useful to them at this time in their development.

We are also aware that young people do not always listen to the guidance of adults and may begin to have intercourse—even in their preteen and early teen years. In these situations, our role is to care, to understand, and to try to help them function in a way that will prevent pregnancy. We do not turn our backs or withhold affection as forms of disapproval. Rather, we are present in an ongoing way to provide guidance and on-site contraceptive services, when necessary, so that unintended pregnancy does not occur.

We have discovered, during the first 36 months of our work, that this type of honest and supportive limit-setting approach is appreciated by young people. It helps them to clarify their thoughts and actions much more than the threat-and-fear-arousing communications that have so frequently characterized the way many adults have chosen to relate with young people.

Our pregnancy prevention efforts are addressed equally to both males and females. Our attitude is that males must also be reached, educated, and positively influenced concerning their roles and responsibilities in relationships. To just teach women to say no continues a sexist double standard. Teaching young men "not to ask" gives our approach balance and also provides them with an important learning opportunity.

THE COMPONENTS OF OUR PROGRAM

The components of our program cover such areas as family life and sex education; physical and mental health services; self-esteem enhancement through the performing arts; lifetime sports; academic assessment and homework-help; job and career awareness; and college admission.

Family Life and Sex Education Program. This is a formal 15-week, two-hours-per-week educational experience for teens and for parents led by the authors, who have been certified by the American Association of Sex Educators, Counselors and Therapists. The program centers on an understanding of sexuality from a holistic viewpoint. While there is discussion of sexual anatomy, reproduction, and contraception, more emphasis is placed on exploring such issues as gender roles, family roles, body images, and patterns of affection, love, and intimacy. Roles, responsibilities, and values in relationships are emphasized. Since increasing the sexual literacy of both young people and the adults in their lives is our goal, we have also included readings, films, role-playing, and lectures for both.

Medical and Health Services are provided four hours each week by the center nurse and by adolescent medicine specialists from Montefiore Hospital in the Bronx and Mt. Sinai Hospital in Manhattan. Every teen has a complete annual physical (and every female a yearly GYN examination), preceded by a thorough social and family health inventory. This becomes a valuable part of each teen's health history.

When necessary, physicians provide confidential contraception counseling and prescription. Each youngster—male and female—who is using a contraceptive has a weekly meeting with a counselor to make sure that the contraceptive is being used regularly and properly. During these sessions, school, family, peer, and employment issues are also explored.

The young people in the program are urged to view the physicians as "their doctors." They can see the doctors and the nurse without an apppointment and can discuss any health or related areas with them.

Mental Health Services. While working with young people and their families on education, health, employment, and support services, we frequently discover, or are told about, interpersonal problems, family discord, and other crises that are affecting their functioning. Often it is the presence of these problems that cause them to act impulsively, and/or to experience repeated failures in school, work, and peer relationships.

Professional social work services and counseling are offered, three days per week, by certified social workers. Because of the "family" quality of this program, referrals are usually made on an informal basis and frequently teens or their family will self-refer.

Clinical assessments are prepared on each individual who is seen for ongoing counseling and the more complex cases are referred to The Children's Aid Society's mental health unit.

Self-Esteem Enhancement Through the Performing Arts. This ongoing self-expression program, taught by professional actors and actresses from the National Black Theatre, is offered to both parents and teens. In weekly two-hour workshops, parents and teens explore issues, through music, dance, role-play, and dramatization which range from conflict resolution—in school and at home—to how to present oneself for a job interview. The sessions also offer a forum for discussing gender roles, family roles, affection, intimacy, culture, values, and racism. This medium enables the youngsters and adults to experiment with various scenarios and conclusions, and allows them to see themselves and their peers from new perspectives. In addition, these workshops provide opportunities for reflection, feedback, recognition, and applause.

Lifetime Individual Sports. In this unusual program component, young people learn skills in lifetime sports such as squash, tennis, golf, and swimming. From a skills development standpoint, these activities are all "unforgiving sports" which require precise mastery and the exercise of self-discipline and self-control. We believe that the skills and the discipline learned in these sports—those that are necessary for having fun, for learning how to play with control, and for achieving success—are transferable to other aspects of the participants' everyday lives and can facilitate their learning to live with greater control over their lives. Moreover, it is our belief that the more opportunities young people have to consistently practice skills which require self-discipline and impulse control, the more likely it is that they will be able to exercise the restraint necessary for delaying early sexual activity. If they should decide to have intercourse, these types of experiences may also help them develop the discipline and control necessary for the consistent and correct use of contraceptives, so that unintended pregnancies can realistically be avoided.

Academic Assessment and Homework-Help Program. Each teen has a thorough academic assessment which is conducted by a team of specialists. Scores are obtained in math, reading, writing, and basic age-appropriate life concepts. After thorough testing, a "prescription" is developed for each teen, which summarizes his or her strengths and deficits and serves as a basic for ongoing individual and small group tutorials. Staff education experts, and a group of volunteers from the New York Junior League, use the academic prescriptions to provide one-on-one and/or small group educational support for the teens several days a week at regularly scheduled times at the Dunlevy Milbank Center.

Separate from the tutorial programs, we also provide a homework-help program, two afternoons a week, during which educators assist young people with homework assignments and/or school-related problems.

The Gannet Foundation funds the educational support structures that assist our young people from junior high school to college.

Job Club and Career Awareness Program. Through this weekly two-hour program, conducted by our employment specialists, young people explore the types of career possibilities available to them and learn, in concrete terms, about the world of work. To date, each youngster in this program has secured a social security card; has accurately completed working papers; and has learned how to complete employment applications in an intelligent fashion. Moreover, they have taken part in several role-playing job interviews—appropriately dressing for each.

Each of the teens participating in this program must secure a part- or full-time summer position. Those who are twelve and thirteen—too young for working papers and typical part-time jobs—participate in our Entrepreneurial Apprenticeship Program. Through this program, they—and older teens who have chosen to be involved—work at various community functions (basketball games, dances, etc.) selling hot dogs, soda, juice and snacks. They earn a minimum hourly wage and participate—at the end of a specific period—in a modest profit-sharing program based on the degree to which they have fulfilled their job responsibilities.

All the young people, who have participated in the employment program at our Central Harlem site in the Dunlevy Milbank Center, have opened bank accounts at the Carver Federal Savings bank at 125th Street in Harlem. They are learning that banks, like college, are a reasonable expectation in their future. In addition, they are learning about interest rates and how to save and spend in a controlled, systematic way. In this unique program component, thrift, self-sufficiency, and planning are emphasized.

College Admission Program. As far as we know, this is the only program of its kind that has received a commitment from a college president of a major university system. Donna Shalala, past president of Hunter College, convened a meeting of all the teens and parents in our program and presented them with certificates. These certificates guaranteed their acceptance, as fully matriculated freshmen in an accredited college (Hunter College), upon completion of high school, participation in our teen pregnancy primary prevention program, and the recommendation of the teen pregnancy project director. This commitment should serve as a concrete incentive to those young people who are interested in furthering their education and should affirm the fact that college is part of their future.

Many of the families of the youngsters in our program receive public assistance. The cost of college, therefore, could still make it impossible for some of these youngsters to attend. To address this situation, major costs at Hunter College will be paid through the numerous aid plans ordinarily available to young people who qualify for financial aid and through The Children's Aid Society's special fund, which supports youngsters who have financial needs that go beyond those supported by federal and state aid plans. Some financial support for education will also be available for those young people who participate in other CAS programs. . . .

THE RESULTS THUS FAR

After 36 months of operation (the program was established in February, 1985), there are 175 young people (90 males, 85 females), ages 10-18, and 75 parents in the program.

• Only two females have become pregnant; and, to the best of our knowledge, only one male has caused a pregnancy.

• All the teens in the program are attending junior and senior high school; and approximately three-quarters of them are at grade level.

• There has been no reported alcohol or drug abuse.

• One hundred teens worked at part-time or full-time jobs last summer; 49 are currently working at part-time jobs after school and on weekends.

• Eighty-nine teens have bank accounts at the Carver Federal Savings Bank.

• Four teens and four parents have begun course work at Hunter College.

NOTES

1. Children's Defense Fund, 1987.
2. Ibid.
3. National Research Council, Panel on Adolescent Pregnancy & Childbearing, 1987.

NO
Sarah Glazer

SEX EDUCATION:
HOW WELL DOES IT WORK?

In the America of the late 1980s, sex education is no longer confined to locker rooms and back alleys—or even to the privacy of the home. Now, according to a major national survey by the Alan Guttmacher Institute,[1] four-fifths of the states either require or encourage the teaching of sex education in the public schools, and nearly nine in 10 large school districts in the United States support such instruction.

But what passes for sex education in U.S. public schools, the institute reported, is often a cursory discussion of human biology and "family life" issues. Most sex education classes place less emphasis on pregnancy prevention than on preventing the spread of AIDS and other sexually transmitted diseases. In fact, many sex education programs include no instruction in birth control methods at all, focusing instead on the importance of abstaining from sexual relations.

Given the survey's findings, it's not surprising that sex education classes have demonstrated little success in preventing teenage pregnancies, reducing students' sexual activity or increasing their use of contraceptives. Indeed, half of America's teenagers have intercourse before the age of 18—and almost a quarter have intercourse before their 16th birthdays. Says the institute's president, Jeannie I. Rosoff: "You cannot expect 13 hours of teaching to affect behavior as complicated as sexual behavior."

But even the more thorough programs have failed to make a dent in teenage sexual activity or pregnancy rates. Nevertheless, those who favor sex education in public schools say the need for such programs goes beyond those goals. They contend that sex education, like other academic subjects, provides students with basic knowledge they will use throughout their lives. "Only 51 percent of those eligible to vote voted in the last election," quips Michael A. Carrera, professor of health sciences at Hunter College in New York City. "I don't hear people saying, 'Let's do away with social studies.' "

Unlike social studies, however, many sex education programs carry a mixed message: On the one hand, they tell students how to protect themselves from pregnancy; on the other hand, they tell students to abstain from sex altogether until they are emotionally ready for the consequences. To some proponents of sex education, that mixed message is of little concern. "In my mind, it's no different than drinking and driving," says Debra Haffner, executive director of the New York-based Sex Information and Education Council, a nonprofit organization dedicated to advancing sex education. "We tell young people not to drink, but we recognize that many teenagers do, so we tell them how to protect themselves so they don't die."

But other observers find this approach ethically unsatisfying and ultimately ineffective. "[A]sking schools to teach morally and ethically neutral sex education asks for failure," says Dr. Donald I. MacDonald, former administrator of the Alcohol, Drug Abuse and Mental Health Administration. "In their efforts to be impartial when offering options, teachers often imply that all options are equally appropriate: that is, that values are not relevant."[2]

Mary Lee Tatum, a renowned family-life educator with 15 years of experience, disagrees. She says it's important to give teenagers options because they are at an age when they have to make decisions for themselves. "Americans believe if we tell teenagers to do something, they'll do it. I want [teenagers] to *conclude* that it's possible to be with someone and love them without having intercourse."

Sitting through one of Tatum's eighth-grade classes in Falls Church, Va., a suburb of Washington, D.C., gives a visitor a picture of how she carries out her philosophy of "active listening." On a hot day near the end of the school year, students are watching a movie about a high-school senior who becomes a father un-

expectedly. One scene in particular shocks them. In the middle of the young man's Spanish exam, his girlfriend walks into the classroom, dumps the squalling infant into his arms and disappears. The movie presents a grim future for the new daddy: Rather than going to the first-rate music school to which he has been accepted, he ends up scooping ice cream after graduation to support his new family.

In a class discussion after the film, the students—with some prompting from Tatum about financial realities—agree with the movie's conclusion that the young man has destroyed his prospects for the future. Some students are critical of the teenage mother for deciding to keep the baby rather than give it up for adoption or have an abortion. (At this point Tatum interjects that, for some people, abortion is not an option because of religious or ethical objections.) Most say the girlfriend harbored an unrealistic vision of the responsibilities entailed in being a mother. The students also say it was irresponsible for the young couple to have had sex without birth control, although they suggest that the couple shared a mistaken belief common among teenagers that they can't get pregnant the first time they have sexual intercourse. But whether these 13- and 14-year-olds think it was a bad idea for the couple to have had sexual intercourse in the first place is not clear.

By presenting movies about the way an early pregnancy can destroy a teenager's career prospects and by following up with discussions about the emotional and financial difficulties of supporting a family at a young age, Tatum hopes to convey the message that "pregnancy is not an acceptable risk." That means, she says, that her students have to understand the statistical effectiveness of each form of birth control.

In the discussion after the film, some students point out that the young father took birth control seriously only after he got his girlfriend pregnant. The film shows him giving a condom to a friend with a word of advice. "Is a condom 100 percent effective?" Tatum asks her class. "No," answers one female student. "You need a condom and foam or a condom and a sponge."

"That's 95 percent effective," Tatum explains. "Is there a 100 percent effective way?" asks one girl. "Abstinence," answers a chorus of voices from one corner of the room.

Tatum, who has a maternal, physically affectionate manner with her students, beams proudly at the answer. After class, she notes that she does not make abstinence the starting point of her class, as some states mandate and some school curricula advise. If she gave abstinence a hard sell, she predicts, it would be dismissed by the students. Instead, the students have learned the practical benefits of abstinence based on information she has given them about different forms of birth control.

Although Tatum won't promise that her method will lead to a statistical reduction in pregnancies, she insists that what she offers—a positive way of thinking about sexuality—is better than doing nothing. "By saying nothing and not allowing teachers to say anything all these years, we've made a very loud statement to kids . . . that this is not an acceptable subject in academia or polite company, and where it is acceptable is in the locker room and the hallways, dirty jokes, pornography, television. . . . Generally the only pronouncements they get about sexuality from responsible adults are negative ones. In order to feel good about this emerging sexual self, they have to turn to the places that are making them feel good, and those places are generally irresponsible."

Like other articulate advocates of sex education, Tatum says her goal is to portray sexuality as a positive part of the human experience. By taking this tack, she hopes to convey the message that sexual relations are something worth saving for a special relationship. Tatum sees it as part of her job, for example, to counsel troubled girls outside of class who she thinks may become sexually involved in a desperate attempt to fill emotional gaps in their lives. "What we haven't done in schools is talk about the serious reasons for taking care of yourself: This is your body and it's wonderful; cherish it and make good decisions for yourself."

But according to Rosoff, many sex education programs put too much emphasis on self-esteem issues and pay too little attention to birth control. The focus on self-esteem, she says, "is another way of saying, 'Nice girls don't do it, and if we fix the self-esteem, they won't want to do it.' . . . In this day and age, I'm not sure that is correct." . . .

SEX EDUCATION IN THE U.S.: IS THE FOCUS CORRECT?

Widespread sex education in American public schools is a recent phenomenon, driven in large part by public concern over AIDS. In 1980, only three states—Kentucky, Maryland, New Jersey—and the District of Columbia required sex education. Today, 17 states require it, 23 other states encourage it, and even more (a total of 46 states and the District of Columbia) support education about AIDS.

"[T]he teaching of sex education, although often very limited, is now the norm in most of the nation's secondary schools," says Rosoff of the Guttmacher Institute. "The prevention of pregnancy, however, falls far behind AIDS and [sexually transmitted diseases] in the attention it receives in the classroom."[5]

"My guess is parents are more concerned about their teenage children getting pregnant than about their teenager getting a sexually transmitted disease," says Asta M. Kenney, the institute's associate for policy development and one of the authors of its study. "After all, sexually transmitted diseases are easily treated with a dose of penicillin quite often. Pregnancy can't be treated quite that easily."

The emphasis on disease prevention is historically consistent with the roots of formal sex education in America, which grew out of concern over the spread of such sexually transmitted diseases as gonorrhea at the turn of the century. In addition, schools appear to be much more comfortable instructing students in the dangers of AIDS than in discussing such topics as pregnancy prevention. The Guttmacher survey found that "while states are developing new and often detailed AIDS curricula, the old sex education curricula . . . still focus largely on the reproductive system, puberty, dating, marriage, pregnancy and the responsibilities of parenthood, rather than on more 'relevant' topics like sexual activity and pregnancy prevention. Moreover, sex education and AIDS education often seem to be viewed by the education system as unrelated, with separate curricula, separate training programs and different standards for teachers."[6]

The Guttmacher researchers found that sex education is almost always offered as part of another subject, usually health education or physical education. Only 10 percent of the schools providing sex education offer it as a separate course. While most teachers said they had taken some kind of training course in sex education, no state requires full-fledged certification in the field. Only three states—Michigan, Ohio and Utah—and the District of Columbia require sex education teachers to take even one course in human sexuality. In states that do require certification in a specialty, certification in such fields as health education or physical education satisfies the requirement. In fact, physical education teachers make up the largest single group responsible for teaching sex education, followed by health educators, home economics teachers, biology teachers and school nurses.

"A variety of people are being thrown into teaching sex education who may not have the health background or be comfortable with the subject," says Ellen Wagman, associate director of ETR Associates Inc., in Santa Cruz, Calif., which conducts teacher-training workshops in sex education. "Most of us didn't have good sex education. We don't have models for communicating about it in a helpful way."

Those who teach sex education have to cope with more than inadequate training and outdated instructional materials. They also face pressures from outside the classroom. The most common problem cited by teachers responding to the Guttmacher survey was lack of support from parents, the community or the school administration. Such concerns contribute to teachers' perceptions that they are restricted in what they can teach, the researchers reported. For example, fewer than half of the surveyed teachers tell students where they can obtain contraceptives even though 97 percent say this information should be provided. Says Kenney: "The teachers are walking a fine line. . . . They know what kids need to protect their health and to protect themselves from getting pregnant, but they are concerned because they feel isolated from administrators and parents."

DOES SEX EDUCATION CHANGE TEENS' BEHAVIOR?

Critics of sex education have long expressed concern that detailed instruction in birth control might encourage students to become sexually active. Researchers generally discount such fears, saying teenagers are no more likely to engage in sexual relations if they take a sex education course than if they do not. On the other hand, teenagers who have taken such courses don't show any greater tendency to delay premarital sex, either.[7]

But sex education advocates offer a number of reasons why this doesn't mean sex education classes aren't worthwhile. For one thing, they argue, it often takes a long time, possibly several generations, to influence people's behavior in any kind of public-health campaign, whether it be smoking habits, nutrition or birth control. Just because people know something is good for them does not mean they will do it. For example, women's favorable opinion of the condom rose from 38 percent in 1982 to 60 percent in 1987 largely as a result of widespread publicity about AIDS and the importance of using a condom for protection against the disease. Yet actual use of the condom remained low—around 16 percent.[8]

Some educators say it's unrealistic to expect sex education alone to solve problems like teenage pregnancy and child abuse, which have deep social and economic roots. To successfully tackle such problems, they say, education programs must reach beyond the schools into the community. "You don't solve a major sociocultural problem . . . with a little teeny pop gun attack," says Murray L. Vincent, a professor at the University of South Carolina School of Public Health. "You have to work hard to change the culture. You have to make bearing a child when you're a teen not very acceptable."

Vincent describes how a community-wide approach worked in a poor, rural South Carolina county that had one of the highest teen pregnancy rates in the state. The program began in 1983 when University of South Carolina researchers, assisted by federal and state funds, hired a community-health educator to orchestrate a pregnancy-prevention marketing campaign. Within three years, pregnancy rates for 14- to 17-year-old girls had dropped to about one-third their previous rate and to about half the rate of neighboring counties with similar populations.[9] According to Vincent, the community has continued to sustain lower pregnancy rates than adjacent counties.

The message the program is trying to sell, Vincent says, is, "You get more out of life if you have children when you want to have them." To help get this message across, the program reaches out to all of the adults and children in the community. For example, it has provided a tuition-free, graduate-level course in sex education to two-thirds of the school district's teachers and staff, who, in turn, have incorporated sex education into the curriculum at all grade levels, frequently as part of other science or social studies courses. The program also recruits clergy, church leaders and parents to attend mini-courses (five two-hour sessions) similar to the teachers' courses. Adults are given tips on communicating with young people, information on the kinds of personal problems that lead to unintended pregnancy and basic biological information. The program also promotes its message in local newspapers, on local radio stations and through special speakers.

Vincent says he's not sure how effective a community-wide program would be outside the kind of homogeneous rural community in which it has been tested, but he is planning to establish a similar program in Columbia, the state capital. He also says it's not possible to tell which elements of the program are responsible for the drop in pregnancies: the advertisements, the cooperation with a nearby family planning clinic or everything put together. "I've said it's a major sociocultural problem so I have to have all my guns blazing—at mom, dad, preacher, etc. . . . As a scientist, I can't tell you which [approach] works best."

Some experts argue that access to contraceptives is the key to turning abstract knowledge about pregnancy into something that teenagers will use. The Johns Hopkins University School of Medicine cooperated in one such venture, providing medical services and counseling out of a storefront clinic to black junior and senior high school students from inner-city Baltimore schools. The program combined classroom presentations and personal counseling for students at the schools with contraceptive services at the clinic. The clinic was located across the street from the senior high school and was open only to students from the participating schools. During the pro-

gram's 28-month existence, pregnancy rates declined 30 percent in the participating schools while rising 58 percent at schools with comparable populations.[10]

A major goal of the program, in addition to providing contraception, was to delay students' first sexual experience. Laurie Schwab Zabin, a professor at the Johns Hopkins University School of Public Health who studied the Baltimore experiment, says the program postponed students' first sexual encounter by about 7 months, compared with the typical age for that population before the program began. In addition, she says, the frequency of sexual activity declined among those who were already sexually active. Those results, she says, "disprove once and for all the claim that you shouldn't give contraceptives because it . . . will make more kids sexually active."

Douglas Kirby, research director of ETR Associates in Santa Cruz, is the author of a 1984 study that found that clinic-linked sex education programs substantially increased teens' use of birth control methods and substantially reduced teenage pregnancies.[11] Kirby's study is widely cited as evidence that access to a family planning clinic is an essential ingredient in successful sex education programs. But Kirby now says he is no longer sure that school-based clinics are essential—or even effective. Distributing contraceptives is only a small part of what these student health clinics do, he says, and many students do not take advantage of them anyway.

SHOULD THE UNITED STATES FOLLOW SWEDEN'S EXAMPLE?

Encouraging abstinence is an important goal of most sex education programs in the United States; 86 percent of the sex education teachers responding to the Guttmacher Institute survey said they taught their students that abstinence is the best way to prevent pregnancy and to avoid sexually transmitted diseases. Most of the teachers said they tried to help students avoid intercourse by providing instruction on how to resist peer pressure and how to say no to a boyfriend or girlfriend.

But most sex educators believe it's unrealistic to focus exclusively on abstinence. They point out that the mean age at which American women now start menstruation is 12½, approximately three years younger than it was in the late 1800s. Not only are women entering puberty earlier, they are waiting longer to get married. This has created "an extended period of time in which people are able and interested in having sex," notes Rosoff of the Guttmacher Institute.

"Nobody's ever died from not having sex," counters Kathleen Sullivan. "It's the one appetite that's not necessary to fulfill." Sullivan is director of Project Respect in Glenview, Ill., which, with the help of federal grants, has developed a sex education curriculum promoting abstinence. Sullivan claims the program—which she says is being used in 26 schools in six Midwestern states—has changed students' attitudes. For example, students were asked whether they agreed with the statement, "It is important for me not to have sex before I get married." Before participating in the program, 38 percent of the students agreed with the statement; after completing the program, 56 percent agreed with it. Sullivan, however, admits she does not yet have any data indicating what effect, if any, her program's curriculum has had on students' sexual behavior or pregnancy rates.

Zella Luria, a professor of psychology at Tufts University, believes that sex education programs that focus exclusively on abstinence could be counterproductive and, ultimately, psychologically damaging. Luria criticizes what she calls the traditional American "anti-pleasure" approach to sex. "In our country, hellfire is still close to sexuality and thus shapes our education and services related to sexuality. Who pays the price? Our children do." Telling girls that their bodies are an enemy within lays the groundwork for "sexual guilt . . . and avoidance of birth control, which requires acknowledgement of a sexual body." When girls think it is improper to seek sexual pleasure, Luria writes, they are "swept away" by passion as a way of dealing with society's double standard. "The script has no room for contraception."[12]

Luria maintains that her positive views of sex can and should be accompanied with a moral message: "I think the message should be [that] sex is a part of intimacy and you're not intimate with just anybody."

Luria and sex educators who share her philosophy point to Sweden's sex education program as one that has produced lower teen pregnancy rates without the "hellfire." In 1975, when a new Swedish law went into effect legalizing abortion on demand, the government intensified its mandatory sex education program at all grade levels and added free distribution of contraceptives for adolescents. From the age of 12 or 13, Swedish children receive formal education in contraception, which may include demonstrations of contraceptives in a classroom or at a family planning clinic. Teachers are trained to answer questions about sexual matters from children from pre-school on.

Between 1975 and 1984, Sweden's teenage pregnancy rate declined by about one-third. The number of abortions also declined, another sign that contraceptives were being used more widely. "The effectiveness [of the country's sex education program] can be measured by the fact that today no child is born in Sweden unless it's planned for," says Christina Engfeldt, deputy director of the Swedish Information Service in New York.

Sweden's sex education program is generally characterized by a non-moralistic tone. Rather than preaching abstinence, Engfeldt says, Swedish teachers present sexuality as a stage of development in becoming an adult. Since 1977, however, Swedish educators have added a new emphasis on ethics to the curriculum. They have incorporated such ethical principles in the teachers' manual as, "Nobody is entitled to regard and treat another human being simply as a means of selfish gratification," and, "Fidelity towards a person with whom one has a permanent relationship is a duty." But the principles make no mention of marriage, reflecting the greater prevalence and social acceptance in Sweden of unmarried couples living together and of children born out of wedlock.

Perhaps because of Sweden's more liberal attitude toward sex, Swedish teenagers have their first sexual relations at an earlier age than American teenagers. By the age of 15, for example, 33 percent of Swedish boys and 41 percent of girls have had their first sexual experience. By contrast, fewer than 17 percent of American boys and 6 percent of American girls report having had intercourse

by that age.[13] (Recent surveys show significantly higher U.S. figures. S. L. Hofferth, J. R. Kahn and W. Baldwin reported in *Family Planning Perspectives* in 1987 that about 15 percent of white American females and about 20 percent of black American females said they had engaged in sexual activity by the age of 15. Still, these numbers are lower than their Swedish counterparts.) Yet the trend toward sexual relations at younger ages is not viewed as a social problem in Sweden. "They're having it earlier because they've learned how to handle it," says Engfeldt. "That's one way of showing your feelings. The risk of getting pregnant is minimal."*

Ronald Moglia, director of the Human Sexuality Program at New York University, says Swedish teenagers actually receive fewer hours of formal sex education than do American students who attend one of the more comprehensive sex education programs in this country. He believes the widespread use of contraceptives by Swedish teens can be attributed more to values in Swedish society than to its sex education program. There is also a big difference in the way the governments of the two countries view their role in making social policies. "Here our government sees itself passing laws that the people want," says Moglia. "Sweden sees the government as passing laws people should

*Like Sweden, most developed countries in Europe experienced a pronounced decline in teenage birth rates during the late 1970s and '80s. One explanation for the decline has nothing to do with sex education. It is that women in these countries are marrying and having children later in life in order to take advantage of wider career and educational options. Because of similar social influences in the United States, teenage birth rates here declined steadily between 1960 and 1976, but the teenage birth rate has since leveled out.

have. That doesn't go over in Washington, D.C. No one would get elected."

For example, many Swedes express astonishment at the "opt-out" option many American school systems offer parents who find sex education courses so objectionable that they prefer to keep their children out of them. Sweden's growing immigrant population, the main source of opposition to sex education in that country, is given no such alternative. "Your parents wouldn't say, 'My child isn't going to take mathematics.' The rest of the curriculum shouldn't be optional either," says Engfeldt.

CAN AMERICANS AGREE ON A SEX ED CURRICULUM?

The wide diversity of views about sexual matters in the United States raises problems that are hard to imagine in a society like Sweden, with its widely shared values. For example, as part of the new Virginia sex education mandate, state regulations require students to be taught that sex outside of marriage violates state laws. Jacquelyn Henneberg of Falls Church is among those who support this approach: "We feel sex is really for marriage, and for marriage alone. Thus, sex should be taught in this context."[14] But another Falls Church citizen, Barbara R. Jasny, finds this part of the curriculum objectionable. For one thing, she says, it doesn't match reality. "By the time students reach the eighth grade, many will be brought face-to-face with a conflict: Despite the curriculum, not all single parents or unmarried adults are celibate." In addition, Jasny believes the approach may create problems of its own: "A consequence of the curriculum as written is that some of our children,

when faced with mounting sexual urges, will be driven into too-early marriages—one reason for the high divorce rate."[15]

Virginia, like other states, finds itself struggling with a difficult dilemma. Claude Sandy, director of the division of sciences and elementary education for the state's Department of Education, believes "it is virtually impossible" to teach sex education without discussing values, as some Virginia citizens have proposed. "What we have stressed is those values should not be the teacher's own values. They should be core values we can agree upon."

But since Virginia's citizens have important disagreements about such issues as abortion, homosexuality and premarital sex, the teacher can be put in the awkward position of trying to represent a common consensus that may not exist. "I don't think these things can be taught without going into some explanation of their perspective," says the Rev. Yates of the Episcopal Church in Falls Church. The best a teacher can do, he suggests, is to reveal his or her perspective and to explain that there are other perspectives so that children from families of different persuasions do not feel uncomfortable in the classroom.

The difficulty in reaching common ground has surfaced even in debates over the opt-out alternative, which Virginia regulations require all schools to offer. According to Virginia education official Sandy, "That has been controversial from the standpoint of whether you can just opt out of sensitive areas. We have difficulty defining what are sensitive areas."

Those Virginia citizens who support a facts-only sex education approach argue

(continued on page 175)

SHOULD SEX EDUCATION BE TAUGHT IN KINDERGARTEN?

Many sex educators believe that children need to learn the facts of life before the onset of puberty and the onrush of new emotions—possibly as early as kindergarten. While kindergarten programs are still extremely rare, a few school systems have picked up on the idea. A new state sex education mandate in Virginia, for example, requires each community to develop a sex education curriculum that starts in kindergarten and continues through 12th grade.

Many of the required topics are probably things that would be covered by a teacher anyway, although not necessarily under the rubric of sex education. Under the state guidelines, for example, kindergarten children will be taught "that physical affection can be an expression of . . . a loving family" and they will learn "how to say 'no' to inappropriate approaches from family members, neighbors, strangers and others."

Not everyone is happy with teaching sex education this early. In Falls Church, Va., for example, some critics have argued that the new curriculum would introduce sensitive material before parents want it presented. "There are many children in our school system who are not ready, physically or emotionally, to be taught the sexual material at the grade level that this program requires," the group said in a written dissent.

The Rev. John W. Yates III of the Episcopal Church in Falls Church is a member of the dissenting group and the father of five children in the local schools. He believes the new curriculum "can be burdensome on some children. In some ways it's like having heavy talks with kids about the Holocaust or world starvation problems."

But Ronald Moglia, director of the Human Sexuality Program at New York University, contends that "you can't tell a child too much at an early age. The only mistake you can make is not telling him enough. . . . If you tell him where babies come from in kindergarten, he'll have a good 10 years before his body is ready. It's a lot different from a 13-year-old under pressure from peers to be sexually active."

Moglia has designed a sex education curriculum for kindergartners that includes a "birthing game." The class chooses a girl to be an "adult mommy," and the teacher asks her when she would like to have her baby. When she is ready, the mommy stands by a plastic tube labeled "mommy's birthing tunnel" and starts the "baby" crawling through. As the baby comes out of the end of the tunnel, labeled "mommy's vagina," a "doctor" and a "nurse" welcome the baby into the world.

Some people are shocked at the idea of teaching 5-year-olds such explicit words as "vagina." But sex educators say students need to learn this kind of information at an early age, before it makes them giggly and embarrassed, "Suppose we didn't talk about the effects of alcohol or smoking before kids came home with their first beer or cigarette?" asks Moglia. "Only in sex do we expect people to get information when they start the behavior." By then, he says, it's too late. Adolescents will already have developed their own values and behavior independently of what adults tell them.

that the curriculum should consciously avoid controversial issues like abortion in order to spare children from religious and ethical conflicts within the classroom. But teacher Mary Lee Tatum says the problem with a stripped-down curriculum is in deciding what you select to teach. She expresses the concern that when sex education is taught outside of a broad discussion of values, sex is presented as a mechanical act. "It gives kids a false message," she says. The right message, in her view, is that sex is "part of who we are instead of what we do."

EVEN IN AN AREA AS POLARIZED AS SEX education there are some areas of agreement. Everyone seems disturbed by the nation's high teenage pregnancy rate and the possibility that young people are exposing themselves to a fatal disease like AIDS through early, unprotected sexual activity. Experts on both sides of the debate seem to agree that parents can be the most important force in transmitting healthy values about sexuality to their children—even if those values vary somewhat—but that many parents are not doing it.

Carrera of Hunter College has urged his fellow sex education proponents to pare down their expectations about what sex education can hope to achieve within the schools. "Everyone is so frightened by the sexual tragedies that we face in our society that they look for some educational remedy. I'm sorry, but . . . sex education is not it. Mommies and daddies are it."

Unfortunately, the most invidious sex education messages children receive are those that are beamed over the airwaves every day. Television, Carrera says, portrays women as "getting what they want by using seduction, not by using their brains" and men as "getting what they want by using force, coercion, money and power." To prevent such messages from becoming the only sexual reality young people ever know will require an intensive effort on the part of parents, religious leaders and educators.

NOTES

1. The survey was conducted in 1988. See Asta M. Kenney, Sandra Guardado and Lisanne Brown, "Sex Education and AIDS Education in the Schools," and Jacqueline Darroch Forrest and Jane Silverman, "What Public School Teachers Teach About Preventing Pregnancy, AIDS and Sexually Transmitted Diseases," *Family Planning Perspectives*, March-April 1989, pp. 56–72.

2. Donald Ian Macdonald, "An Approach to the Problem of Teenage Pregnancy," *Public Health Reports*, July-August 1987, pp. 377–385.

3. *A Minority Report Concerning the Falls Church Ad Hoc Committee's Recommendations on Family Life and Sex Education*, Jan. 20, 1989.

4. The latest poll was conducted in May 1988 by Louis Harris and Associates for the Planned Parenthood Federation of America. It is quoted in Asta M. Kenney et al., op. cit., p. 56.

5. Jeannie I. Rosoff, "Sex Education in the Schools: Policies and Practice," *Family Planning Perspectives*, March-April 1989, pp. 52, 64. Rosoff's previous quotes are from an interview with E.R.R.

6. Kenney et al., op. cit., p. 64.

7. See James W. Stout and Frederick P. Rivara, "Schools and Sex Education: Does It Work?" *Pediatrics*, March 1959, pp. 375–379.

8. Jacqueline Darroch Forrest and Richard R. Fordyce, "U.S. Women's Contraceptive Attitudes and Practice: How Have They Changed?" *Family Planning Perspectives*, May-June 1988, pp. 112–118.

9. Murray L. Vincent, Andrew F. Clearie and Mark D. Schluchter, "Reducing Adolescent Pregnancy through School and Community-Based Education," *Journal of the American Medical Association (JAMA)*, June 26, 1987, pp. 3382–3386.

10. Laurie Schwab Zabin, Marilyn B. Hirsch, Rosalie Streett, Mark R. Emerson, Morna Smith, Janet B. Hardy and Theodore M. King. "The Baltimore Pregnancy Prevention Program for Urban Teenagers," *Family Planning Perspectives*, July-August 1988, pp. 182–192.

11. Douglas Kirby, *Sexuality Education: An Evaluation of Programs and Their Effects*, 1984.

12. Zella Luria, "The Adolescent Years and Sexuality," *Independent School*, Spring 1989, pp. 45–49.

13. Carl Gustaf Boethius, "Swedish Sex Education and Its Results," *Current Sweden*, March 1984, and National Research Council, *Risking the Future*, 1987, p. 97.

14. Quoted in "Minority Members Concerned About Family Prerogatives," *Lasso* (newspaper published by students at George Mason Junior Senior High School in Falls Church, Va.), June 6, 1989, p. 8.

15. *Appendix D: Minority Reports, Ad Hoc Committee's Recommendations on Family Life and Sex Education*, Jan. 20, 1989.

POSTSCRIPT

Does Sex Education Prevent Teen Pregnancy?

A review of the scientific literature in *Pediatrics* (July 1989) by physicians James Stout and Frederick Rivara supports the view that sex education does not affect contraceptive usage, sexual behavior, or teenage pregnancy. The available evidence indicates that traditional sex education programs do not work. Thomas Sowell sounds his agreement in "The Big Lie (Sex Education)," *Forbes* (December 23, 1991). Why do sex education programs lack a measurable effect? One possibility is that we as a society may be asking these programs and our schools to do too much. Teenage pregnancy has been increasing for a variety of complex reasons, including the changing values of our society and the subcultures within it. School-based sex education may improve students' knowledge concerning reproductive health and contraception, but it cannot change sexual behavior in a direction that is opposed to the teens' world, as influenced by the media and peers. Should schools stop teaching sex education? William Bennett, in "Sex and the Education of Our Children," *America* (February 14, 1987), argues that sex education as it is currently taught is not reducing teen pregnancies. Sex education, he believes, fails because it does not teach that premarital sex is immoral. Physician, psychoanalyst, and author Melvin Anchell claims that not only is sex education unnecessary, it also promotes homosexuality and abortion: See "The Case Against Sex Education," *All About Issues* (November/December 1988). James Arata, a public school teacher, in "The Dangerous Trends in Sex Education," *Blumenfeld Education Letter* (February 1988), writes that sex education has not decreased teen pregnancies. The only way to solve this problem, he maintains, is to teach teenagers that sex before marriage is immoral. This belief is supported by Phyllis Schlafly in "The High Cost of Free Sex," *The Phyllis Schlafly Report* (February 1987).

While many experts believe that sex education must focus on morality and abstinence, others argue that it should not even be taught. Carrera and Dempsey maintain that sex education must stay, but not as it is currently being taught. Sexuality education, they say, should be a part of school and community-based programs that help teenagers learn life skills, not just reproductive anatomy and contraceptive information.

ISSUE 11

Can Abortion Be a Morally Acceptable Choice?

YES: Mary Gordon, from "A Moral Choice," *The Atlantic* (April 1990)

NO: Jason DeParle, from "Beyond the Legal Right: Why Liberals and Feminists Don't Like to Talk About the Morality of Abortion," *The Washington Monthly* (April 1989)

ISSUE SUMMARY

YES: Author Mary Gordon believes that abortion is an acceptable means to end an unwanted pregnancy and that women who have abortions are neither selfish nor immoral.

NO: Editor Jason DeParle argues that liberals and feminists refuse to acknowledge that the 3 out of 10 pregnancies that currently end in abortion raise many moral questions.

Few issues have created as much controversy and resulted in as much opposition as has the topic of abortion. Those involved in the abortion debate not only have firm beliefs, but each side has a self-designated label—pro-life and pro-choice—that clearly reflects what they believe to be the basic issues. The supporters of a woman's right to choose an abortion see individual choice as central to the debate. They believe that if a woman cannot choose to end an unwanted pregnancy, a condition that affects her body and possibly her whole life, then she has lost one of her most basic human rights. The pro-choice people feel that although the fetus is a potential human being, its life cannot be placed on the same level with that of the woman. On the other side, the pro-life movement argues that the fetus *is* a human being and that it has the same right to life as the mother. They believe that abortion is not only immoral but murder.

Although abortion appears to be a modern issue, it has a very long history. In the past, women in both urbanized and tribal societies have used a variety of dangerous methods to end unwanted pregnancies. Women sometimes consumed toxic chemicals, or various tools were inserted into the uterus in hopes of expelling its contents. Modern technology has simplified the procedure and has made it considerably safer. Before abortion was legalized in the United States, approximately 20 percent of all deaths from childbirth or pregnancy were caused by botched illegal abortions.

In 1973, the U.S. Supreme Court's decision of *Roe v. Wade* determined that an abortion in the first three months (trimester) of pregnancy is a decision between a woman and her physician and is protected by a right to privacy. During the second trimester, the Court ruled that an abortion could be performed on the basis of health risks. During the final trimester, an abortion could be performed only for the sake of the mother's health.

Since 1973 abortion has become one of the most controversial issues in our society. The National Right to Life Committee, one of the major abortion foes, currently has over 11 million members, who have become increasingly militant. In the summer of 1991, a major battle between pro-life and pro-choice forces took place in Wichita, Kansas. A similar demonstration followed during the spring of 1992 in Buffalo, New York, and others are planned. Largely as a result of these and other efforts, legislators have introduced various proposals to reduce, and eliminate, abortion rights in the United States.

Despite opposition from the right-to-life groups, abortion remains safe and legal in the United States today. However, what continues to kindle the debate are these questions: Does an abortion involve killing what may be a human being? Is abortion moral? Does the fetus have a right to life, liberty, and the pursuit of happiness, as guaranteed by the U.S. Constitution? Or do women have a right to a safe means of terminating an unwanted pregnancy?

In the following selections, Mary Gordon writes that abortion is neither immoral nor selfish. Because abortions usually take place when the embryo is merely a clump of cells and not a developed fetus, Gordon argues that abortion is not immoral and that a woman's life is more important than that of a *potential* human. Jason DeParle argues that there is nothing more vulnerable than the unborn. DeParle cannot understand how liberalism can hope to regain the glory of standing for morality and humanity while finding it humane and moral to extinguish so much life.

YES   Mary Gordon

A MORAL CHOICE

I am having lunch with six women. What is unusual is that four of them are in their seventies, two of them widowed, the other two living with husbands beside whom they've lived for decades. All of them have had children. Had they been men, they would have published books and hung their paintings on the walls of important galleries. But they are women of a certain generation, and their lives were shaped around their families and personal relations. They are women you go to for help and support. We begin talking about the latest legislative act that makes abortion more difficult for poor women to obtain. An extraordinary thing happens. Each of them talks about the illegal abortions she had during her young womanhood. Not one of them was spared the experience. Any of them could have died on the table of whatever person (not a doctor in any case) she was forced to approach, in secrecy and in terror, to end a pregnancy that she felt would blight her life.

I mention this incident for two reasons: first as a reminder that all kinds of women have always had abortions; second because it is essential that we remember that an abortion is performed on a living woman who has a life in which a terminated pregnancy is only a small part. Morally speaking, the decision to have an abortion doesn't take place in a vacuum. It is connected to other choices that a woman makes in the course of an adult life.

Anti-choice propagandists paint pictures of women who choose to have abortions as types of moral callousness, selfishness, or irresponsibility. The woman choosing to abort is the dressed-for-success yuppie who gets rid of her baby so that she won't miss her Caribbean vacation or her chance for promotion. Or she is the feckless, promiscuous ghetto teenager who couldn't bring herself to just say no to sex. A third, purportedly kinder, gentler picture has recently begun to be drawn. The woman in the abortion clinic is there because she is misinformed about the nature of the world. She is having an abortion because society does not provide for mothers and their children, and she mistakenly thinks that another mouth to feed will be the ruin of her family, not understanding that the temporary truth of family unhappiness doesn't stack up beside the eternal verity that abortion is

From Mary Gordon, "A Moral Choice," *The Atlantic* (April 1990). Copyright © 1990 by Mary Gordon. Reprinted by permission of Sterling Lord Literistic, Inc.

murder. Or she is the dupe of her husband or boyfriend, who talks her into having an abortion because a child will be a drag on his life-style. None of these pictures created by the anti-choice movement assumes that the decision to have an abortion is made responsibly, in the context of a morally lived life, by a free and responsible moral agent.

THE ONTOLOGY* OF THE FETUS

How would a woman who habitually makes choices in moral terms come to the decision to have an abortion? The moral discussion of abortion centers on the issue of whether or not abortion is an act of murder. At first glance it would seem that the answer should follow directly upon two questions: Is the fetus human? and Is it alive? It would be absurd to deny that a fetus is alive or that it is human. What would our other options be—to say that it is inanimate or belongs to another species? But we habitually use the terms "human" and "live" to refer to parts of our body—"human hair," for example, or "live red-blood cells"—and we are clear in our understanding that the nature of these objects does not rank equally with an entire personal existence. It then seems important to consider whether the fetus, this alive human thing, is a *person*, to whom the term "murder" could sensibly be applied. How would anyone come to a decision about something so impalpable as personhood? Philosophers have struggled with the issue of personhood, but in language that is so abstract that it is unhelpful to ordinary people making decisions in the course of their lives.

*Ontology refers to the nature of being or existing.—Ed.

It might be more productive to begin thinking about the status of the fetus by examining the language and customs that surround it. This approach will encourage us to focus on the choosing, acting woman, rather than the act of abortion—as if the act were performed by abstract forces without bodies, histories, attachments.

This focus on the acting woman is useful because a pregnant woman has an identifiable, consistent ontology, and a fetus takes on different ontological identities over time. But common sense, experience, and linguistic usage point clearly to the fact that we habitually consider, for example, a seven-week-old fetus to be different from a seven-month-old one. We can tell this by the way we respond to the involuntary loss of one as against the other. We have different language for the experience of the involuntary expulsion of the fetus from the womb depending upon the point of gestation at which the experience occurs. If it occurs early in the pregnancy, we call it a miscarriage; if late, we call it a stillbirth.

We would have an extreme reaction to the reversal of those terms. If a woman referred to a miscarriage at seven weeks as a stillbirth, we would be alarmed. It would shock our sense of propriety; it would make us uneasy; we would find it disturbing, misplaced—as we do when a bag lady sits down in a restaurant and starts shouting, or an octogenarian arrives at our door in a sailor suit. In short, we would suspect that the speaker was mad. Similarly, if a doctor or a nurse referred to the loss of a seven-month-old fetus as a miscarriage, we would be shocked by that person's insensitivity: could she or he not understand that a fetus that age is not what it was months before?

Our ritual and religious practices underscore the fact that we make distinctions among fetuses. If a woman took the bloody matter—indistinguishable from a heavy period—of an early miscarriage and insisted upon putting it in a tiny coffin and marking its grave, we would have serious concerns about her mental health. By the same token, we would feel squeamish about flushing a seven-month-old fetus down the toilet—something we would quite normally do with an early miscarriage. There are no prayers for the matter of a miscarriage, nor do we feel there should be. Even a Catholic priest would not baptize the issue of an early miscarriage.

The difficulties stem, of course, from the odd situation of a fetus's ontology: a complicated, differentiated, and nuanced response is required when we are dealing with an entity that changes over time. Yet we are in the habit of making distinctions like this. At one point we know that a child is no longer a child but an adult. That this question is vexed and problematic is clear from our difficulty in determining who is a juvenile offender and who is an adult criminal and at what age sexual intercourse ceases to be known as statutory rape. So at what point, if any, do we on the pro-choice side say that the developing fetus is a person, with rights equal to its mother's?

The anti-choice people have one advantage over us; their monolithic position gives them unity on this question. For myself, I am made uneasy by third-trimester abortions, which take place when the fetus could live outside the mother's body, but I also know that these are extremely rare and often performed on very young girls who have had difficulty comprehending the realities of pregnancy. It seems to me that the question of late abortions should be decided case by case, and that fixation on this issue is a deflection from what is most important: keeping early abortions, which are in the majority by far, safe and legal. I am also politically realistic enough to suspect that bills restricting late abortions are not good-faith attempts to make distinctions about the nature of fetal life. They are, rather, the cynical embodiments of the hope among anti-choice partisans that technology will be on their side and that medical science's ability to create situations in which younger fetuses are viable outside their mothers' bodies will increase dramatically in the next few years. Ironically, medical science will probably make the issue of abortion a minor one in the near future. The RU-486 pill, which can induce abortion early on, exists, and whether or not it is legally available (it is not on the market here, because of pressure from anti-choice groups), women will begin to obtain it. If abortion can occur through chemical rather than physical means, in the privacy of one's home, most people not directly involved will lose interest in it. As abortion is transformed from a public into a private issue, it will cease to be perceived as political; it will be called personal instead.

AN EQUIVOCAL GOOD

But because abortion will always deal with what it is to create and sustain life, it will always be a moral issue. And whether we like it or not, our moral thinking about abortion is rooted in the shifting soil of perception. In an age inwhich much of our perception is manipulated by media that specialize in the sound bite and the photo op, the anti-choice partisans have a twofold advantage over us on the pro-choice side. The pro-choice moral position is more complex, and the experience we defend is physically repellent to contemplate. None of us in the pro-choice movement would suggest that abortion is not a regrettable occurrence. Anti-choice proponents can offer pastel photographs of babies in buntings, their eyes peaceful in the camera's gaze. In answer, we can't offer the material of an early abortion, bloody, amorphous in a paper cup, to prove that what has just been removed from the woman's body is not a child, not in the same category of being as the adorable bundle in an adoptive mother's arms. It is not a pleasure to look at the physical evidence of abortion, and most of us don't get the opportunity to do so.

The theologian Daniel Maguire, uncomfortable with the fact that most theological arguments about the nature of abortion are made by men who have never been anywhere near an actual abortion, decided to visit a clinic and observe abortions being performed. He didn't find the experience easy, but he knew that before he could in good conscience make a moral judgment on abortion, he needed to experience through his senses what an aborted fetus is like: he needed to look at and touch the controversial entity. He held in his hand the bloody fetal stuff; the eight-week-old fetus fit in the palm of his hand, and it certainly bore no resemblance to either of his two children when he had held them moments after their birth. He knew at that point what women who have experienced early abortions and miscarriages know: that some event occurred, possibly even a dramatic one, but it was not the death of a child.

Because issues of pregnancy and birth are both physical and metaphorical, we must constantly step back and forth between ways of perceiving the world. When we speak of gestation, we are often talking in terms of potential, about events and objects to which we attach our hopes, fears, dreams, and ideals. A mother can speak to the fetus in her uterus and name it; she and her mate may decorate a nursery according to their vision of the good life; they may choose for an embryo a college, a profession, a dwelling. But those of us who are trying to think morally about pregnancy and birth must remember that these feelings are our own projections onto what is in reality an inappropriate object. However charmed we may be by an expectant father's buying a little football for something inside his wife's belly, we shouldn't make public policy based on such actions, nor should we force others to live their lives conforming to our fantasies.

As a society, we are making decisions that pit the complicated future of a complex adult against the fate of a mass of cells lacking cortical development. The moral pressure should be on distinguishing the true from the false, the real suffering of living persons from our individual and often idiosyncratic dreams and fears. We must make decisions on abortion based on an understanding of how people really do live. We must be able to say that poverty is worse than not being poor, that having dignified and meaningful work is better than working in conditions of degradation, that raising a child one loves and has desired is better than raising a child in resentment and rage, that it is better for a twelve-year-old not to endure the trauma of having a child when she is herself a child.

When we put these ideas against the ideas of "child" or "baby," we seem to be making a horrifying choice of life-style over life. But in fact we are telling the truth of what it means to bear a child, and what the experience of abortion really is. This is extremely difficult, for the object of the discussion is hidden, changing, potential. We make our decisions on the basis of approximate and inadequate language, often on the basis of fantasies and fears. It will always be crucial to try to separate genuine moral concern from phobia, punitiveness, superstition, anxiety, a desperate search for certainty in an uncertain world.

One of the certainties that is removed if we accept the consequences of the pro-choice position is the belief that the birth of a child is an unequivocal good. In real life we act knowing that the birth of a child is not always a good thing: people are sometimes depressed, angry, rejecting, at the birth of a child. But this is a difficult truth to tell; we don't like to say it, and one of the fears preyed on by anti-choice proponents is that if we cannot look at the birth of a child as an unequivocal good, then there is nothing to look toward. The desire for security of the imagination, for typological fixity, particularly in the area of "the good," is an understandable desire. It must seem to some anti-choice people that we on the pro-choice side are not only murdering innocent children but also murdering hope. Those of us who have experienced the birth of a desired child and felt the joy of that moment can be tempted into believing that it was the physical experience of the birth itself that was the joy. But it is crucial to remember that the birth of a child itself is a neutral occurrence emotionally: the charge it takes on is invested in it by the people experiencing or observing it.

THE FEAR OF SEXUAL AUTONOMY

These uncertainties can lead to another set of fears, not only about abortion but about its implications. Many anti-choice people fear that to support abortion is to cast one's lot with the cold and technological rather than with the warm and natural, to head down the slippery slope toward a brave new world where handicapped children are left on mountains to starve and the old are put out in the snow. But if we look at the history of abortion, we don't see the embodiment of what the anti-choice proponents fear. On the contrary, excepting the grotesque counterexample of the People's Republic of China (which practices forced abortion), there seems to be a real link between repressive anti-abortion stances and repressive governments. Abortion was banned in Fascist Italy and Nazi Germany; it is illegal in South Africa and in Chile. It is paid for by the governments of Denmark, England, and the Netherlands, which have national health and welfare systems that foster the health and well-being of mothers, children, the old, and the handicapped.

Advocates of outlawing abortion often refer to women seeking abortion as self-indulgent and materialistic. In fact these accusations mask a discomfort with female sexuality, sexual pleasure, and sexual autonomy. It is possible for a woman to have a sexual life unriddled by fear only if she can be confident that she need not pay for a failure of technology or judgment (and who among us has never once been swept away in the heat of a sexual moment?) by taking upon herself the crushing burden of unchosen motherhood.

It is no accident, therefore, that the increased appeal of measures to restrict maternal conduct during pregnancy—and a new focus on the physical autonomy of the pregnant woman—have come into public discourse at precisely the time when women are achieving unprecedented levels of economic and political autonomy. What has surprised me is that some of this new anti-autonomy talk comes to us from the left. An example of this new discourse is an article by Christopher Hitchens that appeared in *The Nation* last April, in which the author asserts his discomfort with abortion. Hitchens's tone is impeccably British: arch, light, we're men of the left.

> Anyone who has ever seen a sonogram or has spent even an hour with a textbook on embryology knows that the emotions are not the deciding factor. In order to terminate a pregnancy, you have to still a heartbeat, switch off a developing brain, and whatever the method, break some bones and rupture some organs. As to whether this involves pain on the "Silent Scream" scale, I have no idea. The "right to life" leadership, again, has cheapened everything it touches. ["Silent Scream" refers to Dr. Bernard Nathanson's widely debated antiabortion film *The Silent Scream*, in which an abortion on a 12-week-old fetus is shown from inside the uterus.—Ed.]

"It is a pity," Hitchens goes on to say, "that . . . the majority of feminists and their allies have stuck to the dead ground of 'Me Decade' possessive individualism, an ideology that has more in common than it admits with the prehistoric right, which it claims to oppose but has in fact encouraged." Hitchens proposes, as an alternative, a program of social reform that would make contraception free and support a national adoption service. In his opinion, it would seem, women have abortions for only two reasons: because they are selfish or because they are poor. If the state will take care of the economic problems and the bureaucratic messiness around adoption, it remains only for the possessive individualists to get their act together and walk with their babies into the communal utopia of the future. Hitchens would allow victims of rape or incest to have free abortions, on the grounds that since they didn't choose to have sex, the women should not be forced to have the babies. This would seem to put the issue of volition in a wrong and telling place. To Hitchens's mind, it would appear, if a woman chooses to have sex, she can't choose whether or not to have a baby. The implications of this are clear. If a woman is consciously and volitionally sexual, she should be prepared to take her medicine. And what medicine must the consciously sexual male take? Does Hitchens really believe, or want us to believe, that every male who has unintentionally impregnated a woman will be involved in the lifelong responsibility for the upbringing of the engendered child? Can he honestly say that he has observed this behavior—or, indeed, would want to see it observed—in the world in which he lives?

REAL CHOICES

It is essential for a moral decision about abortion to be made in an atmosphere of open, critical thinking. We on the pro-choice side must accept that there are indeed anti-choice activists who take their position in good faith. I believe, however, that they are people for whom childbirth is an emotionally overladen topic, people who are susceptible to unclear thinking because of their unrealistic hopes and fears. It is important for us in the pro-choice movement to be open in discussing those areas involving abortion which are nebulous and unclear. But we must not forget that there are some things that we know to be undeniably true. There are some undeniable bad consequences of a woman's being forced to bear a child against her will. First is the trauma of going through a pregnancy and giving birth to a child who is not desired, a trauma more long-lasting than that experienced by some (only some) women who experience an early abortion. The grief of giving up a child at its birth—and at nine months it is a child whom one has felt move inside one's body—is underestimated both by anti-choice partisans and by those for whom access to adoptable children is important. This grief should not be forced on any woman—or, indeed, encouraged by public policy.

We must be realistic about the impact on society of millions of unwanted children in an overpopulated world. Most of the time, human beings have sex not because they want to make babies. Yet throughout history sex has resulted in unwanted pregnancies. And women have always aborted. One thing that is not hidden, mysterious, or debatable is that making abortion illegal will result in the deaths of women, as it has always done. Is our historical memory so short that none of us remember aunts, sisters, friends, or mothers who were killed or rendered sterile by septic abortions? Does no one in the anti-choice movement remember stories or actual experiences of midnight drives to filthy rooms from which aborted women were sent out, bleeding, to their fate? Can anyone genuinely say that it would be a moral good for us as a society to return to those conditions?

Thinking about abortion, then, forces us to take moral positions as adults who understand the complexities of the world and the realities of human suffering, to make decisions based on how people actually live and choose, and not on our fears, prejudices, and anxieties about sex and society, life and death.

NO
Jason DeParle

BEYOND THE LEGAL RIGHT: WHY LIBERALS AND FEMINISTS DON'T LIKE TO TALK ABOUT THE MORALITY OF ABORTION

It's hard to hold these two images—the dismembered body of the fetus and the enveloping body of the mother, each begging the allegiance of our conscience—in mind at the same time. One of the biggest problems with the abortion debate is how rarely we do it, at least in public discourse. While contentious issues naturally produce one-dimensional positions, the remarkable thing about abortion is that many otherwise sensitive, nuanced thinkers hold them. To one side, visions only of women in crisis, terrified and imperilled by an invasive growth; to the other, only legions of innocent children, chased by the steely needle.

The inhumanity that issues from baronies within the right-to-life movement is well known: the craziness of a crusade against birth control; the view of women as second-class citizens; even the descent into bomb-throwing madness. The insistence that an unborn child must always be saved, no matter the cost, isn't compassion but a compassionate mask, and it obscures a face of cruelty.

But what ought to be equally if not more disturbing to feminists, liberals, and others on the Left is the extent to which prominent prochoice intellectuals mirror that dishonesty and denial. One-and-a-half million abortions each year is not the moral equivalent of the Holocaust, precisely because of the way in which fetuses *are* distinguishable: growing inside women, they can wreck the lives of mothers and of others, including her children, who depend upon her. But the fact that three of 10 pregnancies end in abortion poses moral questions that much of the Left, especially abortion's most vocal defenders, refuses to acknowledge. This lowering of intellectual standards offers a useful way of looking at the reflexes of liberals in general, and also reveals much about the passions—many of them just—that underpin contemporary feminism.

WHAT THE SUCTION MACHINE SUCKS

The declaration of a legal right to an abortion doesn't end the discussion of what our attitude toward it should be, it merely begins it. . . . [M]any of the pro-choice movement's writers and intellectuals would have us believe that the early fetus (and 90 percent of abortions take place in the first three months) is nothing more than a dewy piece of tissue, to be excised without regret. To speak of abortion as a moral dilemma, [Barbara Ehrenreich, prolific writer and contemporary feminist and socialist] has written, is to use "a mealy-mouthed vocabulary of evasion," to be compromised by a "strange and cabalistic question."

Yet everything we know—not just from science and religion but from experience, intuition, and compassion—suggests otherwise. A pregnant woman, even talking to her doctor, doesn't call the growth inside her an embryo or fetus. She calls it a *baby*. And she is admonished, by fellow feminists among others, to hold it in trust: Don't drink. Don't smoke. Eat well, counsels the feminist manual, *Our Bodies, Ourselves*: "think of it as eating for three—you, your baby, and the placenta. . . ." Is it protoplasm that she's feeding? Or is it protoplasm only if she's feeding it to the forceps?

Grant for a moment that it is; agree that what the suction machine sucks is nothing more than tissue. Why then the feminist fuss over abortions for purposes of sex selection? If a couple wants a boy and nature hands them the makings of a girl, why not abort and start again? All that matters—no?—is "choice."

It wasn't sex selection but nuclear power that got a feminist named Juli Loesch rethinking her own contradictory views of fetuses. As an organizer attempting to stop the construction of Three Mile Island, she had schooled herself on what leaked radiation can do to prenatal development. At a meeting one day, she says, a group of women issued an unexpected challenge: "if you're so concerned about what Plutonium 239 might do to the child's arm bud you should go see what a suction machine does to his whole body."

In fact, we need neither *The Silent Scream* [Dr. Bernard Nathanson's anti-abortion film, which was widely publicized and debated in the United States during the mid-1980s and which showed, from inside a uterus, an abortion being performed on a 12-week-old fetus] nor a degree in fetal physiology to tell us what we already know: that abortion is the eradication of human life and should be avoided whenever possible. Should it be legal? Yes, since the alternatives are worse. Is it moral? Perhaps, depending on what's at stake. Fetal life exists along a continuum; our obligations to it grow as it grows, but they must be weighed against other demands.

The number of liberals, feminists, and other defenders of abortion eager to simplify the moral questions is, at the very least, deeply ironic. One of the animating spirits of liberalism and other factions on the Left, and proudly so, is the concern for the most vulnerable. But what could be more vulnerable than the unborn? And how can liberalism hope to regain the glory of standing for humanity and morality while finding nothing inhumane or immoral in the extermination of so much life?

The problem with much prochoice thinking is suggested by the movement's chief slogan, "a woman's right to control her body," which fails to acknowledge that the great moral and biological co-nundrum is precisely that another body is involved. Slogans are slogans, not dissertations; but this one is revealing in that it mirrors so much of the prochoice tendency to ignore the conflict in an unwanted pregnancy between two competing interests, mother and embryo, and insist that only one is worthy of consideration. Daniel Callahan, a moral philosopher, has written of the need, upon securing the right to a legal abortion, to preserve the "moral tension" implicit in an unwanted pregnancy. This is something that too few members of the prochoice movement are willing to do.

One fine example of preserving the moral tension appeared several years ago in a *Harper's* piece by Sallie Tisdale, an abortion clinic nurse with a grudging acceptance of her work. First the mothers: "A twenty-one-year-old woman, unemployed, uneducated, without family, in the fifth month of her fifth pregnancy. A forty-two-year-old mother of teenagers, shocked by her condition, refusing to tell her husband. A twenty-three-year-old mother of two having her seventh abortion, and many women in their thirties having their first. . . . Oh, the ignorance. . . . Some swear they have not had sex, many do not know what a uterus is, how sperm and egg meet, how sex makes babies. . . . They come so young, snapping gum, sockless and sneakered, and their shakily applied eyeliner smears when they cry. . . . I cannot imagine them as mothers."

Then the fetus: "I am speaking in a matter-of-fact voice about 'the tissue' and 'the contents' when the woman suddenly catches my eye and asks, 'How big is the baby now?'. . . . I gauge, and sometimes lie a little, weaseling around its infantile features until its clinging power slackens. But when I look in the basin, among the curdlike blood clots, I see an elfin thorax, attenuated, its pencilline ribs all in parallel rows with tiny knobs of spine rounding upwards. A translucent arm and hand swim beside. . . . I have fetus dreams, we all do here: dreams of abortions one after the other; of buckets of blood splashed on the walls; trees full of crawling fetuses. . . ."

It's not surprising that the defenders of abortion don't like pictures of fetuses; General Westmoreland didn't like the cameras in Vietnam either. Fetuses aren't babies, and the photos don't end the discussion. But they make it a more sober one, as it should be. Fetuses aren't just *their* image but our image too, anyone's image who is going to confront abortion.

If the prochoice movement doesn't like the way *The Silent Scream* depicts the fetus, turn to an early edition of *Our Bodies, Ourselves*. Describing an abortion at 16 weeks by means of saline injection, the feminist handbook explains: "Contractions will start some hours later. Generally they will be as strong as those of a full-term pregnancy. . . . The longest and most difficult part will be the labor. The breathing techniques taught in the childbirth section of this book might help make the contractions more bearable. After eight to fifteen hours of labor, the fetus is expelled in a bedpan in the patient's bed."

HEIL MARY

When Suzannah Lessard wrote about abortion in *The Washington Monthly* in 1972 ("Aborting a Fetus: the Legal Right, the Personal Choice"), a year before *Roe v. Wade,* she described what she called a "reaction formation along ideological lines . . . of the new feminist movement" as it related to abortion. This was a time when Gloria Steinem was insisting that a fetus was nothing more than "mass of dependent protoplasm" and aborting it the moral equivalent of a tonsillectomy. "I think a lot of women need to go fanatically ideological for a while because they can't in any other way over-throw the insidious sense of themselves as inferior," Lessard wrote, "nor other-wise live with the rage that comes to the surface when they realize how they have been psychically mauled." This is an observation about the psychology of op-pression that could be applied to any number of righteous rebellions; the path to autonomy tends to pass, by necessity perhaps, through stages of angry de-fiance. "But I don't think that state of mind—hopefully temporary—is the strength of the movement," Lessard wrote. "It has very little to do with work-ing out a new, undamaging way of living as women."

But to judge by much contemporary prochoice writing, the mere-protoplasm camp still thrives. Certainly, there are exceptions, Mario Cuomo's 1984 speech at Notre Dame perhaps being the most famous: "A fetus is different from an appendix or set of tonsils. At the very least . . . the full potential of human life is indisputably there. That—to my less subtle mind—by itself should demand respect, caution, indeed . . . reverence. . . . [But] I concluded that the approach of a constitutional amendment is not the best way for us to seek to deal with abor-tion." And others on the Left have gone even further: Nat Hentoff, who supports a legal ban, has written a number of attacks on abortion in the *Village Voice;*

Mary Meehan, a former antiwar activist, published an article in *The Progressive* that attacked the magazine's own edi-torial stance in favor of legal abortion.

But these are the exceptions. Pick up the past 10 years of *The Nation, Mother Jones,* or *Ms.* Read liberals and feminists on the op-ed pages of *The Washington Post* or *The New York Times*—you're likely to find more concern about the snail darter than the 1.6 million fetuses aborted each year. . . .

LIBERAL PRECINCTS

. . . [T]he point is clear: questioning abortion—not only the legal right but also the moral choice—is often viewed, even by otherwise sensitive and thought-ful activists, as a betrayal of the highest order. (Except, at times, for Catholics, whose antiabortion views are usually dismissed as a quaint if unfortunate quirk of faith.)

A great irony about this public dem-onstration of zeal is that there may be more ambivalence on the Left than is usually acknowledged. When *The Pro-gressive* published Mary Meehan's pro-life piece in 1980, it drew more mail than any article save the famous guide to the workings of the H-bomb. About half were predictable: "your knees buckle at the mere thought of taking a forthright stand for women's rights," "prolife is only a code word representing the neo-fascist absolutist thinking." Etc, etc.

But the others: "I support most of the positions of the women's movement, but I part company with those who insist on abortion as a 'right of women to control their own bodies.' There's a lot more than just one body that is being con-trolled here." "I have no religious objec-tion to abortion, but I do oppose it from a humanitarian point of view." "I was awfully glad to see a liberal publication printing an antiabortion article."

Why aren't there more voices like these heard in liberal precincts? The answers come in two general sets, one pertaining to liberal and progressive values generally and the other connected more specifically to the passions of contemporary feminism.

Right or wrong, abortion helps further values that liberals and progressives generally hold in esteem. Among them is public health. Even those with qualms about abortion tend to back the legal right, if for no other reason than to stem the mutilation that a return to back alleys would surely entail. There's also an equity-between-the-classes argument: if abortion is banned all women may experience trouble getting one, but the poor will have the most trouble of all. For others, there are always planes to Sweden.

Beyond questions of abortion's legality, the Left tends to hold values that encourage the acceptance of abortion's morality too. There's the civil liberties perspective, which argues that the state should "stay out of the bedroom." There's a population control argument; without abortion, wrote one *Progressive* reader, "there will be a more intense scramble for food and all the world's natural resources." There's a help-the-poor strand of thinking; what, liberals constantly ask, about the welfare mother who can't afford another child? And there's a fairness-in-the-marketplace argument, which maintains that without absolute control of their fertility, women cannot compete with men: if two Arnold & Porter associates conceive a child at a Christmas party tryst, bringing it into the world, whether she keeps it or not, will penalize her career much more than his.

These principles—a thirst for fairness between genders and classes, for civil liberties, for economic opportunity—are honorable ones. And they speak well of those who hold them as caring not only for life itself but also for its quality.

Careful, though. Quality-of-life arguments sometimes stop focusing on quality and start frowning on life. Concerns about population control have their place; but whether abortion is a fit means of seeking it raises questions that go well beyond environmental impact studies. One of the most troubling prochoice arguments is the what-kind-of-life-will-the-child-have line. Yes, poverty may appropriately enter the moral calculus if an additional child will truly tumble the family into chaos and despair, and those situations exist. (And there is little cruelty purer than child abuse, which afflicts unwanted children of all classes.) But liberal talk about the quality of life can quickly devolve into a form of cardboard compassion that assumes life for the poor doesn't mean much anyway. That sentiment says to an unborn child of poverty: life is tough, so you should die. Compassionate, that. . . .

THE CHRISTMAS PARTY TRYST

While the values of the Left in general provide one set of explanations for the contours of the abortion debate, the specific passions and experiences of feminists provide another. These concerns don't, finally, answer the question of what our personal, as opposed to legal, obligations toward fetal life need to be. But they do underline the history of injustice that women have inherited.

In rough outline, one persuasive feminist argument for keeping abortion *legal*—an argument I accept—goes something like this: Without the option of abortion, women cannot be as free as men. Not just socially and economically but psychologically as well. And not just those with unwanted pregnancies. As Ellen Willis of the [Village] Voice has put it, "Criminalizing abortion doesn't just harm individual women with unwanted pregnancies, it affects all women's sense of themselves. Without control of our fertility we can never envision ourselves as free, for our biology makes us constantly vulnerable." Vulnerable to failed birth control. To rape or other coercive sex. Or simply to passion. Vulnerable in a way that men are not. And in a society that rightly prizes liberty as much as ours, it's unacceptable for one half of its members to be less free, at an essential level, than the other. Therefore the legal right.

Of course, having the legal right to do something doesn't tell us whether it's a desirable thing to do. Women have the legal right to smoke and drink heavily during pregnancy, but few of us would hesitate to dissuade them from doing so. Why don't more feminists take the same view toward abortion—defending the right, but urging women to incline against it whenever possible? The feminist defenders of abortion I spoke with reacted to that proposal with a litany of past and present injustices against women—economic, social, political, and cultural, all of them quite real. "You can sit around all day talking about what's the morally right thing to do—rights and sacrifices and the sanctity of life and all that—but I don't think it can be divorced from women's lives in this society," [poet and critic Katha] Pollitt said.

Leaving aside for a moment the wrenching emotional issues, one obvious burden is economics. Having a child—even one put up for adoption—costs not only trauma but time and money, and takes them from women, not men. The financial burden is one reason why poor women are more likely to have abortions than others.

But the same inequity is true among professional women. To return to the Arnold & Porter Christmas party tryst, what would happen if the female associate does the right thing by prolife standards and decides to have the child? At $65,000 a year, she can certainly afford to do it, and her insurance is probably blue chip. But in the eyes of some senior partners, the luster of her earlier promise begins to fade. They may be reluctant to keep her on certain accounts, for fear of offending the clients. What's more, even if the clients understand, she'll be missing at least six to eight weeks of work—just, as fate would have it, when she's needed in court on an important case. The long-term penalties may be overestimated—good employees are in short demand in most professions; it's the marginal who will suffer the most—but the fears are nonetheless real. What's more, the burden is unequally shared. Her tryst-ee suffers no such repercussions. The clients love him, he shines in court, and his future seems assured. Unfair? Yes, extremely.

These inequities are one reason why the right-to-life movement has the obligation, often shirked, to support measures that would make it easier for women of all incomes to go through pregnancy—health care, maternity leave, parental leave, day care, protections against employment discrimination. But even if all these things were provided—as they should be—it's unlikely that the strength of feminist feeling on abortion would recede. Economic opportunity is an important facet of the abortion debate, but it's not, finally at its core. Of all the women I spoke with, the one I most expected to forward an economic argument was Barbara Ehrenreich—since she is co-chair of Democratic Socialists of America—but she never mentioned it. When I finally asked her about it she said that no amount of money or servants would change the essential moral equation, which centers, in her mind, on female autonomy. "The moral issue has to do with female personhood," she said.

CRUEL CHOICES

What surprised me in my talks with the female defenders of abortion, was how many of them seemed to view the abortion debate as some sort of referendum by which society judged women's deepest levels of self. Words like *guilt* and *sin*, *punishment* and *shame* kept issuing forth. They did so both about abortion and about sex in general. "The whole debate is more about the value of women's lives and the respect we have for women than it is about the act of abortion itself," said Kate Michelman, the head of the National Abortion Rights Action League.

A few days before my scheduled meeting with Michelman, I got a phone call from her press secretary. "We hear a nasty rumor," she said, "that you're writing something that says abortion is immoral." I mentioned the rumor when I sat down to speak with Michelman, who quickly told me about the very difficult circumstances surrounding her own abortion. Her first husband had walked out on her and her three small children when she was destitute, ill, and pregnant. She had to make a difficult moral judgment, she said, weighing her re-

sponsibilities to her family against those to the fetus. Then, this being 1970, she couldn't even make the decision herself but had to obtain the consent of a panel of doctors and then, to further the pain, get her ex-husband's signature. Call me immoral, she seemed to say, in an I-dare-you way.

But it seemed to me that Michelman's decision, like those, certainly, of a great number of women, had involved a thoughtful handling of difficult questions—as she herself was underlining. "Sure the fetus has interests, absolutely," she said, as do other things, like a woman's commitments to her family and her health. It was only when I began asking why those leading the prochoice movement didn't discuss these moral tensions more often that her reasoning turned curious and defensive.

"The ethical questions are being raised," she said. "And if [a woman] makes a decision [to have an abortion] then she's made the right decision."

I asked her how she knew. With 1.6 million abortions a year, there seems to be a lot of room for error.

Merely asking the question, she said, implied that women had abortions for frivolous reasons. "To even raise the question of when it's immoral," she said, "is to say that women can't make moral decisions."

In considering the way a legacy of injustice fuels the adamance over abortion, it is helpful to consider three generations of women: those who preceded the feminist movement of the late sixties and early seventies; those who soldiered in it; and those who inherited its gains. Each has faced the tyranny of a man's world in a way that primes passions about abortion, but each has done so in a different way.

Women who became sexually active outside of marriage in the days of blanket abortion bans faced a world prepared to hand them the cruelest choice: the life-wrecking stigma of pregnancy out-of-wedlock or the back alley; a "ruined" life or a potentially lethal trip through a netherworld. Men, meanwhile, made the decisions that crafted that world while escaping the brunt of its cruelty. That *was* an unjust life, and the triumph over it is among feminism's proudest achievements. . . .

ACCEPTING FEMALE SEXUALITY

. . . [W]hat's interesting about the observations of male irresponsibility [in casual sexual relationships], as it relates to abortion, is that both sides cite it. Prolife feminists, like Juli Loesch, argue that the acceptance of abortion actually *encourages* exploitation. The "hit and run" artist can pony up $200, send a woman off to a clinic, and imagine himself to have done the gallant thing. "The idea is that a man can use a woman, vacuum her out, and she's ready to be used again," Loesch says."It's like a rent-a-car or something." (In such scenarios, Loesch argues, abortion has the same blame-the-victim effect that the Left is typically quick to condemn, with the victimized mother perpetrating the injustice through violence against the fetus.)

When I asked Katha Pollitt about this, she dismissed it with the argument that men will be just as irresponsible with or without abortion, and that the only difference will be the burden left to women. To some extent she's right: irresponsible sexual behavior—by men and women both—will no doubt continue under any imaginable scenario. Then again, it's not unreasonable to suspect that casual attitudes about abortion, particularly among men, could increase precisely the kind of "stallion" behavior that Pollitt rightly protests. And abortion can become a tool of male coercion in other ways as well. "He said that if I didn't have an abortion, the relationship would be over," a friend recently explained. Many women have experienced the same.

Of course, feminist emotion toward abortion isn't just a reaction to male sexuality but also an assertion that women's own sexual drive is equally legitimate. Feminists argue that antiabortion arguments reflect a larger cultural ambivalence, if not outright hostility, toward female sexuality. This is where words like *guilt* and *shame* and *punishment* continue to arise. I recently sat down with Katha Pollitt for a long conversation about abortion. She cited the many ways in which women (and the children antiabortionists want them to raise) are injured by society: poor health care, poor housing, economic discrimination, male abuse. We talked also about power, politics, religion, and the other forces that play into the abortion debate, like the unflagging responsibilities that come with parenthood. (She is a new, and proud, mother.) But when I asked her which, of the many justifications for abortion, she felt most deeply—what, in her mind, was the real core of the issue—her answer surprised me. "Deep down," she said, "what I believe is that children should not be a punishment for having sex."

Ellen Willis of the *Voice* advances a similar argument. Opposition to abortion, she's written, is cut of the same cloth as the more general "virginity fetishism, sexual guilt and panic and disgrace" foisted on women by a repressive society. The woman's fight for abortion without qualm, she says, is part of the fight for the "acceptance of the erotic impulse, and one's own erotic impulses, as fundamentally benign and necessary for human happiness."

Pollitt agreed. "The notion of female sexuality being expressed is something people have deeply contradictory feelings about," Pollitt said. . . .

BIOLOGY AND DESTINY

What the argument for abortion-without-qualm comes down to is this: the fetus doesn't exist unless we want it to. But the whole crisis over abortion is that we know precisely the opposite to be true. It's there physically, feminists say, but not morally. But how could it be one without the other—there to nurture one day (remember, plenty of fresh vegetables, we're eating for three: you, baby, and placenta), but free to dismember the next? Qualm-less advocates argue that all that finally matters is whether the woman, for whatever reason, desires to bring it into the world. Yet the fetus is already there, no matter what we plan or desire. Forces may conspire against a woman and leave her *unable* to bring it into the world, or unable to do so without a great deal of harm to herself and others. That is, *other* moral obligations may overrule. But it is suspicious in the extreme to argue—as the qualmlessness position does—that our moral obligations are nothing more than what we want them to be, a wish-it-away view of the world. Inconveniently fetuses exist, quite outside our fluctuating emotions and desires.

Finally, Ellen Willis's argument that by giving fetuses any moral status at all we reduce women to vessels breaks down because women *are* vessels. They're not *just* vessels. They're much more than

vessels. But the attempt to reconcile the just desire for full female autonomy with our moral obligations toward fetuses by insisting that we have none attempts to wish away a very real collision; it refuses to acknowledge a (so far) inalterable conflict buried in biology. Willis argues this is precisely the oppressive "biology equals destiny" argument that feminism has fought to overturn. Biology doesn't equal destiny; but it does affect destiny, and it leaves us with the extremely difficult fact that women, for any number of reasons, get burdened with unwanted pregnancies to which there are no easy moral solutions. Something important is lost—female autonomy or fetal life—in either event.

There are two highly imperfect ways of dealing with this conflict. The first is abstinence (since birth control fails). But not much chance of that. The second is adoption—another imperfect solution. The first argument against it is that there aren't enough parents to go around, particularly for minority and handicapped children. Ironically those quickest to point this out tend to be those for whom putting up a child for adoption really is a plausible option—white professionals. George Bush's "adoption not abortion" line brought quick ridicule by Pollitt in *The Nation* and Ehrenreich in *Mother Jones*. He's wrong to suggest it as a panacea—babies would quickly outstrip parents, as Pollitt insists—but right to encourage its wider use. The real challenge for liberals and progressives would be to turn the thought back toward Bush, and demand the governmental support, in health care and other ways, needed to get through pregnancy, and needed to raise a child.

The second argument against adoption focuses not on demand but supply:

nine months of illness culminating in a "physiological crisis which is occasionally fatal and almost always excruciatingly painful," as Ehrenreich has written. . . . "It's almost unimaginable to me to think about giving up the baby," said Ehrenreich. "Talk about misery. Talk about 20 years of grief and ambivalence." The grief is real—particularly for people of conscience, like Ehrenreich. (And people of conscience are the targets of moral suasion in the first place.) But where does that argument lead? That in order to spare a child the risks of an adoptive life, we offer the kindness of a suction machine?

"A VERY SCARY TIME"

A few years ago, I was sharing an apartment with a friend who became pregnant just before breaking up with her fiance. Like many men . . . he just walked away, dealing with the dilemma through denial. My friend dealt with it with a lot of courage. I called her recently to see how the experience seemed in retrospect, and perhaps she should provide the coda, since her view complicates both Ehrenreich's position and my own. Though she said that putting her child up for adoption was "the right thing," she said she "would never, ever, pressure someone to go through the same thing."

It surprised me to hear her say that abortion "crossed my mind several thousand times," since that was the one option she had seemed to rule out from the start. When she realized she was pregnant, she said, she went riding her bicycle into potholes "trying to jar something loose. It was very, very easy for me to think of the sperm and the egg as having just joined. It was like a piece of mucous

to me." She decided against abortion after about a week, "a very lonely, very scary time."

"At some point, I realized I was old enough, and mature enough, that I could do it [have the baby]," she said, but she emphasized that this calculus could have been altered easily by any number of factors—including less support from family and friends, a less understanding employer, or the lack of medical care. She spent months in counseling trying to decide whether to raise the child or put it up for adoption, and the decision to give the baby away "was the most difficult thing I've ever had to do." Since the baby was healthy and white the adoption market was on her side—"I could have dictated that I wanted two Finnish socialists," she said—and her certainty that the new parents would not only love the child but pass on certain shared values was an essential thing to know.

"When I think about her," she said, "just the miracle of being able to have brought her into this life, even if she's not here with me right now, she's with people who love her. It's a miracle."

"When she left to go to her adoptive parents, it was the most devastating and wonderful thing," she said. "I kept thinking this is my child, and I love her."

"It always kept coming back to that—I love her."

POSTSCRIPT

Can Abortion Be a Morally Acceptable Choice?

The abortion issue continues to be complex and polarizing. In June 1983, in a series of decisions, the Supreme Court reaffirmed its support of abortion rights. Similar decisions in 1986 also confirmed the Court's support. However, the Court has become more conservative and pro-life in recent years. With pressure and support from pro-life groups throughout the country, *Roe v. Wade* may continue to come before the Supreme Court for reconsideration. While the majority of Americans favor a woman's right to an abortion, the vocal and well-organized pro-life groups have been successful in keeping the abortion issue in the media and in the political arena.

Media director of the National Right to Life Committee Nancy Meyers agrees with Schwartz and O'Connor that abortion is never justified and that it is a violation of human rights ("Abortion is Morally Wrong," *The World and I*, 1989), as does William F. Buckley, in "Abortion: The Debate," *The National Review* (December 1989). Writing in the *Humanist* (January/February 1991), Planned Parenthood Federation of America president Faye Wattleton argues that women's reproductive rights are inviolable and that no government, court, or politician should ever interfere with these rights.

Many people believe that if abortion becomes illegal again, dangerous self-induced and back alley abortions would reappear. But whether or not legalized abortion has improved women's health is still the subject of controversy. In her book *The Choices We Made* (Random House, 1991), Angela Bonavoglia claims that *Roe v. Wade* made abortion both safe and legal and that legal abortion saves women's lives. She notes that of the 1.6 million legal abortions performed each year in the United States, only six women die from the procedure. In contrast, in Mexico, where abortion is not legal, 140,000 women die annually from the procedure.

David C. Reardon, in his book *Aborted Women: Silent No More* (Loyola University Press, 1987), counters that the legalization of abortion has not improved the health of women. While the number of deaths from legal abortions is low, Reardon claims that the infection and bleeding rates are high. He believes that, overall, since abortion rates have climbed since 1973, the health risks associated with abortion have increased due to the sheer numbers of women having abortions.

While there are literally thousands of articles and books addressing this issue, the following selections debate the moral concerns surrounding abortion: "Life Terms," *New Republic* (July 15, 1991); "A Basic Human Right," *Ms* (August 1989); "Abortion: The Politics—What the People Really Say," *National Review* (December 22, 1989); and "Abortion: The Morality—Is There a Middle Ground?" *National Review* (December 1989).

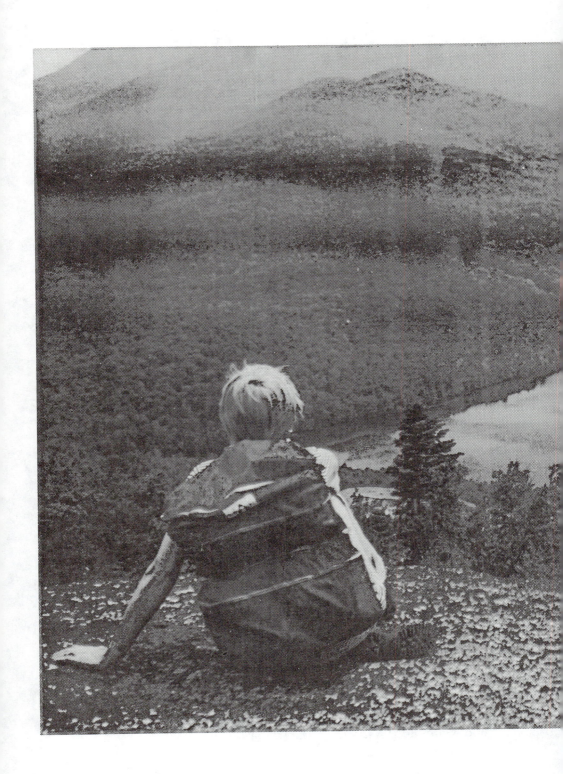

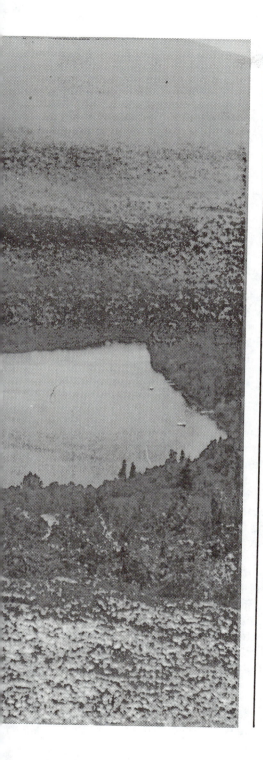

PART 5

Nutrition, Exercise, and Health

Recently, millions of health-conscious individuals have begun exercising, eating low-fat diets, and swallowing vitamin pills in an effort to prevent disease and maintain health and well-being. While most physicians support dietary changes and moderate exercise, critics claim that many people who follow diet and exercise fads may actually develop nutritional deficiencies and increase their risk of physical injury. This section debates some of the controversies that surround diet and exercise claims.

Is Cholesterol Reduction an Important Health Priority?
_____

Can Large Doses of Vitamins Improve Health?
_____

Does Exercise Increase Longevity?

ISSUE 12

Is Cholesterol Reduction an Important Health Priority?

YES: Timothy Johnson, from "The Cholesterol Controversy," *Harvard Medical School Health Letter* (December 1989)

NO: Thomas J. Moore, from "The Cholesterol Myth," *The Atlantic* (September 1989)

ISSUE SUMMARY

YES: Physician Timothy Johnson discusses evidence indicating that the higher one's serum cholesterol is, the greater the statistical risk of having a heart attack.

NO: Journalist Thomas J. Moore argues that there is no legitimate evidence proving that lowering serum cholesterol will prevent a heart attack or affect longevity.

Cholesterol is a white, waxy, fat-like substance that is an essential element in our bodies as well as the bodies of all animals. It is the building block from which the body manufactures sex hormones and bile, which helps digest fats, and it is a component of all animal (and human) cell membranes. The liver manufactures adequate amounts of cholesterol for the body's needs every day; whatever cholesterol is consumed (from animal foods) is added to the overall cholesterol level in the body. When cholesterol becomes a problem, it is usually because the diet leaves an excess of cholesterol in the bloodstream.

For over 100 years scientists have known that cholesterol can accumulate in coronary arteries, reducing the flow of blood to the heart and eventually narrowing the passages so severely that a heart attack occurs. An important investigation that was begun in 1948, known as the Framingham Heart Study, has demonstrated that as blood cholesterol levels rise, the risk of heart attack correspondingly rises. This relationship seems to be strongest for men between the ages of 40 and 59, although women and men of other ages can also be at risk.

Dietary cholesterol comes only from animal foods, such as meat, poultry, fish, eggs, and dairy products; no plant foods contain cholesterol. When foods that are high in dietary cholesterol are eaten, this cholesterol is added to one's own. But *dietary* cholesterol is not a very important risk factor; rather, foods that contain large amounts of saturated fats are of greater concern. Saturated (which refers to the fat's chemical structure) fats are solid at room temperature and are found in fatty meats and whole milk products. Some vegetable foods, such as coconut and palm kernel oils and vegetable shortening, are also high in saturated fats. These fats appear to reduce the liver's ability to remove cholesterol from the blood.

In the following selections, Timothy Johnson discusses evidence, including results from the Framingham Study, that show that the lower the serum cholesterol, the lower the risk of heart disease. He points out that in countries where the average blood cholesterol is very low, heart attack rates are also very low. In the United States and Finland, two countries with very high average blood cholesterol rates, the corresponding heart attack rates are high. Johnson also believes that diet is an important factor. Americans (and Finns) tend to eat diets high in saturated fat, and Johnson claims that they should try to lower their serum cholesterol by reducing their intake of meats, whole milk products, and baked goods.

Thomas J. Moore counters that lowering your serum cholesterol is next to impossible with diet, and even if you manage to do so, there is no real evidence that you will live longer. He also claims that individuals vary widely in diet response. Some can consume large amounts of saturated fat without producing any effect on their blood cholesterol levels. Moore also criticizes various studies conducted on the cholesterol–diet–heart attack relationships. He concludes that heart disease has actually declined from 1960 to 1980, while serum cholesterol levels have remained basically unchanged.

YES

Timothy Johnson

THE CHOLESTEROL CONTROVERSY

THE CHOLESTEROL CONNECTION

Despite the current controversy, almost everyone agrees that some points are settled. (1) The higher your blood cholesterol, the greater your statistical risk of having a heart attack. (2) Middle-aged men with a blood cholesterol above 240 should be especially concerned. (3) In itself, a high cholesterol produces no warning symptoms, so it makes sense to test blood periodically.

The remaining big question is whether the entire population should aim to lower blood cholesterol so as to lower the risk of coronary artery disease. Advocates of this approach say that an accumulation of research has already provided the answer. The evidence they cite includes the following observations:

- In countries where the average blood cholesterol is very low (for example rural China and Japan), heart attack rates are also very low. The Japanese are impressive examples because, even though smoking is common and blood pressure tends to be high in Japan, heart attack rates are low; corresponding to the low blood cholesterol. But ethnic Japanese who live in America and eat the high-fat American diet have higher cholesterol levels and more heart attacks.

- Laboratory animals respond to high-fat diets much as human beings do, by developing higher blood cholesterol and atherosclerosis in their coronary arteries. (Saturated fat in the diet stimulates the liver to raise blood cholesterol levels; this is a much more important influence than cholesterol in the diet. In other words, it's bacon and butter, more than eggs, that raise blood cholesterol.)

- The coronary arteries of people with atherosclerosis have improved after a period of lowered blood cholesterol. This response has recently been demonstrated by the x-ray method known as angiography.

INTERVENTION—A FLOP?

Skeptics, however, hold that no research program to lower blood cholesterol has markedly reduced the frequency of heart attacks or lowered the death rate in a group of experimental subjects. Accordingly, Mr. [Thomas J.] Moore and others argue that these intervention trials have either not demonstrated a benefit, or have found one that was very small.

One of the trials criticized is the MR FIT (Multiple Risk Factor Intervention Trial), which followed two groups of high-risk men for 7 years. One group entered an intensive program to help them quit smoking, lower blood pressure, and reduce cholesterol. The other men were told about their risk status, but then referred back to their private physicians for care. (From the outset, many experts criticized this study for attacking all three risk factors at once; they rightly doubted whether it would be possible to correlate any potential response with change in a specific risk factor.)

In the end, MR FIT subjects differed little from their controls in the rate of heart attacks or total mortality. From this, Mr. Moore concludes, "The trial failed completely." But important information *can* be obtained from this study. Telling the control subjects about their high-risk status and sending them back to their own physicians with that information led to efforts to reduce their risk. The reason the two groups didn't differ much was that the controls, like the subjects, changed. The upshot was that the number of coronary deaths was 40% less than expected in *both* groups. The study failed to prove that the specific MR FIT interventions were more effective than the regular care received by controls. Yet any reasonable interpretation of the results is that the recommendations did help reduce coronary-disease. In criticizing the design of MR FIT, critics miss its real message.

Other experiments in intervention have been more rigorously designed. Two in particular, the Coronary Primary Prevention Trial and the Helsinki Heart Study, did specifically show a modest reduction in heart attacks from lowering cholesterol. The follow-up in these studies was limited to 5–7 years.

Mr. Moore and others have looked at these results and emphasized that the reduction in heart attacks was minimal—and there was no statistically significant decline in overall death rates. These criticisms miss two big points. First, 5–7 years is a relatively short period. Keeping blood cholesterol low for a lifetime would be expected, on many grounds, to have a much larger effect. Even more telling, critics of these trials ignore the finding that those who succeeded in lowering their blood cholesterol levels the most also had the lowest rate of heart disease. Even in these short-term trials, those who lowered their levels by 25% also lowered their rate of coronary events (heart attacks, new onset of angina) by 50%.

THE REST OF THE PICTURE

Advocates of vigorous efforts to lower the population's cholesterol have emphasized the intervention trials in making their case. In so doing, they have left themselves open to the kind of criticism Mr. Moore is making. The cholesterol experts have based their own thinking, however, on a mosaic of evidence—comparison of populations with different cholesterol levels, the animal data, and the results of relatively recent research showing improvement in diseased arteries after cholesterol reduction. Taken together, the pieces come together in a broadly consistent picture: Lower cholesterol is linked to lower risk of coronary artery disease.

The critics have, however, raised some important points.

Americans should not be led to the point of hysteria about cholesterol, to the exclusion of concern about other risk factors, such as smoking and high blood pressure. Even cholesterol experts acknowledge that cigarette smoking is probably the single most important risk factor for coronary artery disease.

It is also true both that dietary changes are difficult to make and that not everyone needs to make them. Some people are blessed with genes permitting them to eat almost anything and keep their cholesterol levels near 200. But it is difficult to make a case that many Americans either need or benefit from a diet that is dense with calories and high in saturated fat. The simple expedient of reducing consumption of saturated fat from meat, dairy products based on whole milk or cream, and baked goods is a reasonable one for the population as a whole, and the majority is likely to benefit from taking these measures.

But then a serious question arises for those who do not respond to diet: Should they take cholesterol-lowering drugs? The short answer is that diet should always be tried first—and should be given at least 6 months to work—unless a cholesterol level is felt to be dangerously high. In addition, many experts believe that the newest cholesterol-lowering drug, lovastatin (Mevacor), is being used too widely and too quickly, simply because it is well-tolerated and usually produces a dramatic reduction in cholesterol. Lovastatin is still a relatively new drug, without a long-distance track record. Before it becomes accepted for widespread use, many conservative physicians feel that long-term follow-up studies should be completed.

FRYING PAN AND FIRING LINE

To the degree that Mr. Moore is taken to prove that Americans need not attempt to minimize their intake of saturated fat, he is doing his audience a real disservice. There is, to be sure, legitimate controversy as to just how low cholesterol levels should be at various ages, about when and how drugs should be used, and about the weight that should be given to levels of HDL (the benign form of cholesterol) in judging the risk of heart disease.

Nevertheless, in my judgment the most important and most practical message to come from studies of cholesterol in this century remains valid: We should all try to cut down our intake of high-fat dairy products and saturated fats from meat and baked goods.

I would like to close with the perspective of Richard Peto, the Oxford epidemiologist who is taken by many as the world's authority on risk factors: "You can't offer eternal life to old people. But what you can do is to avoid death in middle age. At the moment, about a third of all Americans die in middle age, and that isn't necessary. About half of those premature deaths could be avoided if people took smoking, blood cholesterol, and blood pressure more seriously."

NO
Thomas J. Moore

THE CHOLESTEROL MYTH

One morning in early October of 1987 the U.S. health authorities announced that 25 percent of the adult population had a dangerous condition requiring medical treatment. Since there were no symptoms, if would be necessary to screen the entire population to identify those in danger. More than half of those screened would be dispatched to their physicians for medical tests and evaluation. Then for one out of four adults treatment would begin. The first step would be a strict diet under medical supervision. If within three months the dieting had not achieved specified results that could be verified by laboratory tests, a more severe diet would be imposed. The final step for many patients would be powerful drugs to be taken for the rest of their lives.

Considering that this was expected to be one of the most important medical interventions in the nation's history, the formal announcement was deceptively low-key. It was to be called the National Cholesterol Education Program. And while *cholesterol* was surely a household word, the official sponsor was less familiar: the National Heart, Lung, and Blood Institute, a major division of the federal government's National Institutes of Health. Although the heart institute's main job is to coordinate and finance medical research, this departure into medical intervention was not unprecedented. At first glance the program's objective sounded positively innocuous: "To reduce the prevalence of elevated blood cholesterol in the United States and thereby contribute to reducing coronary heart disease morbidity and mortality." But the National Cholesterol Education Program was a medical landmark in several ways.

It was the culmination of an extraordinary and sustained medical-research effort targeting the nation's biggest killer—coronary heart disease. One experiment had taken forty years and was still in progress. Another involved examining 361,622 middle-aged men. A famous experiment by two Nobel Prize winners had penetrated the innermost recesses of the human cell to identify a single gene with a dramatic effect on cholesterol levels. Researchers had studied the arteries of rabbits, given high-fat diets to monkeys, and fed egg yolks to college students. It would be hard to find

From Thomas J. Moore, "The Cholesterol Myth," *The Atlantic* (September 1989). Adapted from Thomas J. Moore, *Heart Failure* (Random House, 1989). Copyright © 1989 by Thomas J. Moore. Reprinted by permission of Random House, Inc.

another medical issue that had been explored with such vigor, by so many researchers, and at such great expense. Just two important experiments took twelve years, cost more than $300 million, and consumed 60 percent of the heart institute's clinical-research budget.

There were serious risks to consider. Not since the introduction of oral contraceptives would so many people be exposed to powerful new prescription drugs over decades. Among the most elusive hazards of any drug are damaging or even deadly side effects that are recognized only after the drug has been administered to thousands of people for years. Nor is dietary therapy quite as simple as it sounds. So complex are the interactions among food compounds, and so varied are the behavior and the chemistry of individuals, that dietary intervention has proved to be one of the most complicated of all medical treatments, subject to unexpected difficulties and disappointing results.

Finally, the National Cholesterol Education Program represented a major change in strategy in the prevention of coronary heart disease. Previous efforts, led mainly by the American Heart Association, had relied on advice and persuasion. Now the federal government was calling on the authority of physicians to prescribe a medically supervised regimen of treatment. This was not just friendly advice from the family doctor to cut down on cholesterol. It was, in the words of the treatment guidelines, a program of "behavior modification" backed by laboratory tests to ensure adherence and measure results. People still might abandon drugs that made them sick—and some cholesterol-lowering drugs were famous for doing so—or refuse to eat foods they didn't like. But now they would be violating explicit doctor's orders.

One would expect a government program of such importance to have survived rigorous examination and review before it moved into high gear. One would suppose that such a far-reaching intervention into the lives of millions of people had been approved by the White House and scrutinized by Congress. In fact the heart institute launched this project on its own authority, consulting panels of hand-picked specialists. One would suppose that before millions of people were put on a medically supervised diet, the diet would have been tested to demonstrate that it was safe and effective. No such tests were conducted. One would suppose that the nation's clinical laboratories could measure cholesterol accurately enough to identify those who needed treatment. In fact laboratory performance was so poor that millions with average or low blood-cholesterol levels would inevitably be misled into believing that their levels were dangerously high. One would suppose that before a program involving billions of dollars in doctors' bills, laboratory tests, and medication was launched, the costs and benefits would have been carefully weighed. In fact officials refused even to guess at the total costs and had no plan to measure the benefits. And one would suppose that it had been conclusively demonstrated that lowering blood-cholesterol levels would save lives. No such evidence existed. . . .

THE CAMPAIGN IS LAUNCHED

Like some ponderous prehistoric beast, the National Cholesterol Education Program slowly surfaced from the bureaucratic swamps of the National Heart, Lung, and Blood Institute.

The program that ultimately came into being was described in detail in 1982, in a major American Heart Association policy statement. By 1983 the heart institute was conducting detailed and expensive surveys of attitudes toward cholesterol, among physicians and members of the public, which it would use as the basis for a public-relations campaign. In late 1984 an NIH-sponsored Consensus Development Conference provided the scientific mandate the heart institute had sought, and in 1985 the National Cholesterol Education Program was officially launched. In 1986 it was unveiled to the medical community, in 1987 to the public.

It is a program of vast scope and consequences. James I. Cleeman, the program coordinator, has said that at least a quarter of all adults would be referred to their physicians for treatment to lower their cholesterol levels. "It's a mammoth intervention and it deserves to be a mammoth intervention."

As heart-institute officials began to plan their anti-cholesterol campaign, it quickly became apparent that the primary obstacle was not public ignorance or apathy but the skepticism of the nation's physicians. Owing mainly to the highly visible and unopposed news-media campaigns of the American Heart Association, the public had long ago been sensitized to the alleged hazards of dietary cholesterol. In 1983, according to a poll by the heart institute, two thirds of the public believed that a high-fat diet had a "large effect" on coronary heart disease, and nearly as many believed that dietary cholesterol was an equally important hazard.

A majority of the nation's physicians disagreed, the institute learned in a re-lated poll. While nine out of ten thought that smoking had a large health effect, only 23 percent were equally concerned about the dangers of saturated fat, and only 39 percent about elevated blood-cholesterol levels. Therefore the nation's doctors became the first target of the heart institute. The slogan that emerged later—"Ask your doctor about cholesterol"—would even exploit the discovery that the public had been easier to convince of the dangers of cholesterol than were the doctors who dealt with heart disease every day.

The public was largely unaware that a lively debate was being waged, mostly out of view, in the nation's medical journals and at scientific meetings, and that expert opinion was never unanimous. In 1980, for example, Thomas N. James, then the president of the American Heart Association, had dissented on diet. "I wish to express some personal reservations about our non-exceptional advice, which is taken by the public as meaning everyone should be deeply concerned about their dietary cholesterol," James said in a broad critique of the emphasis on diet which he delivered at the association's annual scientific meeting. His views were reported in the American Heart Association's medical journal, *Circulation*, with the disclaimer that they were not necessarily those of the association. . . .

Late last year the heart institute acquired powerful new allies. The American Medical Association, a major drug manufacturer, and two huge food companies joined forces to "declare war on cholesterol." The public-relations and advertising campaign began to reach the public early this year and included national and local television programs, special magazine features, cereal-box advertisements, books, videocassettes, brochures, discount coupons, and posters. . . .

THE COALITION AGAINST CHOLESTEROL

So far the dissenters have been overwhelmed by the extravaganza put on not just by the heart institute but by a growing coalition that resembles a medical version of the military-industrial complex. This coalition includes, first, the "authorities"—the experts in the medical schools—most of whom play leading roles in one of the twelve lipid-research laboratories established by the heart institute. Many of these researchers spent many years as principal investigators . . . and their research establishments continue to rely heavily on heart-institute funding. Much of the rest of their funding comes from companies that manufacture cholesterol-lowering drugs. Next is the heart institute itself. Is it possible to imagine a more effective scheme than the National Cholesterol Education Program for raising the institute's public profile? The heart institute, in turn, is tied closely to the drug industry. Not only does it frequently test promising new drugs at no charge to the companies, but it readily endorses products it deems useful. And last comes the American Heart Association, which had long urged just such a cholesterol campaign, as part of its sometimes misdirected but long-standing efforts to modify public behavior. This coalition boasts the authority of the federal government, the money and sales forces of the drug companies, and the reach and

reputation of the American Heart Association. . . .

WHAT EVERYONE IS TOLD TO DO

The National Cholesterol Education Program divides the American public into three groups. People with serum-cholesterol levels of 240 milligrams per deciliter or more have "high blood cholesterol" and require treatment under medical supervision, by drugs or diet or both, for the rest of their lives. There is no quantum leap in risk at this level; it was arbitrarily selected to target 25 percent of the adult population. Next come those with "borderline-high" cholesterol levels, defined as 200–239 mg/dl. Of this group men with one additional risk factor and women with two are said to require medical treatment. (Additional risk factors include smoking, obesity, diabetes, high blood pressure, a family history of heart disease, other vascular disease, and low levels of HDL, or high-density lipoprotein.) The intent of the program's designers to play on fear can be seen in the decision to label as "borderline-high" those levels that are actually average. Finally, those with levels below 200 mg/dl are in the "desirable" range. People in this group can be released with a lecture or a brochure about the dangers of cholesterol, and retested every five years.

Considering that treatment may prove unpleasant, inconvenient, expensive, or all three, it is obviously important to identify correctly those people likely to reap some benefit. Nevertheless, the panel that designed the National Cholesterol Education Program knew that it would result in the treatment of millions of people who had been wrongly classified.

Poor performance by clinical laboratories accounts for part of the problem. The heart institute's lipid-research laboratories proved that serum-cholesterol levels can be measured accurately: a careful series of tests revealed an average error of one to two percent. The equipment in all twelve laboratories had been calibrated to the same reference blood sample. This was a crucial step, because a key danger in measurement is an upward or downward bias in all results from a particular lab. The program's laboratory-standards panel set as a final target a three-percent rate of error which although it would result in some misclassification, would confine the errors to borderline cases. . . .

The failures of the National Cholesterol Education Program grow more severe as a patient whose cholesterol level has been classified as high proceeds with medical treatment. The initial approach calls for a cholesterol-lowering diet of moderate severity, with laboratory tests at six weeks and three months to determine the results of the diet. If little change occurs, a more severe diet is imposed. The principal effect of this therapy will be to introduce 25 million adults and their families to the kind of inconvenience, frustration, and failure that medical researchers experienced in exploring the link between diet and heart disease.

Many observers in the medical community were surprised to discover that the heart institute had made diet the frontline treatment, when sixteen years earlier it had rejected a full-scale diet trial. Given the extensive scientific record on the question of diet, it is remarkable indeed to find dietary intervention once again at the center of attention. The record is replete with evidence that the link between diet and heart disease is weak, and efforts to alter cholesterol levels with diet are maddeningly complicated and fraught with peril. . . .

The final component of the program is the recommendation that millions of Americans take for the rest of their lives an expensive and unpleasant drug that the heart institute's own elaborate tests showed had at best a marginal effect. "The drug of choice," according to the program's treatment guidelines, is cholestyramine (Questran), or the chemically similar colestipol (Colestid). James I. Cleeman, the program coordinator, has estimated that one out of five people treated would ultimately be placed on drug therapy. Early reports at the American Heart Association meeting last November suggested that Cleeman's estimate was proving accurate: in one Iowa community 19.4 percent of the people treated were placed on drugs, in another 18.7 percent.

[Regarding t]he benefits of cholestyramine . . .: giving the drug for 7.4 years to 1,906 men at extremely high risk of heart attack had no effect on life expectancy but did produce a favorable trend toward fewer heart attacks, though this benefit occurred on too small a scale to pass the usual statistical tests of validity. And what about the costs? A total of $23 million in drugs may have prevented thirty-six heart attacks. This works out to $647,205 per heart attack possibly forestalled. Since the heart institute now proposes to give cholestyramine to those at lower risk than the specially selected trial participants, the statistics given above exaggerate the benefits. And although different approaches to cost-benefit analysis may produce somewhat different results, the remarkable fact is that the heart institute steadfastly refused to consider the cost question in any way. . . .

THE DANGERS OF LOW CHOLESTEROL

In 1974 a group of leading epidemiological researchers believed that cholesterol was going to be found guilty of another crime: an association with high rates of colon cancer. Such a trend had already been suggested by the data from entire countries—nations with diets rich in saturated fats also tended to have higher rates of colon cancer. Would people with colon cancer also have elevated blood-cholesterol levels? To find the answer, the research team assembled all the colon-cancer cases it could find among the records of men in six big epidemiological studies, including Ancel Keys's "Seven Countries" and the men in the Framingham study.

The men with cancer did not have high cholesterol levels, as expected. They had the opposite: cholesterol levels that were lower than average for their community or country. The baffled researchers suggested that further study—among other things, a fresh look at polyunsaturated fats, or vegetable oils—was needed. They had good reason to suspect vegetable oils. A few years before, in 1971, Morton Lee Pearce and Seymour Dayton had reported in *The Lancet* an excess of cancer deaths in a diet trial using diets high in polyunsaturated fats. In an action that was to be repeated many times, the researchers who favored lowering cholesterol levels through diet published a rebuttal, saying that Pearce and Dayton's results were likely a result of random chance.

However, the same relationship between low cholesterol levels and cancer was found again in 1978, in the World Health Organization's huge trial of clofibrate. So many cancer cases occurred in the treatment group that they outstripped any beneficial or protective effect of the cholesterol reductions. The findings raised more questions than they answered. Was it the drug or the cholesterol reductions that caused the cancer? The weight of expert opinion favored blaming the drug. Other, smaller studies linking low cholesterol levels to cancer in a variety of sites began to appear, but the authors usually dismissed what they found as "pre-clinical" indications of cancer—a matter of no great importance. . . .

The statistical association found in so many studies neither proves nor disproves that a causal link exists between low cholesterol levels and cancer. Nonetheless, it seems plain that these findings have been unwelcome to many researchers, who have exercised an extraordinary caution that was missing from discussions of the relationship between high cholesterol levels and heart disease. It is not, however, difficult to find a theory to explain the link between low cholesterol levels and cancer. The British heart researcher Michael F. Oliver asks, "How much cholesterol can be depleted from cell membranes over many years without alteration of their function?" In other words, did the membranes' functioning become sufficiently compromised to admit carcinogens?

Cancer is not the only hazard that has been associated with low cholesterol. Studies from Japan raise the question of whether low cholesterol levels increase the risk of stroke. As much as American researchers have admired what seems to be the effect of the Japanese diet in keeping blood-cholesterol levels and heart-disease deaths far below those found in the United States, other effects of the Japanese diet may not be so desirable. Japan experienced far higher rates of stroke and stomach cancer than the United States did. Heart-institute researchers apparently believed that in imitating the Japanese diet they could achieve one effect without incurring the others. But some Japanese epidemiologists weren't so sure. In the journal *Preventive Medicine*, Hirotsuga Ueschima and two colleagues published in 1979 a study showing that in rural communities where the average blood-cholesterol levels were below 180 mg/dl the rates of stroke were two to three times higher than those in areas with higher cholesterol levels. (The Japanese experts described the diets that produced typical serum-cholesterol levels of 167 as "grossly inadequate.") Once again heart-institute researchers greeted the unwelcome news with a torrent of objections.

In fact, the evidence is far from conclusive, in part because so little is known about the low cholesterol levels that the heart institute is aggressively pushing the American public to achieve. Despite decades of clinical trials using a multitude of strategies, the sad fact remains that none of them reduced cholesterol enough to provide an opportunity to understand either the risks or the benefits of low cholesterol levels. The trials have generally selected only subjects with extremely high cholesterol levels, and failed to alter those levels by much. The most aggressive dieting lowered cholesterol levels by only five to seven percent, drugs by only eight to ten percent. . . .

The biggest long-term cost of the National Cholesterol Education Program may be the delay it entails in the search for a better understanding of heart disease. The heart institute has declared

that the major cause of heart disease is elevated levels of serum cholesterol, specifically LDL.

But conflicting evidence has begun to mount. In Helsinki, Finland, a clinical trial recently succeeded in reducing fatal and nonfatal heart attacks by 34 percent and met the usual statistical tests, although, like the other trials, it had no effect on total mortality or life expectancy. The Helsinki trial is the most promising effort yet. It tested a drug called gemfibrozil (Lopid), a chemical relative of clofibrate, and the participants were Finnish men with severely elevated cholesterol levels. Although the Helsinki trial was a success in the battle to prevent coronary heart disease, it was also a distinct setback for the heart institute's official view that LDL is crucial. The most powerful effect of gemfibrozil is to raise levels of HDL, the so-called good cholesterol; it also seems to lower LDL, but its effect is not as powerful or consistent as that of cholestyramine. (Lovastatin appears to raise HDL slightly while lowering LDL by large amounts.) . . .

Other evidence also supports the idea that HDL is important. Framingham researchers found that HDL levels are a more accurate predictor of coronary heart disease than LDL levels. Studies of the positive effects of exercise show that the key benefit is probably the raising of HDL levels. Coronary heart disease begins to develop in young men at puberty primarily because of a sharp drop in HDL levels which does not occur in women.

HDL remains a promising frontier. But whether progress toward more effective prevention of heart disease will come through further trials of lovastatin or through continued research into HDL, it cannot but be slowed by those who have erroneously convinced themselves that they have identified the villain.

WHO WILL LIVE LONGER?

The fear of dying is what will be used to move millions of people into treatment of high cholesterol levels. The language of the cholesterol scare is simultaneously intimidating and vague. "You are at high risk of dying of a heart attack"; "You have dangerously high cholesterol"— these are frightening words indeed. But to probe beneath such generalities is to ask a specific question: What is the actual impact on life expectancy of high or low cholesterol levels? How great a danger to life do we face? Surprising answers to these questions emerge from the same body of heart-institute research that forms the scientific basis for much of what is known about cholesterol.

The elaborate and lengthy MR. FIT trial was quickly forgotten, having failed to demonstrate that following a strict diet, quitting smoking, and lowering blood pressure prevented deaths from heart attack. However, a spin-off project was to have greater influence. A team led by Jeremiah Stamler, of Northwestern University, continued to follow the entire group of 361,662 young and middle-aged men who had originally been screened as possible participants, tallying death rates. Although the team relied on frequently unreliable death certificates and a single cholesterol measurement for each man, the sample was impressive— seventy times as large as that for the Framingham study, twenty years more recent, and consisting of residents of eighteen cities rather than a single Massachusetts town. The MR. FIT spin-off gave rise to one of the most oft-repeated slogans of the campaign for cholesterol

reduction: Each one-percent reduction in cholesterol will lead to a two-percent reduction in the risk of dying of coronary heart disease.

The actual finding was the reverse: for each one-percent increase in cholesterol level, the risk of coronary heart disease increased two percent. The researchers also found no particular threshold at which the danger leaped higher—just a steady increase in the risk of dying of coronary heart disease as cholesterol levels rose. Furthermore, the 20 percent of men with the highest cholesterol levels were about three times as likely to die of heart disease as the 20 percent with the lowest cholesterol levels. The study has since become an important part of the empirical foundation for the assault on cholesterol.

The MR. FIT spin-off report, however, omitted the data needed to answer the critical question of how high or low cholesterol affects life expectancy. The answer can be deduced from a table published in a later article, about the same spin-off group, which was followed for seven years [see Table 1].

When one looks at total mortality and not just deaths from coronary heart disease, the hazards of high cholesterol levels appear quite modest. Further, these figures apply to only a minority of those at risk: young and middle-aged men. . . . [T]he relationship between high cholesterol levels and heart attacks is weak or nonexistent among the elderly, in whom most deaths from heart disease occur, and among pre-menopausal women, in whom the disease is rare.

An answer to the broad question of the benefits to life expectancy from lowering cholesterol levels through diet was found by a team of physicians and re-

Table 1

Serum-Cholesterol Level	Living	Dead From All Causes	Dead From Coronary Heart Disease
Low (202 mg/dl or less)	97.8%	2.2%	0.5%
Average (203–244 mg/dl)	97.3%	2.7%	0.9%
High (245 mg/dl or more)	96.2%	3.8%	1.7%

searchers at Harvard University. Using the risk-factor equations from the Framingham study and the diet results of the MR. FIT trial, the researchers calculated the benefits of a lifelong program of dieting. The team, led by William C. Taylor, published the results in the *Annals of Internal Medicine* in 1987. For persons without other risk factors, such as smoking or high blood pressure, they concluded, "we calculate a gain in life expectancy of 3 days to 3 months from a lifelong program of cholesterol reduction." Taylor and his co-authors also said that they might be overstating the benefits of cholesterol reduction, because they had assumed that no other increased risk would arise from limiting cholesterol intake and offset any reduction in the risk of heart disease. . . .

WHAT THE DATA REALLY SHOW

The evidence on cholesterol shows:

First, while the dangers of high blood-cholesterol levels have frequently been exaggerated, no evidence suggests anything desirable about levels above roughly 240 mg/dl. Among young and middle-aged men such elevated cholesterol levels have been convincingly associated with a greater risk of heart attack. But this relationship cannot be found among the elderly, who experience a majority of the deaths from heart attack, or among women before menopause.

Because the important cholesterol compounds in the blood are synthesized inside the human body, the link between high blood-cholesterol levels and diet is tenuous and indirect. A diet rich in saturated fat, cholesterol, or calories does not necessarily led to high blood-cholesterol levels (though it may be unhealthful for other reasons). Moderately severe dieting, even for years, does not produce a measurable reduction in the risk of dying from a heart attack, as MR. FIT, the government's biggest trial involving diet, convincingly demonstrated.

Individuals vary widely in diet response. Some can consume large amounts of cholesterol and saturated fat—or diet drastically—without producing any effect whatever on their blood-cholesterol levels. At the other extreme, about one in seven people may be highly sensitive to diet; dieting can either elevate or decrease the blood-cholesterol level of such a person by 10 percent or more.

Drugs lower blood-cholesterol levels more consistently and by larger amounts. But the drug the government now recommends—cholestyramine—produced disappointing results when it was tested. Daily treatment of nearly 2,000 men with severely elevated cholesterol for seven and a half years may have lowered the chances of a nonfatal heart attack from eight to seven percent. And while cholestyramine might have reduced the incidence of heart attacks, it did not improve life expectancy at all. The new drug lovastatin achieves even larger reductions in blood cholesterol, but neither its long-term safety nor its ability to prevent heart attacks has been tested.

Laboratory reports on cholesterol are seldom dependable, because of variation within individuals and inadequate quality control in clinical laboratories. The best way to get dependable information is through repeated cholesterol measurements using a laboratory machine known to be calibrated to a standardized national sample.

For most of the people most of the time, the advice of Eliot Corday may be helpful. "Cholesterol should be checked *only* if there are sound clinical indications," he wrote last February in the *Journal of the American College of Cardiology*. "A mixed diet low in calories and saturated fat should be recommended along with some physical exercise. . . . It is irresponsible to force the public into a costly cholesterol-reducing program without firm scientific evidence of the effectiveness of that intervention."

POSTSCRIPT

Is Cholesterol Reduction an Important Health Priority?

Moore and Johnson both present solid data and make intelligent conclusions regarding the role of cholesterol in bringing on heart disease. Is there one right answer? As Moore points out, all individuals respond to diet in different ways. Some people can eat whatever they choose, and their serum cholesterol level remains low; others are not so lucky. For most people, diet will have at least some impact on cholesterol levels. And foods that are high in saturated fats are not only related to elevated serum cholesterol levels; they are implicated in the development of certain cancers as well.

Americans should not be led to the point of hysteria about cholesterol, to the exclusion of concern about other risk factors, such as smoking and high blood pressure. Even cholesterol experts acknowledge that cigarette smoking is probably the most significant risk factor for heart disease. It is also true that dietary changes are difficult to make and that everyone does not need to make them. But it is hard to make a case for the high-fat, high-calorie diets many Americans eat. Most people would see some benefit (weight loss or lowered blood pressure) if they reduced their consumption of fatty meats, whole milk dairy products, and other high-fat foods.

In addition to the classic recommendation of reducing fat intake, other foods that allegedly lower serum cholesterol have recently been promoted. Oat bran became an immediate hit in the late 1980s, as scientific studies seemed to show that this soluble fiber could lower blood cholesterol. A study, published in the January 18, 1990, issue of *The New England Journal of Medicine*, made headlines when it disputed the benefits of oat bran. Olive oil was also highlighted in the media when an investigation associated it with lower serum cholesterol. This report was published in the February 2, 1990, issue of the *Journal of the American Medical Association*. A March 1, 1990, issue of *The New England Journal of Medicine*, however, reported that olive oil was not particularly beneficial. Finally, fish oils may also play a role in the prevention of heart disease. Studies have shown that a diet rich in marine fats may result in lowered serum cholesterol, although there is some dispute over this claim as well; does the benefit come directly from the fish oil or the fact that the fish replaces fatty meat in the diet? See *Mayo Clinic Proceedings* (February 1987).

Additional readings on the cholesterol controversy include: "Hypercholesterolemia: An Assessment of Screening and Diagnostic Techniques," *Modern Medicine* (April 1987); "The Canadian Consensus on Cholesterol: Final Report," *Canadian Medical Association Journal* (1988); and "A Fishy Deal in the Freezer," *Time* (January 16, 1989).

ISSUE 13

Can Large Doses of Vitamins Improve Health?

YES: Linus Pauling, from *How to Live Longer and Feel Better* (W. H. Freeman, 1986)

NO: Editors of *Harvard Medical School Health Letter*, from "Vitamin C— When Is Enough Enough?" *Harvard Medical School Health Letter* (January 1987)

ISSUE SUMMARY

YES: Nobel laureate and biochemist Linus Pauling argues that taking megadoses of vitamins, particularly vitamin C, can help people achieve superior health.
NO: The editors of the *Harvard Medical School Health Letter* acknowledge that humans have a need for vitamin C, but they argue that claims that taking megadoses will prevent colds and cancer and will prolong life are unsubstantiated and that doing so is potentially harmful.

In 1970, Nobel Prize winner Linus Pauling published a book entitled *Vitamin C and the Common Cold*, in which he maintains that huge doses, or "megadoses," of vitamin C can prevent colds by protecting body cells from attack by cold viruses. Pauling believes in taking one or two grams (1,000 to 2,000 milligrams) of vitamin C per day, which is about 20 to 40 times the recommended amount.

Many controlled studies on vitamin C and colds have been performed since Pauling's controversial book first came out. Taken together, they show that the effects of vitamin C, if any, are statistically very small. This does not exclude the possibility that the effects on *some* individuals might be considerable, especially if their vitamin C intakes have previously been low. Research on such effects is not easy to perform because people tend to be influenced by what they believe will be the effects of their medicine. In one now-classic study on the effects of vitamin C, for example, a questionnaire given at the end revealed that participants who received placebos (inert substances) and who thought they were being given vitamin C had fewer colds than the subjects who actually received vitamin C. In addition to curing the common cold, Pauling has also suggested that vitamin C megadoses might be an effective treatment against cancer. However, careful research involving the administration of 10 grams of the vitamin per day to persons with advanced cancer has shown no difference in either symptoms or survival time.

Although the medical establishment has ridiculed Pauling, recent research has shown that vitamin C and vitamin E together appear to be able to inactivate toxic chemicals in the body known as "free radicals." Free radicals, a byproduct of normal metabolism in cells, create problems by damaging the body's genetic material (DNA), altering biochemical compounds, damaging cell membranes, and killing cells. This chemical destruction is believed to play a major role in diseases such as cancer, heart disease, and even premature aging. Vitamins C and E may help reduce the damage from free radicals by inactivating these dangerous chemicals.

Most experts believe a balanced diet can provide enough vitamins to meet our needs. A balanced diet, however, consists of at least three to five servings of vegetables and two to four servings of fruit daily, which is currently consumed by less than 9 percent of Americans. For the remaining 91 percent, who do not eat enough vitamin-rich fruits and vegetables, vitamin pills may be an answer. Although most experts agree that a daily multiple vitamin will not hurt anyone, opinion is divided over whether or not people should take megadoses of vitamins to prevent disease or to delay aging.

In the following articles, Linus Pauling contends that taking megadoses of vitamins and following a few other health practices can extend one's life and years of well-being by 25 to 35 years. The editors of the *Harvard Medical School Health Letter* argue that megadoses of vitamin C have not been shown to prevent cancer and that there may be some serious side effects associated with its use.

YES

Linus Pauling

HOW TO LIVE LONGER
AND FEEL BETTER

I believe that you can, by taking some simple and inexpensive measures, lead a longer life and extend your years of well-being. My most important recommendation is that you take vitamins every day in optimum amounts to supplement the vitamins that you receive in your food. Those optimum amounts are much larger than the minimum supplemental intake usually recommended by physicians and old-fashioned nutritionists. The intake of vitamin C they advise, for example, is not much larger than that necessary to prevent the dietary-deficiency disease scurvy. My advice that you take larger amounts of C and other vitamins is predicated upon new and better understanding of the role of these nutrients—they are not drugs—in the chemical reactions of life. The usefulness of the larger supplemental intakes indicated by this understanding has been invariably confirmed by such clinical trials as have been run and by the first pioneering studies in the new epidemiology of health.

By the proper intakes of vitamins and other nutrients and by following a few other healthful practices from youth or middle age on, you can, I believe, extend your life and years of well-being by twenty-five or even thirty-five years. A benefit of increasing the length of the period of well-being is that the fraction of one's life during which one is happy becomes greater. Youth is a time of unhappiness; young people, striving to find their places in the world, live under great stress. The deterioration in health as the result of age usually makes the period before death a time of unhappiness again. There is evidence that there is less unhappiness associated with death at an advanced age than at an early age.

For such reasons it is sensible to take the health measures that will increase the length of the period of well-being and the life span. If you are already old when you begin taking vitamin supplements in the proper amounts and following other practices that improve your health, you can expect the control of the process of aging to be less, but it may still amount to fifteen or twenty years. . . .

THE IMMUNE SYSTEM

Our bodies are protected from onslaughts from both without and within by our natural protective mechanisms. The most important of these is the immune system. By keeping that system operating as effectively as possible we can make a significant contribution to our own good health.

When vitamins were first isolated and investigated half a century ago it was observed that a deficiency in any one of several of them resulted in impairment of the immune system, such as a decrease in the number of leucocytes in the blood and in a decreased resistance to infection. The vitamins required for good immunity are vitamin A, vitamin B_{12}, pantothenic acid, folacin, and vitamin C. These are also the vitamins that seem to strengthen the immune system when they are taken in amounts larger than those usually recommended. The effect on the immune system is greatest for vitamin C. . . .

There is much evidence that vitamin C is essential for the efficient working of the immune system. The mechanisms of the immune system involve certain molecules, mainly protein molecules that are present in solution in the body fluids, as well as certain cells. Vitamin C is involved both in the synthesis of many of these molecules and in the production and proper functioning of the cells. . . .

THE COMMON COLD

Most people catch several colds each year, usually in the fall, winter, and spring. When you catch a cold, after you have been exposed to cold viruses being spread by some other person, you may sneeze, feel a chill and scratchiness of the throat, develop a runny nose or stopped-up nose, and show other signs of the viral infection. Later, as the cold develops, you may feel rather miserable for two or three days. At this time it is usually wise to stay at home and rest in bed—for your own well-being and to spare your family and your colleagues the risk of exposure to your cold. After a week or ten days you have usually recovered. . . .

It has been known for more than twenty years that most people can keep from having colds, or, if a cold develops, can suppress most of its disagreeable manifestations, by the proper use of vitamin C. There is no need for you to be made miserable by the common cold.

In the medical literature, nonetheless, it continues to be said that no clearly effective method of treatment of the common cold has been developed. The various drugs that are prescribed or recommended have some value in making the patient more comfortable, by giving relief from some of the more distressing symptoms, but they have little effect on the duration of the cold. The fact that doctors have not had a good way of preventing and treating the common cold has been the subject of many jokes. The doctor says to the patient, "You have a cold. I don't know how to treat it, but if it develops into pneumonia, come to see me because I can cure pneumonia." There is another joke that appeared after the first edition of my book *Vitamin C and the Common Cold* was published in 1970. The doctor says to the patient, "You are suffering from an overdose of vitamin C, so I shall give you an injection of cold viruses to counteract it." . . .

I believe that every person can protect himself or herself from the common cold. Catching a cold and letting it run its course is a sign that you are not taking enough vitamin C.

I am convinced by the evidence now available that vitamin C is to be preferred to the analgesics, antihistamines, and other dangerous drugs that are recommended for the treatment of the common cold by the purveyors of cold medicines. Every day, even every hour, radio and television commercials extol various cold remedies. I hope that, as the results of further studies become available, extensive educational efforts about vitamin C and the common cold will be instituted on radio and television, including warnings against the use of dangerous drugs, like those about the hazards of smoking that are now sponsored by the United States Public Health Service, the American Cancer Society, the Heart Association, and other agencies. . . .

CANCER

Cancer, including neoplasms of the lymphatic and hematopoietic (blood-cell-forming) systems, is the cause of 22 percent of all deaths in the United States. Each year about 600,000 people develop cancer, and most of them, more than 420,000, die of the disease. The amount of suffering associated with cancer is much greater than that for most other diseases. It is for this reason that the federal government has emphasized research on cancer and has allocated several hundred million dollars per year for cancer research, reaching $1 billion this year. . . .

One new idea is that large doses of vitamin C may be used both to prevent cancer and to treat it. The most important work along this line has been carried out by Dr. Ewan Cameron, formerly chief surgeon in Vale of Leven Hospital,

Loch Lomondside, Scotland, and now medical director of the Linus Pauling Institute of Science and Medicine. . . .

In 1951 it was reported that patients with cancer have usually a very small concentration of vitamin C in the blood plasma and in the leucocytes of the blood, often only about half the value for other people. This observation has been verified many times during the last thirty years. In 1979 Cameron, Pauling, and Brian Leibovitz listed thirteen studies, all showing large decreases in both plasma and leucocyte concentrations. The level of ascorbic acid in the leucocytes of cancer patients is usually so low that the leucocytes are not able to carry out their important function of phagocytosis, of engulfing and digesting bacteria and other foreign cells, including malignant cells, in the body. A reasonable explanation of the low level of vitamin C in the blood of cancer patients is that their bodies are using up the vitamin in an effort to control the disease. The low level suggests that they should be given a large amount of the vitamin in order to keep their bodily defenses as effective as possible. . . .

The late Dr. William McCormick of Toronto appears to have been the first to recognize that the generalized connective-tissue changes that attend scurvy are identical with the local connective-tissue changes observed in the immediate vicinity of invading neoplastic cells (McCormick, 1959). He surmised that the nutrient (vitamin C) known to be capable of preventing such generalized changes in scurvy might have similar effects in cancer. The evidence that cancer patients are almost invariably depleted of ascorbate lent support to his view.

There are some other interesting associations between scurvy and cancer. The historical literature contains many allusions to the increased frequency of "cancers and tumors" in scurvy victims. A typical autopsy report of James Lind (Lind, 1753) contains phrases such as "all parts were so mixed up and blended together to form one mass or lump that individual organs could not be identified," surely an eighteenth-century morbid anatomist's graphic description of neoplastic infiltration. Conversely, in advanced human cancer, the premortal features of anemia, cachexia, extreme lassitude, hemorrhages, ulceration, susceptibility to infections, and abnormally low tissue, plasma, and leucocyte ascorbate levels, with terminal adrenal failure, are virtually identical with the premortal features of advanced human scurvy.

Epidemiological evidence indicates that cancer incidence in large population groups is inversely related to average daily ascorbate intake. Of the several different published investigations, all giving essentially the same result, I mention the work of the Norwegian investigator Bjelke who in 1973 and 1974 published accounts of the exhaustive studies that he had made of gastrointestinal cancers by means of a dietary survey by mail and a case-controlled study. His work, which involved more than thirty thousand people in the United States and Norway, included a determination of the consumption of various foods, as well as smoking habits and other factors. He found a negative correlation between the consumption of fruits, berries, vegetables, and vitamin C and the incidence of gastric cancer, whereas starchy foods, coffee, and salted fish were positively correlated. The two most important factors were, he concluded, the total intake of vegetables and the intake of vitamin C. The greater the

intake of vegetables and of vitamin C, the smaller is the incidence of cancer. . . .

Better results are obtained with intakes greater than 10 g per day.

In our book *Cancer and Vitamin C*, Cameron and I stated our conclusion that "This simple and safe treatment, the ingestion of large amounts of vitamin C, is of definite value in the treatment of patients with advanced cancer. Although the evidence is as yet not so strong, we believe that vitamin C has even greater value for the treatment of cancer patients with the disease in earlier stages and also for the prevention of cancer." . . .

THE LOW TOXICITY OF VITAMINS

Physicians, these days, are armed with increasingly potent drugs, which they must prescribe and administer with great care, keeping their patients under alert surveillance. In extension of this chary attitude, I think, they are cautious about vitamins. It is easy to develop an exaggerated and unjustified fear of the toxicity of vitamins. During recent years it has become the practice of writers on medical matters and on health to warn their readers that large doses of vitamins may have serious side effects. For example, in *The Book of Health, a Complete Guide to Making Health Last a Lifetime* (1981), edited by Dr. Ernst L. Wynder, president of the American Health Foundation, it is said that "So-called megavitamin treatment—taking massive doses of a particular vitamin—should be avoided. Vitamins are essential nutrients, but high dosages become drugs and should only be taken to treat a specific condition. Large doses of the fat-soluble vitamins A and D have well-recognized ill effects, and this must be true of others, too. Large doses of vitamin C are mainly excreted in the urine. In the absence of certainty that 'megavitamins' are safe, they are better avoided."

The authors of this book on health are depriving their readers of the benefit of the optimum intakes of these important nutrients, the vitamins, by creating in them the fear that any intake greater than the usually Recommended Daily Allowances (RDA) may cause serious harm.

I believe that the main reason for this poor advice is that the authors are ignorant. They make the false statement that large doses of vitamin C are mainly excreted in the urine. They give no indication that they know that the RDAs of the vitamins are the intakes that probably would prevent most people in "ordinary good health" from dying of scurvy, beriberi, pellagra, or other deficiency disease but are not the intakes that put people in the best of health. They seem not to know that there is a great span between the RDAs and the toxic amounts of those that exhibit any toxicity and that for several vitamins there is no known upper limit to the amount that can be taken. These authorities on health should show greater concern about the health of the American people. . . .

Nobody dies of poisoning by an overdose of vitamins.

I have credited the physician with caution for the patient, even though the caution is entirely misplaced. Several people have suggested another possible explanation to me. It is that the drug manufacturers and the people involved in the so-called health industry do not want the American people to learn that they can improve their health and cut down on their medical expenses simply by taking vitamins in the optimum amounts.

The bias against vitamins may be illustrated by an episode that occurred a few years ago. A small child swallowed all the vitamin-A tablets that he found in a bottle. He became nauseated and complained of a headache. His mother took him to an East coast medical-school hospital, where he was treated and then sent home. The professors of medicine then wrote an article about this case of vitamin poisoning. The article was published in the *New England Journal of Medicine*, the same journal that had rejected a paper by Ewan Cameron and me on observations of cancer patients who received large intakes of vitamin C. The *New York Times* and many other newspapers published stories about this child and about how dangerous the vitamins are.

Some child in the United States dies of aspirin poisoning every day. These poisonings are ignored by the medical-school doctors, the medical journals, and the *New York Times*.

There are seven thousand entries in the index of the *Handbook of Poisoning* by Dr. Robert H. Dreisbach, professor of pharmacology at Stanford University School of Medicine. Five of these seven thousand are about vitamins. These five entries refer to vitamins A, D, K, K_1 (a form of K), and the B vitamins.

You do not need to worry about vitamin K. It is the vitamin that prevents hemorrhage by promoting coagulation of the blood. It is not often put into vitamin tablets. Adults and children usually receive a proper amount, which is normally supplied by "intestinal bacteria." The physician may prescribe vitamin K to newborn infants, to women in labor, or to people with an overdose of an anticoagulant. The toxicity of vitamin K is a problem of interest to the physician who administers it to a patient.

Vitamin D is the fat-soluble vitamin that prevents rickets. It is required, together with calcium and phosphorus, for normal bone growth. The RDA is 400 International Units (IU) per day. It is probably wise not to exceed this intake very much. Dreisbach gives 158,000 IU as the toxic dose, with many manifestations of toxicity: weakness, nausea, vomiting, diarrhea, anemia, decreased renal function, acidosis, proteinuria, elevated blood pressure, calcium deposition, and others. Kutsky (*Handbook of Vitamins and Hormones*, 1973) states that 4000 IU per day leads to anorexia, nausea, thirst, diarrhea, muscular weakness, joint pains, and other problems.

Vitamin A is usually mentioned as a prime example in any discussion of the toxicity of vitamins. Thus in her 1984 *New York Times* article "Vitamin Therapy: The Toxic Side Effects of Massive Doses," the writer about foods, Jane E. Brody, stated that "Vitamin A has been the cause of the largest number of vitamin poisoning cases." She did not mention that the patients did not die (as do many of those poisoned by aspirin and other drugs), but she did give two case histories, presumably the worst that she could find.

A 3-year-old girl was hospitalized with confusion, dehydration, hyperirritability, headache, pains in the abdomen and legs, and vomiting, the result of daily ingestion of 200,000 I.U. of vitamin A a day for three months (2,500 is the amount recommended for a child her age, theoretically to prevent respiratory infections).

A 16-year-old boy who took 50,000 I.U. daily for two and a half years to counter acne developed a stiff neck, dry skin, cracked lips, swelling of the optic nerves, and increased pressure in the skull.

These reports indicate that the long-continued daily intake of doses of vita-min A ten to eighty times the RDA may cause moderately severe effects. Dreisbach in his book on poisons says that twenty to one hundred times the RDA may in time cause painful nodular periosteal swelling, osteoporosis, itching, skin eruptions and ulcerations, anorexia, increased intracranial pressure, irritability, drowsiness, alopecia, liver enlargement (occasionally), diplopia, and papilledema....

Until 1983 it was thought that none of the water-soluble vitamins had significant toxicity even at very high intakes. Then a report was made that seven persons who had been taking 2000 to 5000 mg per day (one thousand to three thousand times the RDA) of vitamin B_6 for between four months and two years had developed a loss of feeling in the toes and a tendency to stumble (Schaumberg et al., 1983). This peripheral neuropathy disappeared when the high intake of the vitamin was stopped, and the patients showed no damage to the central nervous system.

We may conclude that there is an upper limit, one thousand times the RDA, to the daily intake of vitamin B_6. The authors of the report were far more cautious, however; they recommended that no one take more than the RDA of this vitamin, 1.8 to 2.2 mg per day. To follow this recommendation would deprive many people of a means for improving their health by taking 50 or 100 mg or more every day. . . . Many orthomolecular psychiatrists recommend 200 mg per day to their patients, with some patients taking 400 to 600 mg per day (Pauling, 1983). Hawkins reported that "In more than 5,000 patients we have not observed a single side effect from pyridoxine administration of 200 mg of vitamin B_6 daily." (Hawkins and Pauling, 1973).

Single doses of 50,000 mg of vitamin B_6 are given without serious side effects. These large doses are given as the antidote to patients suffering from poisoning with an overdose of the antituberculosis drug isoniazid (Sievers and Harrier, 1984).

No fatal doses are known for folacin (folic acid), pantothenic acid, vitamin B $_{12}$, and biotin. These four water-soluble vitamins are described as lacking in toxicity, even at very high intakes. The values of the RDA for adult males are 400 micrograms (µg) for folacin, 7 mg for pantothenic acid, 3 µg for vitamin B_{12}, and 200 µg for biotin. . . .

There is no known fatal dose of vitamin C. As much as 200 grams (g) has been taken by mouth over a period of a few hours without harmful effects. Between 100 and 150 g of sodium ascorbate has been given by intravenous infusion without harm.

There is little evidence of long-term toxicity. I know a man who has taken over 400 kilograms (kg) of this vitamin during the last nine years. He is a chemist, working in California. When he developed metastatic cancer, he found that he could control his pain by taking 130 g of vitamin C per day, and he has taken this amount, over a quarter of a pound per day, for nine years. Except that he has not succeeded in ridding himself completely of his cancer, his health is reasonably good, with no indication of harmful side effects of the vitamin. . . .

TAKE THE OPTIMUM SUPPLEMENTARY AMOUNT OF EACH OF THE ESSENTIAL VITAMINS EVERY DAY.

No matter what your present age is, you can achieve significant benefit by starting the regimen now. Older people can benefit greatly, because they have special need for optimum nutrition. Steadfast adherence is essential. It is fortunate that the regimen imposes few restrictions on the diet, so that for the most part you can add to the quality of your life by eating foods that you enjoy. What is more, you can, and it is even recommended that you do, enjoy the moderate intake of alcoholic beverages. . . .

[B]y keeping in the best of health, in particular by maintaining optimum intake of the vitamins, we can resist the entire long list of illnesses that afflict mankind. The list begins with the afflictions laid upon us by deficiencies of the vitamins, deficiencies so easily cured by restoring the functions in the biochemistry of the body; the vitamins help us to fend off infection and fortify our tissues against the self-assault of cancer and the auto-immune diseases. With the best understood vitamin, vitamin C, as our example, we have been able to envision a new kind of medicine, the orthomolecular medicine that uses substances natural to the body both to protect it from, and to cure, illness. Already, orthomolecular medicine has shown how vitamin C can prevent and cure and may yet eliminate from human experience the illness most familiar and most baffling to the old medicine, the common cold. . . .

The physicians and the old-fashioned professors of nutrition have for fifty years been urging that everyone adopt a diet that is described as healthful. For two or three decades we were all urged to eat a well-balanced diet, with servings of the four categories of food: meat or fish or fowl; cereals; fruits and red or yellow vegetables; and dairy products. This dietary regimen was urged on us whether or not we liked all these foods. Recently much of the enjoyment of life has been taken away from many of us by additional strong recommendations by these authorities. We are told that we should not eat a succulent steak, because of the animal fat. We are told that we should not eat eggs, because of the cholesterol they contain; instead, we are urged to eat a sort of factory product, a preparation, probably not very appealing to the taste, that is made by treating eggs with some chemical solvent to remove some of the cholesterol. We are told not to eat butter. Going to a fine restaurant then is not a pleasure, but a source of worry and a cause of a feeling of guilt.

Why are these recommendations being made to us? A part of the reason is that good health depends on a good supply of vitamins. In the past, to obtain even a passable supply of vitamins, leading to even ordinary poor health, required a moderately large intake of fruits and vegetables. In every culture in countries other than the tropical ones some special foods, such as sauerkraut and pickles, had to be eaten in order for us to survive the winter. Even with the best selection of foods the health of most people has in the past not been very good.

The revolution that is taking place now liberates us from this obsession to restrict our diet, to refrain from eating those foods that we like. The only limitations that I suggest are that you not eat large amounts of food and that you limit your intake of the sugar sucrose. This nutritional freedom has become possible because of the availability of vitamin and mineral supplements.

Moreover, it is now possible to take these important nutrients in the optimum amounts, far larger than can be obtained in foods, and in this way to achieve a sort of superhealth, far beyond what was possible in earlier times. We can be grateful to the organic chemists and biochemists of the past 140 years who laboriously solved the riddles of the nature of the compounds of carbon and the way that they interact with one another in the human body. Because of their efforts, we are now able to get greater enjoyment of life.

NO

**Editors of *Harvard Medical
School Health Letter***

VITAMIN C—
WHEN IS ENOUGH ENOUGH?

It is now 16 years since Linus Pauling's book *Vitamin C and the Common Cold* appeared. This very successful little volume converted ascorbic acid from a deservedly popular vitamin into one of the nutritional superstars of our time. In 1970, Dr. Pauling opined that the average person needs 1–2 grams a day of vitamin C for "optimum health." By 1986, Pauling was advocating a routine daily intake of 6–18 grams, as a way not only to prevent colds but to treat cancer and prolong life.

That's a lot of vitamin C. The average American diet supplies 60–70 milligrams a day, or about one fifteenth of a gram; 25% of the population consumes a good deal more, but even at that the amount ranges between 130 and a little over 200 milligrams. In the United States, the recommended dietary allowance (RDA) has been set at 60 milligrams—very near the typical intake. Someone who regularly consumes this amount of vitamin C is well protected from scurvy.

And the reason everyone *must* take in at least some vitamin C is to prevent scurvy. Unlike all but a few other animal species, human beings are incapable of producing ascorbic acid from sugar (which the vitamin chemically resembles). As a result, connective tissue breaks down, because collagen, a crucial structural protein, can't be manufactured. Easy bruising or bleeding, loosening of teeth, failure of wound healing, and feeling thoroughly miserable are among the major signs of this nasty deficiency disease. Unless vitamin C comes to the rescue, sudden death from uncontrollable bleeding follows. However, 10 milligrams a day is all it takes to cure or prevent scurvy. By consuming 60 milligrams a day, the average American maintains body stores adequate to stave off the illness for a month or two if suddenly switched to a diet with no vitamin C whatever.

Nobody is really arguing that point. The live controversy is whether vitamin C has some benefit other than preventing scurvy, and whether a larger intake than average is needed to obtain it. Yes, says Dr. Pauling, who has received one Nobel prize for his work in basic chemistry and another for his efforts to reduce the risk of nuclear warfare. An effective writer and skilled debater, Dr. Pauling has won many converts to his point of view. Where does the evidence now stand?

COLDS

Dr. Pauling's 1970 book presented the case that taking large amounts of vitamin C would reduce the number of colds people get, or make the symptoms milder when a cold managed to break through defenses presumably enhanced by the vitamin. In the next 10 years several tests of his hypothesis were conducted. The results of these trials have been quite consistent. There is no measurable reduction in the frequency of colds when people take vitamin C at these levels, and specific symptoms, such as sneezing or runny nose, are not affected. On the other hand, people who take extra vitamin C do seem to feel better during the cold and are likely to take less time off work. According to the Canadian investigator, Terence W. Anderson, who conducted three studies on more than 5,000 adults, the sense of well-being that comes from taking additional vitamin C is probably achieved with a daily dose of 200 milligrams or less. People who don't regularly take extra vitamin C may get some benefit if they take as much as 1 gram a day for up to 4 days at the beginning of a cold.

Dr. Pauling criticized most of the studies conducted to test his hypothesis on the grounds that not enough vitamin C was given. (This is, of course, a conveniently elastic criticism.) In general, much larger doses of the vitamin were given than anyone normally receives in the diet. The design of the research projects was not air-tight, but on the whole these studies were carefully executed on enough subjects to warrant the conclusion that vitamin C does not have the dramatic effect predicted in the 1970 book. On the other hand, it's fair to say that a modest increase of vitamin C taken during a cold often makes people feel better, even when they don't know they are taking vitamin C. The effect is enhanced if subjects know or guess that they are taking the vitamin.

CANCER

Dr. Pauling and some colleagues subsequently put forth a more startling claim for vitamin C: that it could improve survival in cancer—particularly cancer of the colon, which has been highly resistant to chemotherapy. The basis for this claim was the reported experience of terminal cancer patients at a Glasgow hospital. These patients were given 10 grams a day of vitamin C. Their length of survival was then compared with that of other patients who had not been so treated. An important flaw in this study was that the investigators picked their control cases (10 for every patient given vitamin C) from hospital records. This procedure is notoriously unreliable. If the people selecting control cases unconsciously chose records of patients with more advanced disease, the effect attributed to vitamin C could have been completely spurious.

Two careful investigations at the Mayo Clinic have attempted to test vitamin C as an anti-cancer agent. Patients with incurable bowel cancer were selected and randomly assigned to vitamin C or a placebo. Neither the patients nor the investigators knew who was getting what. Vitamin C was given as long as the patient could take oral medication or until the disease had progressed, as measured by a 50% growth in the diameter of the tumor, a weight loss of at least 10%, or marked worsening of symptoms. Neither study showed any benefit to the patients receiving vitamin C.

The first Mayo investigation was conducted on patients who had received prior treatment, such as chemotherapy. Dr. Pauling objected that chemotherapy weakens the immune system and thus had probably undermined the potential effectiveness of vitamin C, so the second study was conducted on patients who had received no previous chemotherapy for their disease. Dr. Pauling criticized this study on the grounds that it did not exactly reproduce his procedure, which was to give vitamin C in very high doses until the patient died (and he objected when the HMS Health Letter failed to mention this difference in its April 1985 account of the Mayo report). Dr. Pauling speculated that the Mayo result came about because withdrawal of the vitamin led to a kind of "rebound" in which the patient was made worse. There was, however, no evidence for such a rebound in the Mayo subjects, whose experience after withdrawal of the vitamin was no different from that of the control patients after the placebo was withdrawn.

On the basis of evidence currently available, vitamin C seems highly unlikely to be effective at controlling cancers that resist other forms of therapy. On the other hand, vitamin C may play a useful role in preventing some kinds of cancer.

The reason for thinking so is based partly on laboratory results, which indicate that vitamin C prevents formation of nitrosamines (potent carcinogens) in the digestive tract. Many foods, especially cured and charcoal-broiled meats, contain nitrates and nitrites, which can be converted by bacteria to nitrosamines. Vitamin C inhibits this process. Vitamin C also has been found to inhibit formation of a carcinogenic substance in the bladders of female mice. In several recent epidemiologic studies from Australia, southern Louisiana, and Hawaii, people with diets high in vitamin C appeared to be protected from bowel, stomach, or bladder cancer, respectively. These results are only suggestive, though; they are not conclusive.

LONGEVITY

In his latest book, *How to Live Longer and Feel Better* (1986), Dr. Pauling advocates taking 6–18 grams of vitamin C supplements a day as the keystone of a program to prolong life by 25–35 years. Readers must decide for themselves whether this promise is credible or extravagant. There is hardly any evidence on which to base a discussion.

One study, however, has attempted to assess the relationship between life expectancy and use of vitamin C supplements. The subjects were a group of 479 elderly subscribers to *Prevention* magazine, all of whom were living in California. These people were questioned about their dietary and other health practices—including vitamin intake. Six years later, differences between those who had died and those who survived were compared. There was, as the authors summarized, "no clear reduction in total mortality because of high levels of vitamin intake *per se*." The authors were James E. Enstrom and Linus Pauling (*Proceedings of the National Academy of Sciences,* October 1982, p. 6023).

MINIMUM, OPTIMUM, MAXIMUM

The human body is remarkably adaptable. It seems capable of getting by on relatively small amounts of vitamin C, and it protects itself quite well from overdoses of this vitamin. On the other hand, in some people large doses could be something between a nuisance and a health hazard.

The main nuisance from very large doses is diarrhea, but many people seem capable of adapting to high intake of the vitamin without much difficulty. There's a theoretical possibility that people whose bodies have grown accustomed to eliminating excess vitamin C would develop scurvy if for any reason the high doses were abruptly stopped. This doesn't seem to be a common occurrence. Pregnant women are advised not to take large quantities of the vitamin to avoid inducing such a rebound in their babies after birth. High intake of vitamin C may slightly increase the risk of forming kidney stones in some people. Because vitamin C favors the absorption of iron, people who suffer from an excess of iron storage in their bodies would be harmed by taking large doses. On the other hand, people who need iron probably are helped by this effect.

Taking high doses of vitamin C can interfere with certain standard laboratory tests, including those that check for blood in the stool (which will be falsely negative) and tests for urine sugar (results on Tes-Tape® and Chemstrip uG® can be falsely lowered, whereas Clinitest® gives a falsely high result). Skepticism about vitamin C should be tempered by the recognition that standard recommendations for intake (such as the RDA) may not be high enough to account for all the potential benefit that vitamin C could offer. By and large, these recommendations are based on the quantity known to prevent scurvy and provide a margin of safety. The useful amount beyond that is anybody's guess. Ours is that the range is somewhere between the current RDA of 60 milligrams and, at the very most, 250 milligrams a day. The main reason for choosing the higher figure is that this is around the dose that will saturate the body's ability to store vitamin C. Amounts in excess of 250 milligrams daily do not produce significantly higher tissue levels; most of the dose is lost in the urine. On the whole, people probably would do better to get their vitamin C from food than from supplements, because the foods that are high in vitamin C have other good things as well.

Though most people taking supplements of up to 1 gram or so a day probably won't be harmed, the long-term consequences of taking this amount of vitamin C really aren't known. And anyone who is taking medications or needs regular medical testing should check with a physician to make sure that the excess vitamin won't interfere with his or her care.

POSTSCRIPT

Can Large Doses of Vitamins Improve Health?

A recent article in the *Journal of the National Cancer Institute* (April 17, 1991) provides an overview of a 1990 symposium sponsored by the National Cancer Institute and the National Institute of Diabetes and Digestive and Kidney Diseases on the biological functions of vitamin C and its possible relation to cancer. These organizations report that vitamin C is protective against cancers of the esophagus, larynx, oral cavity, pancreas, stomach, rectum, lung, breast, and uterus. In a *Time* magazine article (April 6, 1992), research is presented that links several different vitamins to the prevention of many diseases. The article cites a number of scientists who believe that vitamins may be much more important than previously thought in warding off heart disease, cataracts, cancer, and even aging.

While many respected scientists involved with vitamin research maintain that these nutrients may be the answer to disease prevention and treatment, there are many skeptics who disagree. Victor Herbert, a professor of medicine at New York City's Mount Sinai medical school, believes that vitamin pills do not do any good. He feels that Americans get all the vitamins they need in their diets and that taking supplements is a waste of money. This opinion is echoed by Elizabeth M. Whelan and Frederick Stare in *The One-Hundred Percent Natural Purely Organic, Cholesterol-Free, Mega-vitamin, Low-Carbohydrate Nutrition Hoax* (Atheneum Publishers, 1983). Whelan and Stare contend that taking large amounts of vitamins is costing people unnecessary millions of dollars and may be costing people their health. They believe that "the human body is simply not equipped to handle on a daily basis the amount of vitamin C equivalent to an entire carload of oranges or the vitamin A from a carload of carrots." The opinions of Whelan, Stare, and Herbert are also endorsed by many reputable agencies, such as the American Medical Association and the National Institutes of Health. These organizations maintain the position that Americans, in general, eat a healthy diet that provides all the necessary nutrients for good health and well-being.

While experts disagree, consumers continue to be confused about exactly how much of specific vitamins is needed and what is the best way to get them—from food or from pills? Although it is probably preferable to get needed vitamins and minerals from the diet, many American diets do not provide an adequate amount of the necessary foods, particularly fruits and vegetables. Supplements could certainly furnish the nutrients missing from the diet. However, supplements can only supply certain nutrients, such as vitamins, minerals, and amino acids; pills do not contain the fiber, carbohydrates, or calories necessary for maintaining the body and supplying energy. While in theory these nutrients could be put into pill form, it would be an impractical and tasteless substitute! Real food also supplies a variety of other, more obscure, nutrients which may have some value.

Additional readings on the subject may be found among the following: "Vitamin C Gets a Little Respect," *Science* (October 18, 1991); "$2.9 Billion for Vitamins," *FDA Consumer* (April 1987); "Santa Barbara Physician Warns of Vitamin Overdosing," *California Council Against Health Fraud Newsletter* (March/April 1983); "Nutrition Insurance: A Skeptical View," *Nutrition Forum* (May 1987); and "Food Versus Pills Versus Fortified Foods," *Dairy Council Digest* (March/April 1987).

ISSUE 14

Does Exercise Increase Longevity?

YES: Joel Gurin, from "Linking Exercise With Longevity," *Runner's World* (April 1985)

NO: Henry A. Solomon, from *The Exercise Myth* (Harcourt Brace Jovanovich, 1984)

ISSUE SUMMARY

YES: *American Health* editor Joel Gurin claims that there is conclusive evidence that regular exercise will increase longevity.
NO: Cardiologist Henry A. Solomon argues that longevity is based on a complex interaction of genetics and life-style and that claims that exercise is a major variable in increasing longevity are exaggerated, unsubstantiated, and based on conflicting data.

Many Americans are involved in an exercise and fitness revolution that began over 20 years ago. In the early 1970s, medical reports linked Americans' sedentary life-styles with rising incidences of heart disease and cancer, both of which contribute to decreased longevity. As a result, millions of Americans began jogging and aerobic dancing to achieve fitness and to possibly add years to their lives. Although many people continue to work out on a consistent basis, currently only 10 percent of Americans over 18 exercise on a regular basis.

In the past, the healthiest form of exercise was thought to be a daily constitutional—a modestly brisk walk that could be accomplished without any special equipment or overexertion. As the fitness movement of the 1970s and 1980s gained momentum, millions began not only doing strenuous exercise (no pain, no gain!) but spending millions of dollars on sporting equipment, sweat suits, and expensive athletic shoes.

Most believers in strenuous exercise claim that it leads to better health and longer life. They believe, specifically, that exercise promotes cardiovascular health and protects against heart attack, the leading cause of death in the United States and other industrialized nations. This belief is supported by the American Heart Association, as well as many other health organizations, and by most physicians. In the early 1950s, the result of a now-classic study of London transit workers was that the more sedentary bus drivers experienced more heart disease than the physically active conductors (Morris and Heady, "Mortality in Relation to the Physical Activity of Work: A Preliminary Note on Experience in Middle Age," *British Journal of Industrial Medicine*, 1953). The authors of the study concluded that physical activity offers protection from coronary heart disease. Although there was little public reaction to this early report, there was considerable impact on the medical profession. To this day, this report is considered by doctors to be a landmark study proving that a relationship exists between exercise and the prevention of disease and premature death.

In the following selections, Joel Gurin argues that the evidence is clear that exercise increases longevity by lowering blood pressure, cancer risks, and other illnesses that affect life span. Henry A. Solomon, however, does not support data claiming exercise increases longevity. He believes that exercise can help make people feel and look better but that heredity and other factors determine longevity and that the evidence in favor of exercise is overblown.

YES
Joel Gurin

LINKING EXERCISE WITH LONGEVITY

Dr. Ralph S. Paffenbarger Jr. is a patient man. A *very* patient man. He's worked for more than 20 years to find convincing evidence that people who exercise live longer than those who don't. And now, finally, he's succeeded.

Paffenbarger isn't a slow worker; far from it. But his medical field—epidemiology, the study of disease in populations—makes you take the long view. Methods vary, but each is glacially slow. Paffenbarger sent out questionnaires to thousands of people, followed up on them every few years, and waited to see who died first, and of what diseases. Then he tallied the numbers and reached his conclusions.

Since 1960, Paffenbarger has been studying the effects of exercise in groups as diverse as Ivy League alumni and San Francisco longshoremen. But the people who really proved his case were 17,000 men of Harvard—16,936, to be exact. Paffenbarger has followed the Harvard alumni long enough to reach a stunning conclusion. "It really is the first demonstration that people who exercise vigorously live longer than those who don't," says Dr. Peter Wood, associate director of the Stanford Center for Research in Disease Prevention.

Paffenbarger admits with a smile that his is not the *very* first research to prove this crucial point. "You can go way back in history to Bernardino Ramazzini in 1700, who compared tailors with people more active and found that the tailors didn't live as long," he says. But Paffenbarger insists that his study is "the first adequate one . . . in a scientific sense."

The news is welcome at a time when runners may wonder whether they're doing themselves more harm than good. The deaths of Jim Fixx and Jacques Bussereau (the Frenchman who collapsed in the New York Marathon) started a scare over exercise and health. At the same time, a popular book, Dr. Henry Solomon's *The Exercise Myth*, claimed that the evidence in favor of exercise had been vastly overblown.

Paffenbarger's work provides the best answer to the skeptics. He's taken the care and time to build a solid case. "There's no question that Ralph Paffenbarger is thorough and hardworking—what they call in the business a shoeleather epidemiologist, who really does it the old way, the hard way, with huge numbers of people and long periods of time," says Wood.

Paffenbarger became interested in exercise long before it was fashionable. In 1958, he decided to do research on heart disease, and came to Boston to talk to Paul Dudley White, the charismatic cardiologist who treated Dwight Eisenhower. White had been promoting exercise as rehabilitation for cardiac patients, and thought it might help prevent heart attacks in the first place. But he couldn't prove it, because really good data didn't exist. So when Paffenbarger asked him what aspect of heart disease was worth studying, White's answer was clear: its relationship with physical activity.

Two years later, in 1960, Paffenbarger joined the famous Framingham study. An ongoing survey of more than 5000 people in a Massachusetts town, this study has been critical in revealing the risk factors for coronary heart disease: high blood pressure, cigarette smoking and high cholesterol.

When Paffenbarger arrived, the researchers at Framingham were collecting relatively little information about the role of physical activity, so he decided to study a group outside the town. Paffenbarger and his colleagues liked the idea of focusing on an alumni group, and began going from college to college. They were looking for several things. "It takes a university that keeps its records," Paffenbarger says. "A university that has a very active alumni organization that keeps track of its survivors. And it takes a university that has the insight to make important documents available."

Paffenbarger tried the University of California, Ohio State, the University of Wisconsin, the military academies and many others—and rejected them. In the end, he settled on the University of Pennsylvania and Harvard. It's the Harvard alumni who have provided the bulk of the evidence on exercise and health. (Though Paffenbarger has studied these men, and is now on the Harvard faculty, he is not an alumnus himself.)

His survey included men who came to Harvard between 1916 and 1950. Paffenbarger went back to their records to see what sports, if any, they had taken part in during college and high school. Then he sent out a questionnaire to find out how active they were decades after graduating. Finally, he sat back and waited to see how their history of activity would affect their health.

In order to compare all the men on an equal basis, Paffenbarger translated their activity levels into use of kilocalories—known to nonscientists simply as calories. The calorie is nothing more than a measure of energy. A piece of candy containing 100 calories gives the body that much energy as fuel. If running a mile burns 100 calories, that means it takes that long to work off the candy (see box).

After a decade, the Harvard men showed a clear pattern. Those who burned fewer than 2000 calories a week in climbing stairs, walking, or sports had a *64 percent higher* risk of heart attack than their more active classmates. Exercise clearly offered people some protection.

It was only when the men had been followed for six more years, however, that Paffenbarger could really prove his case. The data were analyzed and broken down a dozen different ways. Finally, in the *Journal of the American Medical Association* (July 27, 1984), Paffenbarger and his colleagues published the

---

CALORIES BURNED PER MILE

The first figure is weight; the second is the number of calories you'll burn each mile you run, depending on your weight: 120/80; 130/87; 140/93; 150/99; 160/106; 170/112; 180/119; 190/125; 200/131; 210/137; 220/144.

---

best evidence yet that exercise can not only prevent heart disease, but extend life.

The researchers divided the Harvard men into three groups: those who got less than 500 calories worth of exercise a week (only about 15 percent of the group), those who did 500 to 2000 calories of activity, and those who did more than 2000. The results were clear: The more exercise they did, the longer they lived. The men in the most active group had a death rate 39 percent lower than those in the least active group.

The link between exercise and health was no accident. You might guess that a man who had a stronger constitution by birth would be more likely to exercise and less likely to develop heart disease or other illnesses. In other words, people who were healthy by nature might be more likely to exercise, rather than the other way around.

But Paffenbarger found that exercise helped whether a man's parents had died young or old, a rough measure of his genetic constitution. He also showed that even men who had been healthy in college—healthy enough to be varsity athletes—weren't protected unless they worked out later in life.

The study also uncovered some real surprises. Exercise not only lowered the risk of death from coronary heart dis-

ease, it also lowered the risk of dying from respiratory illness. Though Paffenbarger is confident of his finding, he still puzzles over why it's true. There's also a hint that the overall risk of cancer may drop with exercise, though Paffenbarger finds this less convincing.

Most remarkable, however, was the way exercise overshadowed other factors that influence health. Exercise dramatically lowered the risk of heart attack even if a man had high blood pressure, was a smoker, was overweight or had parents with heart disease.

Paffenbarger also ran the numbers through a computer to compare the risk of a sedentary lifestyle—less than 2000 calories of exercise a week—with other risk factors. A sedentary life turned out to be less of a risk than high blood pressure. But within this group of men, a sedentary lifestyle was *more* dangerous than being overweight, having a family history of heart disease, or even smoking.

Paffenbarger estimates that going from a sedentary to an active lifestyle could reduce the average man's heart attack risk by 33 percent. And he believes that getting more than 2000 calories a week of exercise would be even more protective. As a rough estimate, it looks like 2500 or 2750 calories a week provide an even greater benefit.

No study, even one as extensive as Paffenbarger's, offers definitive proof of the benefits of exercise. But many researchers take Paffenbarger's work as strong evidence, largely because it matches other major, recent studies.

One is another study of Paffenbarger's of a very different group of men: San Francisco longshoremen. In 1969, while the Harvard study was under way, Paffenbarger moved to California to head the Bureau of Chronic Diseases in the state health department. (Today he shuttles back and forth between California and Massachusetts, holding appointments at both Stanford and Harvard.)

The bureau had been conducting a study of longshoremen, analyzing their smoking and the incidences of obesity and diabetes, but neglecting the energy outputs of their jobs. Paffenbarger analyzed the old job-assignment records of about 6000 longshoremen, going back to 1951. With the help of these records, he was able to estimate the amount of energy they'd spent on the job.

The results, published in the mid-1970s, were striking. The burly cargo handlers burned more than 8500 calories a week on the job—roughly the equivalent of running three marathons. They turned out to have roughly half as many fatal heart attacks as less active men.

It's a nice counterpart to the Harvard study. The longshoremen were lower-middle-class, the Harvard men middle-to-upper. The longshoremen had extremely active jobs. The Harvard men "spend no energy whatsoever" at work, says Paffenbarger. "They sit at a desk, walk to the water cooler, etcetera." But since both groups manifested the benefits of exercise, they must be benefits that cross socioeconomic lines, and accrue whether you're active on the job or in your spare time.

Other epidemiological surveys have shown that exercise can lower the risk of heart disease. The Framingham study had accumulated some good data on exercise by the late 1970s. As you might expect, once again, sedentary people had much higher rates of heart disease than active people.

Heart disease is still the main ailment that has been linked to inactivity—and seems to be prevented by exercise. It makes sense. Exercise has been shown to control most of the major risk factors that lead to heart disease. For example, several studies have shown that exercise reduces blood pressure, and that a fitness-oriented lifestyle can keep blood pressure down as a person ages.

Exercise also helps balance your blood cholesterol. A Boston University study showed that monkeys on a high-cholesterol diet lived longer and healthier lives if they were forced to exercise. And exercise seems to increase blood levels of high-density lipoprotein, or HDL, the so-called "good" cholesterol that clears out the arteries.

Despite all the data, though, there are still some unanswered questions. For one thing, it's not certain how much exercise per week is the best amount. For another, Paffenbarger would still like to prove that exercise boosts longevity whenever you start—even late in life.

"I think we have some excellent, unquestioned data on the effect of physical activity on cardiovascular disease," he says. "But what we haven't done is look at individuals who have been sedentary until recently, and then have converted to a more active way of life."

Paffenbarger knows that many of the Harvard alumni have been swept along by the fitness boom; a larger proportion are active now than were in the 1960s. With time, he should be able to show whether even a late start has its benefits, as he suspects it does. "That's the next important area for all of us to be concerned with," he says.

The answer won't come overnight. But Paffenbarger still has time. After all, he says, "we've been involved in this since 1960. I hope we'll be involved another 24 years."

A CRITIC'S COMPLAINTS

Though Paffenbarger's results are striking, some critics still question whether exercise can lead to a longer life. Perhaps the most vocal is Cornell cardiologist Henry A. Solomon, author of *The Exercise Myth.* Through talk shows, Solomon has spread the word that exercise isn't all it's cracked up to be. And his critique of studies like Paffenbarger's is basic to his case.

In his book, Solomon writes that "despite the widespread notion that physical exercise can add years to your life, there is no reliable evidence to prove it."

Paffenbarger's latest study was published after *The Exercise Myth* was written, but Solomon finds the latest report, like the earlier ones, unconvincing. "It's lousy evidence," he says. "And lousy evidence shouldn't be given credence."

Solomon's criticism is based on a number of questions about Paffenbarger's research methods. In general, however, the questions he raises are ones that Paffenbarger has considered very carefully—and has answers for.

One potential problem, for example, is the risk of getting inaccurate information in a mailed questionnaire. Paffenbarger only followed men who told him at the start of the study that they had never had heart disease. Suppose that many of these men actually did have heart disease, and just hadn't realized it or admitted it.

People with heart disease are less likely to be physically active, and more likely to have heart attacks later on. So, says Solomon, an apparent link between inactivity and heart attacks might be explained by the number of men who had undiagnosed heart disease at the beginning.

Paffenbarger, however, was concerned about this potential problem from the start, and checked the questionnaire's results in three different ways. "First, we invited some of the alumni back to Cambridge, and matched their questionnaire responses against what we found in our own examinations with our own physicians," he says. "Second, we did personal interviews with some 800 subjects. And third, we wrote to the physicians of 2200 subjects."

With these cross-checks, Paffenbarger found that the mailed responses were accurate 85 to 98 percent of the time. "It was a well thought out set of questionnaires," he says, "pretested, pilot-tested, and used because they were proven to be reliable and valid measures of activity and health."

Solomon has other complaints about Paffenbarger's work. He points out that many alumni never answered the request for information (though the number who did, about 70 percent, is quite respectable for a study like this). Paffenbarger collected no data on cholesterol level, now known to be a major risk factor for heart disease—"A glaring omission," says Solomon. And so on.

It's so difficult to conduct a large-scale, long-term study that it may never be possible to do one that could answer everyone's objections. By Solomon's standards, would it *ever* be possible to answer the question of whether exercise prolongs life?

"I don't know," says Solomon. "Perhaps the question isn't answerable. All I've said in *The Exercise Myth* is that what you've been told about the benefits of exercise isn't proven." That seems to depend on your standards of proof.

HOW ACTIVE
ARE YOU?

If you want to know how you compare with 17,000 Harvard alumni or how close you are to the 2000-calories-a-week mark, there are a few rules of thumb you can follow.

• The simplest, says Paffenbarger, is this: If you spend about 2½ hours a week running at a moderate pace, that's worth about 2000 calories.

• If you want a more precise measurement, you can use the same guidelines Paffenbarger did in his questionnaire. Just figure out how much of the following activities you do per week, and add up the calories:

Flights of stairs climbed (10 steps per flight): four calories per flight.

City blocks walked (12 blocks per mile): eight calories per block.

Strenuous activities—Running, swimming, cross-country skiing, singles tennis or racquet sports, basketball, soccer, bicycling: 10 calories per minute.

Moderate activities—Doubles tennis, brisk walking, downhill skiing: 7½ calories per minute.

Light activities—Boating, dancing, golf, yard work, bowling, baseball: five calories per minute.

• If you want a more precise estimate of the calories you burn in your running program, use the accompanying figures. The more you weigh, the more calories you'll burn per mile. Your running speed, however, has surprisingly little effect on the calories you burn in a given distance. If you run a mile in six minutes instead of eight, you'll only burn about five additional calories. The chart shows how many calories people of different weights would burn in a 7:20 mile.

NO

THE CASE AGAINST LONGEVITY

Longevity is the most compelling of the promised protections of exercise. Millions of today's exercise enthusiasts, seduced into the latest warm-up gear, designer labels sticking to their sweating bodies, run, dance, stretch and strain in the hope and expectation of living longer lives. But despite the widespread notion that physical exercise can add years to your life, there is no reliable evidence to prove it.

Biological aging is a fact of life. Although some researchers conclude that we have a biological potential of up to 110 or 120 years, living that long is so rare that most scientists settle for a biological limit of about 80 years, barring extraordinary new and fundamental discoveries about the human organism and the aging process itself.

We think of ourselves as living longer than our forebears, but in fact the biological limit hasn't changed. Tombstones in eighteenth- and nineteenth-century cemeteries are witness to the frequency then of infant and childhood mortality, deaths in epidemics and death in childbirth. But the ages of those who did reach "old age" are not different from ages today. Advances in medicine and public health have primarily extended the *average* life expectancy by allowing more people to reach the upper limit of their biological potential. A larger proportion of the population reaches old age these days, but the upper limit of life expectancy has not been dramatically altered. If the two leading causes of death today—cardiovascular disease and cancer—were conquered, overall life expectancy would still increase by only a few years.

Given the biological limit to longevity, the likelihood of attaining that age depends upon many things. Diseases, although different ones from those that took our forebears to early graves, are still important. But other, less tangible, circumstances, generally lumped under the label "psychosocial variables," seem to matter as much, since they affect mortality to a large degree. For example, at any given age more than twice as many people from the "lowest" social class die as from the "highest" social class. And men with less than eight years of schooling have a 50 percent higher death rate than those completing one or more years of college.

Because psychosocial variables can exert a large influence on any analysis of mortality, a valid study of the relationship between physical activity and

From Henry A. Solomon, *The Exercise Myth* (Harcourt Brace Jovanovich, 1984). Copyright © 1984 by Henry A. Solomon. Reprinted by permission of Harcourt Brace Jovanovich, Inc. Notes omitted.

longevity must take a long list of them into account. Studies that don't—and that is nearly all of them—are simplistic and unreliable.

Besides social group and educational status, the best-documented psychosocial variables that influence longevity are income, occupational status, work satisfaction, social activity and life satisfaction. People who are more prosperous, who hold higher-level positions, who find their work and their social lives interesting and gratifying live longer! . . .

Heredity, nutrition, habits and environment are other factors that affect the length of our lives. If your parents, your Great-Aunt Matilda and your Grandfather Jones all lived to be ninety, you can make a fair guess that longevity "runs in the family." What you eat and whether you smoke or drink alcohol in more than moderate amounts affect health in general, and therefore longevity. Mortality rates vary by where a person lives, partly because of such factors as industrial pollution, but also because of such measures as the pace of life, the social integration possible and the extent of community support systems of all kinds.

Clearly, the issue of longevity is enormously complex. So many things—many of which are poorly understood and very difficult to measure—are involved that predicting the life span of any individual is virtually impossible. If marriage itself is protective, does a "bad" marriage work just as well? And if not, how happy must the marriage be, and how do you measure that? A person might be delighted with his job as a coal miner, but easily contract "black lung" in his forties. Mrs. Smith might volunteer for every committee in sight out of strident contempt for the incompetence of her co-

workers, so that the fact of her membership is a poor measure of her social interaction.

Into this morass of ill-defined and unquantifiable elements has been dropped the complicated question of exercise and *its* relationship to longevity. However ill-founded, the idea that exercise is protective and life-enhancing is compelling. Children, who can run about all day, strike us as "full of life," and we say of an active older person that she is "brimming with vitality." When we are full of life, it often brims over in the form of activity. What is more logical, then, than to build from this the notion that exercise *puts* more life into a person? The idea is accepted by most people as a biological "given." There is an almost unassailable belief that exercise adds more life, and that we will therefore not die so early. The idea has a simple and intuitive logic, a seductive, magical quality.

Studies of the relationship between physical activity and mortality deal almost exclusively with death from coronary disease, and with good reason. Cardiovascular disease is the leading cause of death in industrialized societies, and any measurable impact on life expectancy would have to affect a major cause of death. Physical activity is, moreover, dependent upon the cardiovascular system at least to the extent that the heart pumps the blood and the arteries carry it around the body so the cells can use the oxygen in it to provide energy for activity. No one has even suggested a link between physical activity and other major causes of death, such as cancer or car accidents.

Research in this area is thoroughly confused. In study after study of physical activity and mortality, results are so contradictory that any conclusion that could be drawn from them amounts to no more than unsubstantiated opinion. . . .

No doubt these studies could also be picked apart to reveal their flaws. All such rather unsophisticated uses of statistics are powerless to explain so complicated a thing as why one person dies of a heart attack at fifty, and his neighbor lives on to be one hundred. Studies that claim that physical activity confers longevity are inevitably faulty in design, and just as much contradictory data can be accumulated by the same methods. Jeremy Morris, who maintained his belief that physical activity protected against coronary heart disease, was nevertheless a candid man. "The evidence on this problem is quite conflicting," he admitted. "In several studies coronary heart disease has been found to be associated with physical activity/inactivity in the expected way. In as many, no relationship was demonstrated, or an equivocal or opposite one; and why this is so is still quite unclear."

There is one simple explanation of why the relationship between activity and longevity is unclear. They may not be related. How much you exercise and how long you live may not be connected at all.

If you start with the belief that exercise is beneficial to life, then contrary or conflicting data will certainly be troubling and puzzling. But if you start with no particular assumption, if you approach the subject with an open mind, suddenly there is no problem. Some people who exercise live a long time, some don't; some sedentary people die young, others live to their biological limit. There is about the same relationship between activity and longevity as you might find if you were to compare the amount of

chocolate pudding children eat with the likelihood of their coming down with chicken pox—that is, no relationship at all. That's the most reasonable interpretation of the "conflicting" results from all the studies.

Unfortunately, little reason has lit this murky subject. If Morris's London transit worker study had shown either no protection from exercise or actual deleterious effects, as later studies did, then the dilemma of today would not exist. The burden of proof would be on those trying to establish a protective effect of exercise, something they in all likelihood couldn't do. Instead, however, the protective effect of exercise is widely accepted as a biological fact, and the burden of proof falls on those, like me, who doubt it.

Faulting the methodology of studies that purport to show life-extending benefits of exercise and laying out an equal array of data contradicting that notion is still not enough to dispel the ingrained idea that exercise must somehow be good. The exercise believers have a fallback position: Since coronary disease is an insidious affair, usually unfelt and undiagnosed until it is well advanced, perhaps exercise cannot really undo it once it is well established. But maybe exercise can affect its course, delay its appearance, retard its progression. Perhaps exercise benefits us in a less obvious but nevertheless important way. If we could just find, for example, that exercise did something to the way fats pile up in our arteries, or to the way our arteries respond to damage, or to anything else we know contributes to coronary artery disease, we might then still have a treatment we should respect and recommend.

POSTSCRIPT

Does Exercise Increase Longevity?

There seems to be a continuing debate over the benefits of exercise, particularly strenuous exercise, such as running. In 1977, running advocate James Fixx wrote *The Complete Book of Running* (Random House). The book, which claims that running can help individuals become healthier and happier, sold nearly 1 million copies in hardcover alone. Fixx, a former smoker and "couch potato," became highly visible in the media, promoting both his book and the sport of running. Unfortunately, Fixx died at age 52 of a heart attack (while running). His followers claim that since premature heart disease ran in Fixx's family, he actually prolonged his life by running; had he continued his former unhealthy habits, he would have died much sooner than 52.

Other sources of controversy surrounding running involve the risk of injury. In one extensive survey of the records of over 1,600 runners in Vancouver, British Columbia, doctors identified over 1,800 injuries over a two-year period (Clement, Taunton, and Smart, "A Survey of Overuse Running Injuries," *Physician and Sports Medicine*, May 1981). Injuries in other sports and various kinds of exercises are also common. Skiing accidents, for instance, are so common that they are almost expected. Contrary to popular belief, better and more experienced athletes tend to acquire more serious and disabling injuries. This may be because these athletes play harder and take more risks.

While running may or may not have been beneficial for Fixx, and while exercise-related injury is always a concern, several studies carried out during the past few years have attempted to prove that regular exercise is not only beneficial but that it will also add years to one's life. In 1988, researchers Siegfried Heyden and George Fodor reviewed the literature linking exercise and life expectancy ("Does Regular Exercise Prolong Life Expectancy?" *Sports Medicine*, June 1988). They found that exercise will indeed prolong life expectancy but that smoking and other risk factors may be more important issues. In early 1989, Steven Blair, the leader of the largest study ever carried out to measure fitness, suggested that even modest amounts of exercise can substantially reduce a person's chance of dying prematurely (*Journal of the American Medical Association*, November 1, 1989). A report in *American Health* (March 1992) identifies several studies that indicate exercise may help prevent cancer by enhancing the immune system. Other articles supporting the relationship of exercise and longevity include "Exercise and Longevity: A Little Goes a Long Way," *The New York Times* (November 3, 1989); "You Can Reverse Aging," *Family Circle* (October 16, 1990); and "Exercise and Longevity," *Time* (March 17, 1986).

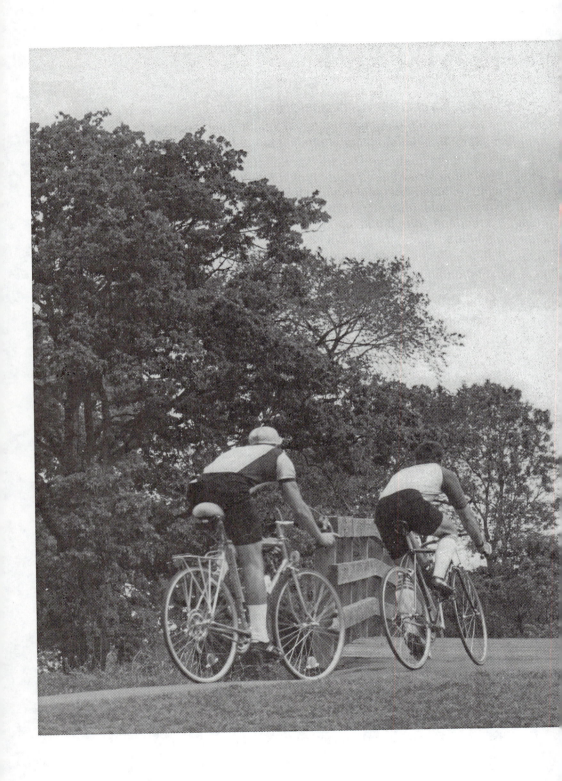

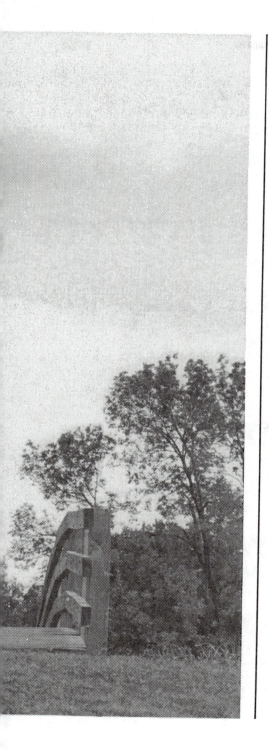

PART 6

Environmental Health Issues

Many of today's environmental concerns are related to modern technology. Since World War II, thousands of new chemicals have been developed for the manufacturing and agricultural industries. Energy needs have increased, resulting in the release of environmental pollutants. As the world population continues to grow, how can food production keep pace without increasing environmental degradation and exposure to toxic substances? This section discusses controversies related to environmental health issues.

Are Pesticides in Foods Harmful to
   Human Health?

Is Acid Rain a Serious Environmental
   Problem?

ISSUE 15

Are Pesticides in Foods Harmful to Human Health?

YES: Lawrie Mott and Karen Snyder, from "Pesticide Alert," *Amicus Journal* (Spring 1988)

NO: Bruce Ames, from "Too Much Fuss About Pesticides," *Consumers' Research* (April 1990)

ISSUE SUMMARY

YES: Pesticide researchers Lawrie Mott and Karen Snyder maintain that the very foods consumers are trying to eat more of—fresh fruits and vegetables—are those that are most contaminated with harmful pesticide residues.
NO: Professor of biochemistry and molecular biology Bruce Ames argues that any risks from pesticides in foods are minimal and that fears are greatly exaggerated.

Throughout history, farmers and other food growers have fought with insect and weed pests that invade the food supply and cause disease and discomfort. Early attempts to reduce pest damage included purely physical attacks—burning and stepping on the pests, as well as saying prayers and performing ritual dances. A few more effective measures were discovered before modern times. These included sulfur compounds, plant extracts, wood ashes, and natural pest enemies.

For the past 50 years, the battle against pests has escalated, and some of the most lethal and sophisticated chemicals ever invented have been used against them. Modern pesticides, such as DDT, were first introduced in the late 1940s, upon which scientists proclaimed total victory against the destruction and diseases carried by insects. While many dispute this victory, the evidence of these chemical weapons against insects is present in streams, rivers, soils, and our bodies. Most of us carry traces of several chemical pesticides in our body tissues. Moreover, although pesticides are used specifically to kill insect pests, many of them are quite toxic to humans as well. Pesticides are responsible for an estimated 25 million human poisonings each year, mostly of children under 10.

To cause harm to humans, a pesticide must be taken internally through the mouth, skin, or respiratory system. Eating unwashed fruits or vegetables that were recently sprayed with pesticides or entering a field too soon after pesticide application are examples of ways in which pesticides may enter the body. Symptoms of acute or one-time exposure include headache, fatigue, abdominal pain, coma, and death. Long-term exposure may cause cancer, mutations, or birth defects.

Pesticide poisoning from sprayed fruits and vegetables became a national issue when reports of the contamination of the apple crops made headlines. Since 1968 some red varieties of apples have been sprayed with a chemical growth regulator that prevents the apples from dropping off trees before they ripen, improves color and firmness, and extends shelf life. The chemical, known as daminozide, is marketed under the trade name Alar. Alar penetrates the pulp of the apple and cannot be washed, cooked, or peeled off. In 1986, processors and stores, bowing to consumer pressure, vowed not to accept apples treated with the chemical. It appears that a breakdown product of Alar, which is formed when treated apples are heated, is a low-level cancer-causing agent.

In addition to the risk of Alar, a report released in the spring of 1987 by the National Academy of Sciences claimed that pesticides may be responsible for as many as 20,000 cases of cancer a year. In their report, the academy identified 15 foods (tomatoes, beef, potatoes, oranges, lettuce, peaches, pork, wheat, soybeans, beans, carrots, chicken, corn, grapes, and apples) treated with a small group of pesticides that pose the greatest risk of cancer. While these figures are certainly frightening, many scientists believe that too much fuss is being raised about pesticides. They point out that many foods contain natural cancer-causing agents, and they argue that people are still better off with a high intake of fruits and vegetables—ironically because they contain nutrients that may help prevent cancer.

In the following articles, Lawrie Mott and Karen Snyder contend that a lot of what is sold in supermarkets is not safe and that the government does not adequately test the fruits and vegetables that are sold to the public. Bruce Ames feels that while it is good for consumers to be concerned about what they eat, the hysteria about pesticide residues may not be warranted by the actual risk they pose.

YES

Lawrie Mott and Karen Snyder

PESTICIDE ALERT

If you are like most Americans, when you go to the supermarket, you try to choose foods that are healthy. Instinctively, you steer your shopping cart towards the produce section. The typical produce section currently stocks over five times the number of items displayed a decade ago. The increased availability and variety of fresh fruits and vegetables is due, in part, to the extensive use of chemical fertilizers and pesticides. Yet, residues of these agricultural chemicals can remain in our food. The fruits and vegetables in your supermarket may contain invisible hazards to your health in the form of residues of pesticides.

All of us are exposed to pesticides on a regular basis. The food we eat, particularly the fresh fruits and vegetables, contains pesticide residues. In the summer of 1985, nearly 1,000 people in several western states and Canada were poisoned by residues of the pesticide Temik in watermelons. Within two to twelve hours after eating the contaminated watermelons, people experienced nausea, vomiting, blurred vision, muscle weakness, and other symptoms. Fortunately, no one died, though some of the victims were gravely ill. Reports included grand mal seizures, cardiac irregularities, a number of hospitalizations, and at least two stillbirths following maternal illness.

In 1986, the public grew increasingly concerned over the use of the plant-growth regulator, Alar, on apples. Primarily used to make the harvest easier and the apples redder, Alar leaves residues in both apple juice and apple sauce. The outcry led many food manufacturers and supermarket chains to announce they would not accept Alar-treated apples.

Also in 1986, approximately 140 dairy herds in Arkansas, Oklahoma, and Missouri were quarantined due to contamination by the banned pesticide, heptachlor. Dairy products in eight states were subject to recall. Some milk contained heptachlor in amounts as much as seven times the acceptable level. Those responsible for the contamination were sentenced to prison terms.

Last year, the National Academy of Sciences issued a report on pesticides in the food supply which concluded that pesticides in our food may cause

From Lawrie Mott and Karen Snyder, "Pesticide Alert," *Amicus Journal*, vol. 10, no. 2 (Spring 1988). Copyright © 1988 by Natural Resources Defense Council. Reprinted by permission.

more than 1 million additional cases of cancer in the United States over our lifetimes. Although some have argued that this theoretical calculation is excessively high, the number was based on the presence of fewer than thirty carcinogenic pesticides in our food supply (many more pesticides applied to food are carcinogens) and does not consider potential exposure to carcinogenic pesticides in drinking water.

The repetition of the Temik, Alar and other stories suggests that the government programs designed to protect us from pesticide residues may be inherently flawed. These events also demonstrate the need for information on a series of fundamental issues concerning pesticide residues in food. As it now stands, you have no way of knowing if your food contains dangerous residues or whether the amount of residue you are eating is hazardous. Not only is government testing of food for residues spotty and inadequate, not only are some levels of pesticides allowed in food being challenged by leading scientists as too high, but no state or federal government agency really attempts to answer your most basic questions about pesticide residues in food—questions such as what pesticides are found in your food, what level of residue is safe, and who should make these decisions.

Each year, approximately 2.6 billion pounds of pesticides are used in the United States. Pesticides are applied in countless ways throughout the United States, not just on food crops. They are sprayed on forests, lakes, city parks, lawns, and playing fields, and in hospitals, schools, offices, and homes, and are contained in a huge variety of products from shampoos to shelf paper, mattresses to shower curtains. As a consequence, pesticides may be found wherever we live and work, in the air we breathe, in the water we drink, and in the food we eat. A former director of the federal government's program to regulate pesticides called these chemicals the number one environmental risk, because all Americans are exposed to them.

By definition, pesticides are toxic chemicals—toxic to insects, weeds, fungi, and other unwanted pests. Most are potentially harmful to humans and can cause cancer, birth defects, changes in genetic material that may be inherited by the next generation (genetic mutations), and nerve damage, among other debilitating or lethal effects. Many more of these chemicals have not been thoroughly tested to identify their health effects.

Pesticides applied in agriculture—the production of food, animal feed, and fiber, such as cotton—account for 60 percent of all U.S. pesticide uses other than disinfectants and wood preservatives. Pesticides are designed to control or destroy undesirable pests. Insecticides control insects; herbicides control weeds; fungicides control fungi such as mold and mildew; and rodenticides control rodents. Some of these chemicals are applied to control pests that reduce crop yields or to protect the nutritional value of our food; others are used for cosmetic purposes to enhance the appearance of fresh food.

As a result of massive agricultural applications of pesticides, our food, drinking water, and the world around us now contain pesticide residues; they are literally everywhere—in the United States and throughout the world. In fact, though all these chemicals have been banned from agricultural use, nearly all Americans have residues of the pesticides DDT, chlordane, heptachlor, aldrin, and dieldrin in their bodies. Ground water is the source of drinking water for 95 percent of rural Americans and 50 percent of all Americans; yet, according to a 1987 Environmental Protection Agency (EPA) report, at least twenty pesticides, some of which cause cancer and other harmful effects, have been found in ground water in at least twenty-four states. In California alone, fifty-seven different pesticides were detected in the ground water. The banned pesticide DBCP remains in 2,499 drinking water wells in California's San Joaquin Valley—1,473 of these contaminated wells are not considered suitable for drinking water or bathing because the DBCP levels exceed the state health department's action level. As more states conduct ground water sampling programs for pesticides, more pesticides are expected to be found. Surface water supplies have also been found to contain pesticides. For example, the herbicide alachlor, or Lasso, has contaminated both ground and surface water in the midwest, primarily as a result of use on corn and soybeans. The federal government must provide financial assistance to cotton and soybean farmers because enormous surpluses of these crops exist in the United States.

The extent of contamination of our food is unknown. The federal Food and Drug Administration (FDA) monitors our food supply to detect pesticide residues. Between 1982 and 1985, FDA detected pesticide residues in 48 percent of the most frequently consumed fresh fruits and vegetables. This figure probably understates the presence of pesticides in food because about half of the pesticides applied to food cannot be routinely detected by FDA's laboratories, and the agency samples less than one percent of our food.

The cumulative effect of widespread, chronic low-level exposure to pesticides is only partially understood. Some of the only examples now available involve farmers and field workers. A National Cancer Institute study found that farmers exposed to herbicides had a six times greater risk than nonfarmers of contracting one type of cancer. Other studies have shown similar results, with farmers exposed to pesticides having an increased risk of developing cancer. Researchers at the University of Southern California uncovered startling results in a 1987 study sponsored by the National Cancer Institute. Children living in homes where household and garden pesticides were used had as much as a sevenfold greater chance of developing childhood leukemia.

Another frightening consequence of the long-term and increasing use of pesticides is that the pest species farmers try to control are becoming resistant to these chemicals. For example, the number of insects resistant to insecticides nearly doubled between 1970 and 1980. Resistance among weeds and fungi has also risen sharply in the last two decades. In order to combat this problem, greater amounts of pesticides must be applied to control the pest, which in turn can increase the pest's resistance to the chemical. For example, since the 1940s pesticide use has increased tenfold, but crop losses to insects have doubled.

Pesticides can also have detrimental effects on the environment. The widespread use of chlorinated insecticides, particularly DDT, significantly reduced bird populations, including bald eagles, ospreys, peregrine falcons, and brown pelicans. DDT is very persistent and highly mobile in the environment. Animals in the Antarctic and from areas never sprayed were found to contain DDT or its metabolites. Though most of the organochlorines are no longer used in the United States, continuing use in other nations has serious environmental consequences. Other types of pesticides now applied in the United States have adverse effects on the environment.

A FEBRUARY 1987 EPA REPORT, ENTITLED *Unfinished Business*, ranked pesticides in food as one of the nation's most serious health and environmental problems. Many pesticides widely used on food are known to cause, or suspected of causing, cancer. To date, EPA has identified fifty-five pesticides that could leave residues in food as being carcinogens. Other pesticides can cause birth defects or miscarriages. Some pesticides can produce changes in the genetic material, or genetic mutations, that can be passed to the next generation. Other pesticides can cause sterility or impaired fertility.

Under today's scientific practices, predictions of the potentially adverse health effects of chemicals on humans are based on laboratory testing in animals. Unfortunately, the overwhelming majority of pesticides used today have not been sufficiently tested for their health hazards. The National Academy of Sciences estimated, by looking at a selected number of chemicals, that data to conduct a thorough assessment of health effects were available for only ten percent of the ingredients in pesticide products used today.

A 1982 congressional report estimated that between 82 percent and 85 percent of pesticides registered for use had not been adequately tested for their ability to cause cancer; the figure was 60 percent to 70 percent for birth defects, and 90 percent to 93 percent for genetic mutations. This situation has occurred because the majority of pesticides now available were licensed for use before EPA established requirements for health effects testing.

In 1972, Congress directed EPA to reevaluate all these older chemicals (approximately 600) by the modern testing regimens. Through reregistration, EPA would fill the gaps in required toxicology tests. By 1986, however, EPA still had not completed a final safety reassessment for any of these chemicals. Roughly 400 pesticides are registered for use on food, and 390 of these are older chemicals that are undergoing reregistration review. To make matters worse, scientists are uncovering new types of adverse health effects caused by chemicals. For example, a few pesticides have been found to damage components of the immune system—the body's defense network to protect against infections, cancer, allergies, and autoimmune diseases. Yet testing for toxicity to the immune system is not part of the routine safety evaluation for chemicals. In short, pesticides are being widely used with virtually no knowledge of their potential long-term effects on human health and the human population is unknowingly serving as the test subject.

The lack of health effects data on pesticides means that EPA is regulating pesticides out of ignorance, rather than knowledge. This poses particularly serious consequences for EPA's regulation of pesticides in food. Pesticides may only be applied to a food crop after EPA has established a maximum safe level, or tolerance, for pesticide residues allowed in the food. However, EPA's tolerances may permit unsafe levels of pesticides for five reasons:

1. EPA established tolerances without necessary health and safety data.

2. EPA relied on outdated assumptions about what constitutes an average diet, such as assuming we eat no more than 7.5 ounces per year of avocados, artichokes, melons, mushrooms, eggplants or nectarines, when setting tolerance levels.

3. Tolerances are rarely revised when new scientific data about the risks of a pesticide are received by EPA.

4. Ingredients in pesticides that may leave hazardous residues in food, such as the so-called "inert" ingredients, are not considered in tolerance setting.

5. EPA's tolerances allow carcinogenic pesticide residues to occur in food, even though no "safe" level of exposure to a carcinogen may exist.

The EPA is not solely responsible for the flaws in the federal government program to protect our food supply. The FDA monitors food to ensure that residue levels do not exceed EPA's tolerances. Food containing pesticide residues in excess of the applicable tolerance violates the food safety law and FDA is required to seize the food in order to prevent human consumption. However, FDA is not always capable of determining which foods have illegal pesticide residues. For instance, FDA's routine laboratory methods can detect fewer than half the pesticides that may leave residues in food. Some of the pesticides used extensively on food that cannot be regularly identified include alachlor, benomyl, daminozide and the EBDCs. Furthermore, FDA's enforcement against food with residues in excess of tolerance is ineffective: according to a 1986 General Accounting Office report, for 60 percent of the illegal pesticide residue cases

identified, FDA did not prevent the sale or the ultimate consumption of the food.

TO GET A BETTER PICTURE OF THE PESTICIDES that occur in the foods most commonly eaten, NRDC analyzed representative federal and state pesticide monitoring data. From 1982 to 1985, FDA analyzed 19,515 samples of the twenty-six types of fruits and vegetables nationwide. Forty-eight percent contained detectable residues. In the same period, the California Department of Food and Agriculture (CDFA) analyzed 17,237 produce samples. Pesticide residues were detected in 14 percent of the samples. These numbers most likely understate the amount of pesticides in food because the laboratory tests cannot detect all the chemicals applied to our food. The discrepancy between FDA and CDFA results is probably due to FDA's ability to detect a greater number of chemicals in lower amounts and the greater number of imported samples analyzed by FDA.

Over 110 different pesticides were detected in all these foods between 1982 and 1985. Of the twenty-five pesticides detected most frequently, nine have been identified by EPA to cause cancer (captan, chlorothalonil, permethrin, acephate, DDT, parathion, dieldrin, methomyl, and folpet). And two of these carcinogens, DDT and dieldrin, are now banned from use in the United States (DDT and dieldrin were banned in 1972 and 1974, respectively, due to their carcinogenicity and environmental persistence); residues occurring in food result either from the continued use of these chemicals in foreign nations exporting food to this country, or from contamination by trace levels of the chemicals persisting in the U.S. environment.

PEACHES

Over half of all fresh peaches sampled were found to contain residues of one or more pesticides. Altogether, thirty-six different pesticides were detected. (The routine laboratory method used by the federal government can only detect fifty-five of the nearly 100 pesticides that can be applied to peaches.) Dicloran residues were detected in 30 percent of all samples, and captan residues were detected in 20 percent of the FDA samples. Here are the five pesticides detected most frequently in order of decreasing occurrence:

Pesticide	Health Effects	Can residue be removed by washing?	Residue removal
Dicloran *DCNA, Botran*	No observed reproductive toxicity in one animal study. According to EPA, has not been sufficiently tested for carcinogenicity, birth defects, or mutagenic effects.	YES	Residues remain on surface following foliar treatment but are absorbed and translocated to edible tissue, following soil treatment. Incorporation of dicloran into wax formulations reduces the effectiveness of washing. Washing, peeling, cooking, or heat processing may reduce residues.
Captan *Merpan, Ortho-cide*	Probable human carcinogen. Some evidence of mutagenic effects in laboratory test systems. EPA initiated Special Review in 1980 due to carcinogenicity, mutagenic effects, and presence of residues in food.	YES	Residues remain primarily on the produce surface. However, the metabolite THPI, a suspected carcinogen, may be systemic. Washing, cooking, or heat processing will reduce residues.
Parathion *Phoskil*	Possible human carcinogen. Some evidence of mutagenic effects in laboratory studies. No observed reproductive toxicity or birth defects in animal studies.	UNKNOWN	Residues remain primarily on the produce surface. Washing, peeling, cooking, or heat processing may reduce residues slightly.
Carbaryl *Sevin*	Some evidence of adverse kidney effects in humans, and mutagenic effects in laboratory test systems. No observed carcinogenicity or reproductive toxicity in animal studies.	YES	Residues remain primarily on the produce surface. Washing, peeling, or cooking will reduce residues.
Endosulfan	Some evidence of adverse chronic effects including liver and kidney damage and testicular atrophy in test animals. No observed mutagenic effects in laboratory test systems.	UNKNOWN	Residues remain on the produce surface; however, endosulfan metabolites may be systemic. Peeling, cooking, or heat processing may reduce residues slightly. No information on removal with water.

Certain fruits and vegetables are more likely to contain pesticides more frequently than others. For some fruits and vegetables, including strawberries and peaches, high standards about the cosmetic appearance of the food result in greater pesticide use. Foods with edible portions grown directly in contact with soil, such as celery, carrots and potatoes, may act as sponges and absorb chemical residues from the soil. Other fruits and vegetables have naturally occurring barriers to some pesticide residues, including thick skins on bananas, husks on corn, and wrapper leaves on cauliflower.

Between 1982 and 1985, approximately 40 percent of all FDA's sampling of these fruits and vegetables was of imported foods. Of the imported foods analyzed, pesticide residues were detected in 64 percent; in comparison, 38 percent of the domestic foods were found to have pesticide residues.

For all but six of the individual food commodities, imported foods contained more pesticide residues than the domestically grown foods. In some cases, the imported foods had pesticide residues over twice as frequently. For example, 23 percent of the domestically grown tomatoes contained pesticides, whereas 70 percent of the imported tomatoes had residues. Thirty percent of the domestic cucumbers had residues, while 80 percent of the imported cucumbers contained residues.

In the short run, here are a few tips on how to limit your exposure to pesticides in fresh foods:

• Wash all produce. This will remove some but not all pesticide residues. A mild solution of dishwashing soap and water will help remove additional residues.

• Peel produce when appropriate. Unfortunately, this may reduce the nutritional value of some produce and will not help if the pesticide has been absorbed.

• Grow your own vegetables.
• Buy organically grown fruits and vegetables.
• Buy domestically grown produce.
• Buy produce in season.
• Beware of perfect-looking produce.

You can accelerate the transition to a less chemically dependent method of agriculture by meeting with your supermarket manager and alerting him to your concerns. Also, write your congressional representatives, the FDA, and EPA.

In the long run, we need to reduce agriculture's reliance on chemicals substantially. Methods to produce food with little or no pesticides have existed for many years. But more research needs to be done to expand these techniques, and the nation's food producers must be encouraged to switch to these methods. You can participate directly in resolving the problems posed by pesticide residues in food. If consumers begin to look for and demand safer food, farmers will be forced to reduce their use of pesticides and make changes that will significantly benefit our health and protect the environment.

Through your choices in the supermarket of foods with less chemicals, you can send a direct message to the food industry that will speed the transition away from hazardous pesticides in agriculture. Even food companies can now take steps to reduce the levels of pesticides in their products. The H.J. Heinz Company, in a March 13, 1986, letter to growers, announced that food treated with any of thirteen pesticides EPA is reviewing as a potential health hazard will not be used to manufacture baby food. You can also make the government do a better job of protecting your food supply and regulating these chemicals.

The ideal solution to the current problems posed by pesticide residues in our food has five different components:

• Organic food should be made available in regular supermarkets. You should have the right to choose between different types of produce.

• All produce should be labeled to identify where the food was grown and what pesticide residues it contains. This information would allow you to make more informed choices when purchasing produce.

• The Environmental Protection Agency should regulate pesticide use more stringently, and set tougher limits on pesticide levels in food.

• The Food and Drug Administration should improve and expand its monitoring for pesticides in food.

• Agricultural production methods should be modified to reduce reliance on chemical pesticides. Food should be grown without chemicals used to improve the cosmetic appearance of our fruits and vegetables. Sustainable agriculture—farming that renews and regenerates the land—would be better for our health and the environment.

THESE CHANGES WILL NOT COME OVERnight, but some already are occurring. Several California supermarkets have adopted an independent program to identify pesticides in the produce sold in their stores. Organic produce is available in certain Boston food stores. Some national chain stores have said they would offer organic produce if requested by customers. By our efforts individually and together, we can ensure that these goals become reality.

NO
Bruce Ames

TOO MUCH FUSS ABOUT PESTICIDES

In the wake of the Alar-in-apples scare last year [1989], consumers have become highly concerned about the threat posed to their health by the ingestion of trace amounts of man-made pesticides. While it is good for consumers to be concerned about what they eat, the hysteria about pesticide residues may not be warranted by the actual risk they pose. In helping consumers develop a fuller picture of the true risk of man-made pesticides (or other chemical additives to food), we present below an excerpt of a letter from Dr. Bruce Ames to Consumer Reports *magazine. The letter was in response to an article run in that magazine (October 1989), which, according to Dr. Ames, "distorts my views and misstates facts." . . .—Ed. [of* Consumers' Research.]

Consumer Reports' four-page attack on my scientific work both distorts my views and misstates the facts on which they are based. Good scientists are committed to challenging assumptions rigorously, and this is particularly important in the prevention of cancer, a murky, complex, multidisciplinary field to which I have devoted much of my scientific career. Sound public policy should be based on sound science, and new data or theory may require altering some prevailing assumptions.

In our efforts to prevent human cancer, it makes no sense to apply a double standard for human exposures to natural vs. synthetic chemicals. My colleagues and I have therefore attempted to provide an overview of possible carcinogenic hazards.

The following points clarify my views and their factual and theoretical basis:

1) Discovering the Causes of Cancer. Epidemiologists are continually coming up with clues about the causes of different types of human cancer, and these hypotheses are then refined by animal and metabolic studies. This approach will, in my view, lead to the understanding of the causal factors for the major human cancers during the next decade. Current epidemiologic data point to the major risk factors for human cancer as cigarette smoking (which is responsible for 30% of cancer), dietary imbalances, hormones, viruses, and lifestyle factors—not to such factors as water pollution or synthetic pesticide residues.

For example, epidemiologists in many countries have identified excessive salt as a risk factor for stomach cancer, one of the major types of cancer. Extensive experimental work in rodents on salt as a co-carcinogen supports the epidemiology. Yet *Consumer Reports* unfairly criticized Edith Efron for saying that salt is a carcinogen.

Consumer Reports criticized me for calling alcohol a carcinogen, yet alcoholic beverages, of numerous types, are carcinogenic in humans at a level of 5 drinks/day. Alcohol itself was positive in one rat test and also was co-carcinogenic in other tests. Acetaldehyde, the main metabolite of alcohol, is a carcinogen in rodents. Most of the leading scientists in the field believe that the active ingredient in alcoholic beverages is alcohol itself. I think that chronic high doses of alcohol are active by causing cell proliferation and inflammation and that, therefore, low doses are not of much interest.

2) Animal Cancer Tests. There are three fundamental problems with the use of animal cancer tests in trying to prevent human cancer from low-dose human exposures.

a) There are millions of chemicals in the world that we are exposed to in low or moderate doses, 99.9+% of which are natural. To identify significant risks, we need to identify the right chemicals to test in rodents.

b) About half of the chemicals tested in long-term bioassays in both rats and mice have been found to be carcinogens at the high doses administered, the maximum tolerated dose (MTD). Synthetic industrial chemicals account for almost all (82%) of the chemicals (427) tested in both species. However, despite the fact that humans eat vastly more natural than synthetic chemicals, only a small number (75) of *natural* chemicals have been tested in both rats and mice. For the 75 natural chemicals the proportion of positive results (47%) is similar, also about *half*. While some synthetic or natural chemicals were selected for testing precisely because of suspect structures, most chemicals were tested because they were natural or synthetic food additives, colors, high volume industrial compounds, pesticides, or natural or synthetic drugs. Thus, the high proportion of carcinogens among synthetic test agents in rodent studies is not simply due to selection of suspicious chemical structures, and the natural world of chemicals has never been looked at systematically. Recent research into the mechanism of carcinogenesis (see #4 below) supports the idea that when tested in rodents at the MTD, a high proportion of all chemicals we test in the future, whether natural or synthetic, will prove to be carcinogenic.

(c) The problem of knowing whether there is any risk at all from the very low doses of human exposure to chemicals causing tumors in rodents at very high doses has been argued by toxicologists and regulators for years, precisely because one cannot measure effects at low doses. Regulators have opted for worst-case estimates, using assumptions that increasing scientific evidence suggests may be incorrect.

Because conventional risk assessment is focused mainly on man-made chemicals and is based on worst-case assumptions that we believe are proving to exaggerate hazard greatly, many leading scientists have argued that it is misleading to the public to try to present estimates of "worst-case risk" from animal studies in terms of expected numbers of human cancers. Our HERP [Human Exposure/Rodent Potency, Dr. Ames's index for estimating carcinogenic risk] uses essentially the same information as that in conventional risk assessment, but is explicitly intended as a relative scale. We have attempted to achieve some perspective on the plethora of possible hazards to humans from exposure to known rodent carcinogens by establishing a scale of the possible hazards for the amounts of various common carcinogens to which humans might be chronically exposed. We view the value of our calculations not as providing a basis for absolute human risk assessment, but as a guide for priority setting.

Carcinogens clearly do not all work in the same way, and as we learn more about the mechanisms, HERP comparisons can be refined, as can risk assessments.

Thus, if the public is told that the possible hazard of the UDMH residue [the breakdown product of Alar] in a daily glass of apple juice (about 30 parts per billion) is 1/18 that of aflatoxin (a mold carcinogen) in a daily peanut butter sandwich (the Food and Drug Administration [FDA] allows 10 times that residue level), 1/50 that of a daily mushroom, and 1/1,000 that of a daily beer, it puts these items in perspective. The possible relative hazard of a daily apple is at least 10× less than the apple juice. This is quite different from showing a witch's hand holding an apple [as was depicted on the May 1989 *Consumer Reports* cover on Alar—Ed].

3) Pesticides, 99.99% All Natural. All plants produce toxins to protect themselves against fungi, insects, and animal predators such as man. Tens of thou-

sands of these natural pesticides have been discovered, and every species of plant contains its own set of different toxins, usually a few dozen. In addition, when plants are stressed or damaged, such as during a pest attack, they increase their natural pesticide levels many fold, occasionally to levels that are acutely toxic to humans. We estimate that Americans eat about 1,500 mg/day of natural pesticides, 10,000 times more than man-made pesticide residues, which FDA estimates at a total of 0.15 mg/day. Their concentration is usually measured in parts per thousand or million, rather than parts per billion (ppb), the usual concentration of synthetic pesticide residues and pollutants in water. We estimate that Americans are ingesting 5,000 to 10,000 different natural pesticides and their breakdown products, a subset of the tremendous number of natural chemicals we ingest. For example, there are 49 different natural pesticides (and breakdown products) ingested in eating cabbage.

Surprisingly few plant pesticides have been tested in animal cancer bioassays, but among those tested, again about *half* (25 out of 47) are carcinogenic. A search for the presence of just these 25 carcinogens in foods indicates that they occur naturally in the following (those at levels over 50,000 ppb are listed in parentheses); anise, apples (50,000+ ppb), bananas, basil (4 million ppb), broccoli, Brussels sprouts (500,000 ppb), cabbage (100,000 ppb), cantaloupe, carrots (50,000+ ppb), cauliflower, celery (50,000+ ppb), cinnamon, cloves, cocoa, coffee (brewed) (90,000 ppb), comfrey tea, fennel (3 million ppb), grapefruit juice, honeydew melon, horseradish (4 million ppb), kale, lettuce (300,000 ppb), mushrooms, mustard (black) (40 million ppb), nutmeg (5 million ppb), orange juice (30,000 ppb), parsley, parsnips (30,000 ppb), peaches, black pepper (100,000 ppb), pineapples, potatoes (50,000+ ppb), radishes, raspberries, strawberries, tarragon (1 million ppb), and turnips.

There is every reason to expect that we will continue to find mutagens and carcinogens among nature's pesticides if we ever test them systematically. In short-term tests for detecting mutagens, the proportion of natural pesticides that turn up positive is just as high as for synthetic industrial chemicals. In a compendium on the ability of 950 chemicals to break chromosomes in animal tests, there were 62 natural pesticides: half of them were positive. Thus, it seems highly probable that almost every plant product in the supermarket will contain natural carcinogens at much higher levels than those of man-made pesticides. We have suggested that many more natural pesticides (and chemicals from cooking of food) be tested in long-term bioassays.

Additionally, there is a fundamental trade-off between nature's pesticides and man-made pesticides. We can easily breed out many of nature's pesticides to protect our crops from being eaten by insects. In contrast, growers are currently breeding some plants for insect resistance and unwittingly raising the levels of natural pesticides. A new variety of insect-resistant celery that is being widely sold is almost 10× higher in carcinogens (6,200 ppb) than standard celery.

4) Mechanisms of Carcinogenesis. In the rapidly advancing field of mechanisms of carcinogenesis, there is now evidence to suggest that cell proliferation is extremely important. A large number of the major human carcinogens such as hormones, chronic viral infection, salt, asbestos, and alcohol are likely to be primarily active through causing cell proliferation. A cell is at considerably greater genetic risk during division, so chronic cell proliferation in itself is a mutagenic and carcinogenic stress. Cancers induced in animal cancer tests done at high doses seem to be primarily caused by cell proliferation, in part due to chronic cell killing, and inflammation that results from high toxic doses. This would be in agreement with the high proportion of all chemicals that are turning out to be carcinogens at high doses and the relation of toxicity to carcinogenic potency. The induction of cell proliferation is restricted to high doses, and this strongly suggests that low doses of carcinogens are of no risk, or are very much less hazardous than has been assumed.

In addition, humans, who live in a world of natural toxins, are well protected by many layers of inducible general defenses against low doses of toxins—defenses that do not distinguish between synthetic and natural toxins. Therefore, even the high levels of natural plant pesticides may not be of much concern in a balanced diet.

5) Trade-offs. Identifying and controlling the major causes of human cancer are not a matter of blame. We have tried in our scientific work to put into perspective the tiny exposures to pesticide residues by comparing them to the enormous background of natural substances. Minimizing pollution is a separate issue, and is clearly desirable, aside from any effect on public health, but it involves economic trade-offs. As a society, efforts to regulate pesticides or other synthetic rodent carcinogens down to the ppb level inevitably involve understanding these trade-offs. Synthetic pesticides (and

chemicals such as Alar) have markedly lowered the cost of our food, a major advance in nutrition and, thus, health. Every complex mixture from gasoline to cooked food to orange juice contains rodent carcinogens. When people drive to work, put logs on a fire, or make a barbecue they are putting carcinogens into the air. There are costs and benefits to all of these. Exaggerating the risks from man-made substances, ignoring the natural world, and converting the issue to one of blaming U.S. industry does not advance our public health efforts. If we spend all our efforts on minimal, rather than important, hazards, we hurt public health. The Environmental Protection Agency (EPA) is trying to prevent hypothetical risks of 1 in a million at enormous economic cost. Yet the leading scientists trying to prevent cancer are working on numerous possible carcinogenic risks in the 1 in a 100 to 1 in 10 range: my lab is working on 4 that we think are in this range.

POSTSCRIPT

Are Pesticides in Foods Harmful to Human Health?

Increased consumer fear of pesticide residues on food has encouraged many activists to push for a ban on their use. While doing so might provide some limited health benefits, Ronald Knutson, director of the Agricultural and Food Policy Center at Texas A & M University, believes that such a ban would cause a significant rise in food prices ("Pesticide-Free Equals Higher Food Prices," *Consumers' Research*, November 1990). Knutson and his colleagues argue that if there were a complete ban on the use of pesticides, food bills would rise at least 12 percent, crop yields would fall, and there would need to be a 10 percent increase in cultivated acreage, which would result in a corresponding rise in soil erosion.

An investigation by Constance Matthiessen challenges the opinions of Knutson and others. Matthiessen, writing in *Mother Jones* (March/April 1992), takes the position that despite the widespread use of pesticides, insects and weeds seem to be doing as much damage as ever. The reason: Insects and weeds have the ability to adapt and evolve to become pesticide-resistant. As a result, the share of crop yields lost to pests has almost doubled over the last 40 years. Environmentalist Shirley A. Briggs agrees that pesticides have failed to decrease crop losses while causing widespread environmental damage. In "Silent Spring: The View from 1990," *The Ecologist* (March/April, 1990), Briggs argues that we must find ways to reduce pesticide dependence.

Robert J. Scheuplein, a scientist with the Office of Toxicological Sciences at the Food and Drug Administration, shares the opinions of Ames. In "The Risk from Food," *Consumers' Research* (April 1990), Scheuplein argues that the public has an unrealistic view of pesticides and that other factors, particularly overall diet, contribute much more to the development of different cancers than do pesticide-treated foods.

Most scientists agree that pesticide residues can affect human health to *some* degree. Many experts, however, maintain that current levels of residues are insignificant and that our food supply is safe. Others argue that pesticides pose health risks, are environmentally unsound, and do not work in the long run, because many pests have become resistant to them. Researching alternatives to pesticides, as described in "A New Crop of Pest Controls," *New Scientist* (July 14, 1988) and "Getting Off the Pesticide Treadmill," *Technology Review* (November/December 1985), may be a safer, more ecologically sound, and ultimately more successful approach to limiting pest damage than is maintaining a total reliance on chemicals.

ISSUE 16

Is Acid Rain a Serious Environmental Problem?

YES: Jon R. Luoma, from "Acid Murder No Longer a Mystery," *Audubon* (November 1988)

NO: William M. Brown, from "Hysteria About Acid Rain," *Fortune* (April 14, 1986)

ISSUE SUMMARY

YES: Science writer Jon R. Luoma believes that there is convincing evidence implicating acid rain as a long-term threat to some aquatic ecosystems, forests, and public health.

NO: William M. Brown, director of energy and technological studies at the Hudson Institute in Indianapolis, argues that the dangers of acid rain have been greatly exaggerated by the media and that scientists really do not know exactly what has caused the decline of some forests and waterways.

Acid rain, by definition, is any precipitation containing more acidity than what is considered normal. It is not a new concern, since it has been observed as a local phenomenon in the area surrounding coal-burning plants for over a century. The term *acid rain* was first used by English chemist Robert Angus Smith to describe the corrosive rain that fell on Manchester, England, in the late 1800s.

Acid rain forms when two chemicals, sulfur dioxide and nitrogen dioxide, are converted into acids. This conversion can take place either within clouds or rain droplets or on the surface of soil or water. Sulfur dioxide is discharged into the atmosphere mainly from coal- and oil-burning power plants and industrial smelters and boilers. Nitrogen dioxide comes primarily from auto emissions, power plants, and industry. Unlike sulfur emissions, which have somewhat stabilized in recent years, the amount of nitrogen dioxide emissions continues to rise.

Acid rain does not just pollute the area immediately surrounding power plants; prevailing winds can carry sulfur and nitrogen oxides for hundreds of miles. Power plants in midwestern United States release these chemicals, which are often carried to Ontario, Canada, and the Northeast, where they are released as acid rain.

The effects of acid rain are a subject of controversy, particularly the extent to which it can be blamed for the decline of forests in both the United States and Europe. The high acidity of the rain and snow appears to alter soils and increase surface water acidity, resulting in the decline of many species of trees. Acid precipitation has also been linked to damage involving aquatic ecosystems. There are numerous documentations of "dead" lakes that were teeming with fish only a few decades ago.

With regard to human health, acid rain is related to the mobilization of toxic metals from water. Contact with acidified water can cause tightly bound toxic metals, such as aluminum, lead, mercury, copper, and cadmium, to dissolve out of soils and bottom sediments and leach into the aquatic environment. These metals can accumulate in fish tissues, making the fish dangerous for humans to eat. Mobilization of poisonous metals also presents a direct threat to human health; some acidified lakes are sources of drinking water. In some areas, acidified water that was originally free of toxic metals has become contaminated by passing through lead or copper plumbing. The acidity of the water causes corrosion of the pipes, which results in the leaching of these toxic metals into the drinking water.

While there is a growing consensus among scientists that sulfur and nitrogen emissions are a principal cause of acid rain, there are also denials from the coal and oil industries. In the following articles Jon R. Lumoa supports the theory that man-made pollution is responsible for the decline of lakes and forests. William M. Brown takes the position that scientists cannot specifically pinpoint acid rain as the cause for the decline of lakes and forests. Brown claims that the threat of acid rain is exaggerated and that more research is needed in order to determine the exact causes of these problems.

YES

Jon R. Luoma

ACID MURDER NO LONGER
A MYSTERY

It's been nearly a decade since acid rain surged into news media and public consciousness with reports from scientists that the rains and snows—once symbols of purity—could quite literally poison entire freshwater ecosystems. Captured in huge weather systems, acid-forming pollutants could travel hundreds, or even thousands, of miles from their sources to pollute waters across state or national boundaries.

Now, a near-decade and hundreds of millions of research dollars later, concerns about acid rain have broadened to include threats to wider regions of freshwater lakes and streams, threats to forests, and threats to public health. A clear scientific consensus that acid rain is at least a long-term threat to some aquatic ecosystems has solidified.

In many other ways, very little has changed. The key sources of acid rain remain sulfur dioxide from poorly controlled fossil-fuel-burning power plants and nitrogen oxides from a range of combustion sources, including industrial furnaces and cars. The responsible industries, citing high costs, steadfastly oppose tighter controls, instead calling for more research.

Attempts at federally legislating new controls may have faltered because the pathways of acidification are initially so subtle that widespread damage is not evident. Chemical compounds naturally present in even some of the most sensitive lakes, streams, and watersheds can neutralize acids, often for many years. Only when those neutralizers are used up will a lake quite suddenly begin to turn acid. And although lakes with little remaining neutralizing capacity number in the tens of thousands in North America, lakes actually acidified to date number only in the hundreds. Similarly, research scientists have learned that visible symptoms of forest destruction become obvious only after damage is well under way.

What follows is a compendium of new developments on the acid rain front.

NEWS FROM MOUNT MITCHELL

When Audubon last visited Mount Mitchell in North Carolina ("Forests Are Dying, But is Acid Rain to Blame?" March 1987), plant pathologist Robert I. Bruck was speculating that it might be many years before he had enough data to make clear projections about whether acid rain—or any kind of air pollution—was causing the forest devastation there, so complex was the issue. He said that he'd let us know when he felt scientifically confident to make a bold statement—maybe a decade hence.

"Time's up," Bruck fairly growled in a telephone interview from his prefab headquarters on the 6,684-foot mountain this summer. "You would not believe how this place has changed even in the time since you were up here."

As it turns out, Bruck and a team of scientists, with their networks of towers, collectors, monitors, tubes, and wires laced through the skeletal trees, have discovered persistent high levels of pollutants—notably ozone and atmospheric acids—that appear to correlate strongly to a forest die-off that has increased by some 30 percent since we visited the mountain.

"It's plain," he says, "that no one has proved, or ever will, that air pollution is killing the trees up here. But far more quickly than we ever expected, we've ended up with a highly correlated bunch of data—high levels of air pollution correlated to a decline we're watching in progress."

A trip up Mount Mitchell, eastern North America's highest peak, is a thumbnail experience of the kind of biotic transition one might see on a 1,500-mile automobile journey northward from the sultry southeastern United States to frigid Labrador. Although Mount Mitchell sits at about the same latitude as California's Mojave Desert, the trees on and around the blustery mountaintop are hardy near-Arctic species, red spruce and Fraser fir.

And like many of the ridgetop trees along the entire stretch of the Appalachians—like trees in many of the forests of Europe—they are in evident decline. During my 1986 visit, the fir forest at the summit was eerily dominated by death—stark, brown hulks and deadfalls creaking in the ever-present wind.

According to Bruck, it has gotten worse. The damage extends even further down the mountain into more of the pure red spruce stands and, in some cases, all the way down to the line where hardwood forests begin. According to other reports, Appalachian spruce-fir forests from the White Mountains in New Hampshire to the Great Smokies south of Mount Mitchell are showing signs of reduced growth and general decline.

The information gathered during the federally funded mega-study that Bruck has been coordinating on Mount Mitchell has him saying that he is "ninety percent certain" that air pollutants are killing the southern Appalachian ridgetop spruce and fir forests.

Two years ago Bruck was wondering if some other factor or complex of factors—insects, fungi, climate, or even forest management practices—might be responsible.

But his data now shows that more than half of the time ozone levels on the mountain exceed those at which tree damage has been proven to occur in contolled laboratory studies. Frequently, levels increase to more than double the minimum damage limit. Acidity in the clouds that bathe the summit of the mountain eight out of every ten days has also been extraordinary: ranging from a worst case of pH 2.12 to a best case of 2.9. In other words, on the *best* days of cloud cover, acidity has been somewhat more than that of vinegar.

"Let me tell you about an experiment thirty yards from where I'm sitting on top of the mountain," Bruck said. He described a set of large outdoor chambers, sealed in clear plastic to create a controlled greenhouse, in which young trees have been placed. The usual, and apparently polluted, mountain air is pumped into one chamber without alteration. A second chamber receives mountain air filtered though activated carbon, which removes ozone and some other pollutants. "We set up that experiment only six weeks ago. We're already getting fifty percent growth suppression in the chamber receiving ambient [unfiltered] air."

He also reports that the research team noted widespread burning of new needle-tips on conifers after particularly acid air masses passed through. Analysis of the burnt needles in Environmental Protection Agency laboratories revealed extremely high levels of sulfate, a compound associated with acid rain.

Mountaintops are subject to greater pollutant deposits because they are frequently bathed in polluted cloud water. Extensive forest destruction in Europe began in the 1970s on the mountaintops but has extended to stands at lower altitudes. Many scientists studying the problem feel that air pollution does not kill trees directly but rather weakens them to the point where, like punch-drunk fighters, they are no longer able to withstand normal episodes of moderate drought or insects or diseases that they could otherwise easily resist.

KILLER MOSS, ACID SOILS

Now come reports from field reseachers of problems stemming from acid mosses and acid soils.

Lee Klinger, working with the National Center for Atmospheric Research in Boulder, Colorado, claims to have correlated forest diebacks with the presence of three kinds of mosses: sphagnum, polystrichum, and aulocomnium. He says that the mosses alone are not killing trees but were virtually always present in more than a hundred dying forests that he examined, and that they appear to be a key part of a forest death syndrome.

The mosses produce organic acids which appear to gang up with inorganic acids in polluted rain to mobilize aluminum naturally present but harmlessly bound up in most soils. Additional aluminum appears to be falling out of the atmosphere bound to dust particles. The mobilized aluminum is toxic to the fine feeder roots of most trees. In fact, says Klinger, mats of killer mosses inevitably overlay networks of dead feeder roots. Furthermore, sphagnum acts as a sponge, saturating the soil just beneath the moss and creating an anaerobic, or oxygen-starved, soil environment, which also helps kill roots. The mosses, he says, occur naturally in forests and may even be part of an extremely slow plant succession process that, over centuries or millennia, turns old forests to bogs. But the present moss invasion appears to be promoted and greatly speeded up by acidic rainfall.

"In general," Klinger says, "mosses require acid conditions for their establishment—so it appears that as the soils become acidified, there are more places for the mosses to get established." He also suggests that nitrates that form from nitrogen oxide pollutants in the rain fertilize the mosses, which have no roots but are entirely nourished by atmospheric chemicals.

Meanwhile, some scientists have begun to change their minds about acid soils. Until recently, most researchers looking into acid rain's terrestrial effects have assumed that trees and other plants growing in naturally acid soils—including trees found in many northern coniferous forests—had more resistance to pollutants.

But now Daniel Richter of Duke University reports that his laboratory experiments show that naturally acid soils, such as those often found at high elevations in parts of the Appalachians, are highly sensitive to chemical imbalances caused by the addition of more acids from precipitation. According to Richter, highly acid forest soils that become further acidified can become virtually "infertile" through a complex series of chemical reactions that deprives them of nutrients. At the same time, the soils are assaulted by an overload of mobilized and root-toxic aluminum.

IT KEEPS GETTING WORSE

New York was one of the first states to become deeply concerned about the effects that acid rain could have on its surface waters, and particularly on the pristine but poorly buffered lakes of the huge and beautiful Adirondack Park. In the 1970s the New York Department of Environmental Conservation jolted the conservation community by reporting that more than two hundred lakes, most of them in the western Adirondacks, had already become too acidic for fish to

survive, and that many more appeared to be threatened.

In a new study, three years in the making, the New York DEC reports that fully 25 percent of the lakes and ponds in the Adirondack Mountains are now so acidic that they cannot support fish life. Another 20 percent have lost most of their acid-buffering capacity and therefore appear doomed if acid input continues.

Massachusetts has reported that almost 20 percent—or about eight hundred—of the state's ponds, lakes, and rivers are vulnerable to acid deposition and could become acidified within the next forty years. Already, according to Environmental Affairs Secretary James Hoyte, surveys have located 217 acidified bodies of water that cannot support natural communities. Particularly alarming to state officials is data showing that more than 50 percent of the state's thirty-four drinking-water reservoirs have lost much of their acid-buffering capacity since 1940. The largest of these, Quabbin Reservoir, has lost about three-fourths of its buffering capacity, and the Massachusetts Executive Office of Environmental Affairs now estimates that twenty years remain before the reservoir loses all of its capacity to handle acids. Acidification tends to occur within a few years after buffering capacity is lost.

Meanwhile, Environmental Protection Agency researchers, in a recent report, have identified new and surprising acidification sites in the mid-Atlantic states of Virginia, Delaware, Pennsylvania, Maryland, and West Virginia. The report shows that 2.7 percent of sampled stream miles in the mid-Atlantic region are already acidic, with the afflicted number as high as 10 percent at higher elevations. Despite the fact that rain acidity levels in the region are among the highest in the nation, it has long been assumed that soils in much of the mid-Atlantic could buffer the acidity effectively. The study notes that the stream damage is "probably associated with atmospheric acid deposition."

The Pennsylvania Fish Commission estimated in 1987 that half the state's streams will not be able to support fish life by the year 2000 unless acid deposits decline. Now seventy-eight of the two hundred members of the Pennsylvania House of Representatives are cosponsoring a bill to slash emissions of sulfur dioxide by more than half, in a program that would be phased in over a period of thirteen years.

Pennsylvania has long been in an acid rain quandary. Its emissions of sulfur dioxide are the second worst in the nation, and both its industrial emitters and its powerful coal industry have strongly opposed regulation. But unlike many other high-emission areas, which contain few easily acidified waters, the state has long recognized that many of its woodland streams are acid-sensitive. Pennsylvania government insiders expect vigorous opposition from the pollution lobby on the bill: The state coal association issued a statement immediately after the bill was introduced pointing to government "facts" that watershed acidification was not going to get any worse.

FERTILIZING CHESAPEAKE BAY

Two-thirds of the excess acidity in precipitation falling on the eastern United States comes from sulfur dioxide. So SO_2 has long occupied the attention of most of those concerned with the problem.

But a new study from the Environmental Defense Fund points out that there are plenty of reasons to be concerned about oxides of nitrogen, which not only produce the other one-third of the acid rain problem but are key to the formation of ground-level ozone. (While ozone in the stratosphere is, indeed, necessary to shield the Earth from excess ultraviolet radiation, low-level ozone is not only a health hazard but a proven multibillion-dollar destroyer of agricultural crops and, possibly, forests.)

The EDF study looked at neither of those aspects of nitrogen oxides, but rather at their ability also to function as fertilizers—in this case, unwanted fertilizers of the already pollution-ravaged Chesapeake Bay. The resulting report, based on data from government studies, calculated that one-fourth of the total nitrogen entering Chesapeake Bay comes from excess atmospheric nitrogen oxides, which are produced by combustion in automobile engines, in power plant furnaces, and in virtually all high-temperature burners.

The deposited nitrogen, in turn, is one of the key nutrient pollutants feeding algae in the waters of Chesapeake Bay—to such an extent that biological oxygen demand is up and water quality and fish and shellfish survival are down. The entire process is accelerating eutrophication, a rapid and premature aging process in the bay.

According to the EDF's analysis, the nitrogen input to the bay from air pollution exceeds the contribution from the sewage-treatment-plant effluents and, in fact, exceeds the contribution from all sources but agricultural fertilizer runoff. Although the study was limited to Chesapeake Bay, it suggests that other bays and estuaries may also be suffering from the fertilizing effects of nitrogen raining from the skies.

AN HONEST FEDERAL SUMMARY?

In the history of acid rain research, surely the strangest few days came in September 1987, when the National Acid Precipitation Assessment Program finally released a long-awaited "interim report."

NAPAP, set up late in the Carter Administration to coordinate federal acid rain research, had already been criticized by the General Accounting Office for foot-dragging. When the interim assessment was finally released—two years late—it ignited a veritable firestorm of scientific protest.

There are few complaints about the veracity of the three main volumes of the study. But the slim fourth volume, an "executive summary" was at the heart of the heat. J. Lawrence Kulp, then the NAPAP director and a former Weyerhaeuser executive appointed by Ronald Reagan, had written much of the summary himself.

Critics were especially disturbed that the summary's tally of "acid lakes" counted only those so acid that adult fish could not survive, with far less emphasis on the more numerous acidified waters where amphibian and insect life are harmed, fish reproduction is destroyed, and ecosystem food webs are disrupted.

Further, some critics were outraged that the summary promoted as fact an unproven chemical "steady state" theory, favored by Kulp, that lakes in the Northeast would not become more acidic.

Some prominent researchers spoke out, including several vociferously in the pages of *Science*, which had obtained a pre-release copy. Just days after the summary's release, J. Lawrence Kulp resigned.

The new NAPAP director is one James R. Mahoney. Last April, Mahoney offered a pleasant surprise to many conservationist observers. Testifying before a congressional subcommittee, he offered to prepare a new summary. "I believe the executive summary can and should be expanded to be more representative of all the data available," he said, adding that he "would not subscribe . . . at this time" to Kulp's assertion that acid rain would not harm more northeastern lakes.

Mahoney and Representative James Scheuer, chairman of the subcommittee, later agreed that a shorter report responding to the scientific criticisms would make more practical sense than a wholly republished "interim" summary. That because Mahoney has agreed to gear up his staff to accelerate the massive final assessment to meet the original 1990 deadline, despite the previous delays.

NAPAP plans, this time around, to be more active in soliciting criticisms and comments, according to staff ecologist Patricia Irving. "We want this to be a [scientific] consensus document in every sense," she says.

Scheuer, the congressman, appears to agree that the summary, at least, needs some work. He called that 1987 version "intellectually dishonest."

WAIT FOR CLEAN COAL?

A broad and bipartisan coalition of representatives and senators has introduced compromise legislation in an attempt to break through the political blockade that has stalled all attempts to control acid rain at its source. The new legislation scales back on earlier calls for an annual reduction of 12 million tons of sulfur dioxide. The new target would be 10 million tons per year, or about a 35 percent decrease from current levels.

Connie Mahan of National Audubon Society's government relations office says the society is supporting the bill "even though we are not happy with scaling back by two tons. We went into the 100th Congress believing that the political will for solving this problem was finally taking shape. We continue to hope that by the 101st Congress we'll have acid rain legislation."

The coal and electric power lobbies are continuing to fight legislation which would require them to reduce sulfur dioxide emissions at costs that could exceed $100 million for each poorly controlled fossil-fuel-burning power plant. Instead, they are promoting "clean coal technologies" now in the research and testing stage that could control pollution in the combustion process at much lower costs. However, they have not suggested that large-scale clean coal technology will be available in the foreseeable future.

"We're very suspicious that the promise of future technological improvements is being used as an excuse for not introducing technology that's already known," says Jan Beyea, National Audubon Society senior staff scientist. Beyea points out that the dirtiest power plants, in terms of acid gas emissions, are pre-1980s facilities that were grandfathered at high emission rates by the Clean Air Act. "The real need is for control technology on these older plants. A technology that's useful by the year 2010 isn't going to be of much use. And we don't want to see North America's forests go the way of the European forests."

From his mountaintop headquarters in western North Carolina, Bob Bruck would seem to agree. "People are going to have to start understanding that this is not like some kind of disease where we're going to give all the trees a pill and cure it. We are going to have to decide as a society how to come up with the most logical and reasonable way of implementing what looks like the best solution."

NO
William M. Brown

HYSTERIA ABOUT ACID RAIN

A reasonably attentive follower of the acid rain controversy might well have concluded in March that the case was closed—that there was no longer a scientific controversy. The Reagan Administration was certainly acting as though it had reached some such conclusion. After years of insisting that more research was needed before it would act, the Administration formally accepted the view that acid rain is a big problem, that it is rooted in industrial emissions, and that something must be done to prevent these emissions from drifting over the Canadian border. Ronald Reagan has also bought a proposal, previously endorsed by the Canadian government, that the U.S. spend $5 billion over five years to develop ways of limiting emissions. In recounting this story the other day, the *New York Times* had this to say about our knowledge of acid rain: "A scientific consensus says these [emissions] are considered responsible for damage to freshwater lakes and streams. They may also damage trees and plant life and human health."

To those who have monitored the scientific evidence about acid rain's environmental effects, the goings on in Washington are astonishing. Much is still unknown about acid rain's dimensions and effects, and that "consensus" in the *Times* is nonexistent. But to the extent that science has been participating in the debate, it has been telling us we have *less* reason to be concerned about those industrial emissions than previously supposed.

Some recent analyses have suggested that acid rain is only a minor contributor to the environmental damage (the extent of this damage being itself a matter of great uncertainty). So far as the lakes are concerned, the principal sources of damage are likely to be natural sources of acid. In fact, acid rain has never been conclusively shown to be the principal cause of *any* of the environmental problems it's accused of causing. These are among the findings of a major Hudson Institute study published several weeks ago.

It has always been clear to the scientific community that the claims of acid rain damage were based on circumstantial evidence: you could point to industrial emissions and you could point to acidified lakes. Efforts to gain a more direct knowledge of cause and effect have repeatedly been frustrated.

In the U.S., the federal government established a National Acid Precipitation Assessment Program (NAPAP) in 1980. Initially budgeted at $17 million—a figure that has grown to a proposed $85 million in fiscal 1987—NAPAP has made the first serious effort to determine the degree to which acid rain may be responsible for damage; most earlier research *assumed* that acid rain was the cause of environmental damage and was concerned only to ascertain how the process worked. The findings of the new program have called into question the accepted earlier notion that rivers, lakes, trees, and forests were being "killed" by acid rain.

The media have repeatedly served up certain simple images about acid rain—images that are easy to understand, and therefore easy to believe. We are all familiar with the image of acid rain falling on the land area above some lake, after which it flows into and acidifies the lake, killing the fish. All very clear, simple, and misleading.

The NAPAP scientists and others have focused on three main questions about the acidification of U.S. lakes: (1) Has there been a significant increase in lake acidity over time? (2) Might something other than acid rain be contributing to lake acidification? (3) Might something other than acidity be affecting the survivability of the fish?

Getting solid answers to these questions is not easy. For example, a lake's acidity can vary with the time of day, the season, the amount of prior rainfall, the temperature and cloud cover, the depth and distance from the shore at which samples were taken, and much more. Not surprisingly, successive acidity measures of a particular lake can vary by a factor of 100.

BUT WHAT ABOUT THOSE RELATIVELY ACIDIC lakes without any fish populations? Don't they support the claim linking acid rain to stresses in aquatic systems? It is not clear that they do. For one thing, nobody seems able to prove that the number of lakes without fish is greater now than it was several decades ago. Nor has it been proven that where fish populations clearly have disappeared, the change reflects acidification. A major problem confronting researchers is the paucity of past data to use as a base line.

And there is some evidence that fishless lakes in the Adirondacks were a major concern over 60 years ago. Has the number of fishless lakes in the U.S. increased since then? We simply do not know. In any case, only about 200 such lakes have been identified—all of them in the Adirondack Mountain region of New York. It happens to be a region in which the vegetation and geology predispose aquatic systems toward *natural* acidification.

The amount of acid generated by nature is now known to be far greater than that contributed by industrially generated acid rain. Take bird droppings, which are a relatively minor contributor to the problem. A calculation based on Audubon Society data shows that the droppings hit the U.S. at a rate of about one million per second, and the 150 million tons of droppings per year outweigh sulfur dioxide emissions by something like six to one.

Soil scientists, largely ignored in acid rain research before 1980, have long known that the acidity of water in soil is essentially determined by properties of the soil through which it moves, not by the acidity of the rainfall. Precipitation that gets down to the mineral layers of watersheds before entering a lake tends to lose acidity; conversely, precipitation that makes contact only with the topsoil tends to become more acidic. The humus layer in Eastern watersheds can increase the acidity of rainfall tenfold.

What about the effect of acid rain on our forests? Here again the media have given a simple and misleading story. The story tends to take its direction from a widely publicized hypothesis offered in 1982 by botanist Hubert Vogelmann of the University of Vermont, who suggested acid rain as the reason for a so-called dieback among spruce trees on Camels Hump, a Vermont mountain peak. But since 1982 the international scientific community has registered skepticism about the basic hypothesis, and many investigators today even doubt that acid rain is the primary suspect in the claimed forest damage. Some investigators even question whether any unusual amount of damage is occurring. But even assuming that the damage is abnormal, scientists today tend to look also at the impact of such natural stresses as droughts, frosts, insects and pathogens, combined with ozone, heavy metals and other air pollutants.

Several other accusations have been leveled against acid rain, including its possible detrimental effect on human health, on crops, and on building materials. It is understandably easy to confuse the damage attributed to acid rain with that caused by ozone, sulfur dioxide, ammonia, nitrogen oxide, and other pollutants. To what degree are such claims improperly directed against acid rain? NAPAP's huge research program does not yet have all the answers to that question, but the preliminary findings are suggestive.

Clearly we can reject the claims about acid rain causing many premature deaths.

The claim that acid rain damages important crops appears almost as frivolous. Of the many experiments performed, only a rare few gave any support at all to the claim. These experiments have led the Environmental Protection Agency to conclude that the effects of acid rain on crops are as likely to be positive as negative but are minimal in either case.

Many scientists in the past found it plausible that acid rain significantly degrades various exposed structures and materials. But most of the NAPAP analyses dispute this view, suggesting instead that natural weather conditions (especially freeze-thaw cycles) and several air pollutants cause the damage.

One important finding of the NAPAP scientists is that most urban pollution comes from local emissions, not from distant emissions borne by rainfall. The evidence suggests that attempts to reduce the impact of pollutants on exposed structures in urban areas should focus on local automobiles and buildings and on nearby industries.

NONE OF THE ABOVE IS MEANT TO SUGGEST that the scientific community is agreed about acid rain's environmental impact. If anything scientists are more polarized than ever about the issue. Debates reflecting that polarization within the National Academy of Science evidently caused a delay of about ten months in the publication of its most recent report on acid rain issues, which ended up being endlessly hedged and qualified about major matters.

I believe that the urge to control acid rain stems from beliefs that once seemed intuitively plausible but that have been made obsolete by most of the recent evidence. I do not know why the Reagan Administration is bowing now to the political pressures to "do something" about acid rain. Perhaps the Administration is simply recognizing that just about everybody wants to reduce industrial emissions and that the steps contemplated under the new $5-billion program (half of which will be financed by the private sector) could be justified even if those emissions are not rally acidifying our lakes and forests. Perhaps the program is viewed as a reasonable accommodation to a conservative Canadian government; there is no doubt that the acid rain issue, propelled in some measure by anti-Americanism, has a lot of emotional firepower behind it in Canada. Whatever the President's reasons, Americans shouldn't read the news as evidence that acid rain is the monstrous problem it's made out to be.

POSTSCRIPT

Is Acid Rain a Serious Environmental Problem?

In 1991, a 10-year, $500 million, federally sponsored investigation concluded that acid rain causes some significant environmental damage but far less than initially feared. Some of the study's findings, however, are filled with uncertainty. Scientists from both the United States and Canada maintain that the report understated the problem in their countries ("Worst Fears on Acid Rain Unrealized," *The New York Times*, February 19, 1991). A final draft of the study revealed that many scientists' concerns about the environmental damage caused by acid rain are valid but that the problem is not of crisis proportions. This conclusion is discussed in *The Great Acid Rain Mystery*, by William M. Brown (Hudson Institute Press, 1986). The coal and oil industry claimed that the report showed that damage from acid rain was less than feared and that there was no need to rush into expensive control measures (National Coal Association, Statement before the Subcommittee on Environmental Protection, Committee on Environment and Public Works. U.S. Senate, June 17, 1987; "Acid Rain Report Confirms Concern," *The New York Times*, September 5, 1991). Environmentalists contend that the report did not address long-term effects on forests, lakes, and human health.

The issue of whether or not human health risks can be associated with acid rain is documented by Luoma in the preceding selection. In 1990, Luoma offered additional documentation into the acid rain–human health connection in "Acid Rain?" *Audubon* (February 1990). Further reading on acid rain can be found in "Acid Rain: How Great a Threat?" *Consumer Research Reports* (March 1986); "Our Polluted Environment," *Science* (May 1991); "The Problem of Acid Rain," *Scientific American* (August 1988); *Acid Rain* (Chelsea House Publishers, 1992); "Acid Rain," *The Amicus Journal* (Winter 1983); "Acid Rain's Political Poison," *The New York Times* (April 8, 1985); "Our Trees Are Dying," *Science Digest* (September 1984); "An International Storm Over Acid Rain," *The Christian Century* (May 7, 1986); and "Science Hot on the Trail of Answer to Acid Rain," *U.S. News & World Report* (January 14, 1985).

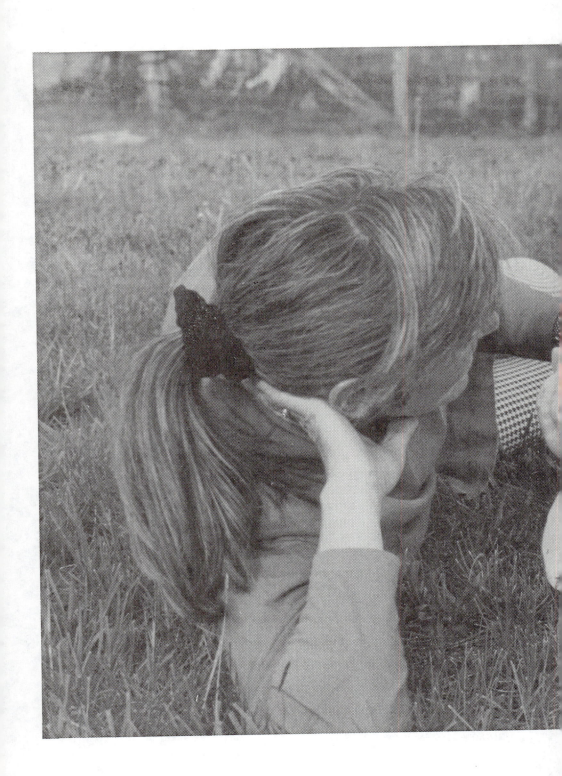

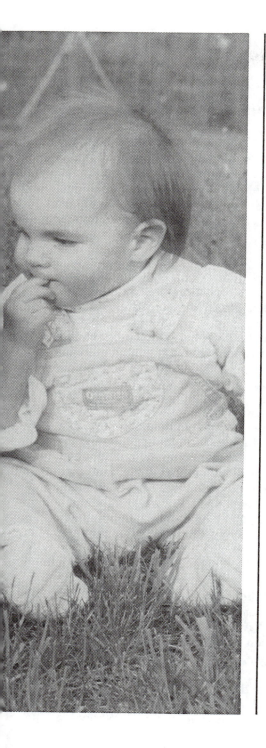

PART 7

Making Choices

A shift is occurring in medical care toward informed self-care: People are starting to reclaim their autonomy, and the relationship between doctor and patient is changing. Many patients are asking more questions of their doctors, considering a wider range of medical options, and becoming more educated about what determines their health. Some individuals are rejecting traditional medicine altogether and seeking alternative health providers, while others are rejecting only some aspects of traditional medicine, such as immunizations. This section debates some of the choices consumers may make regarding their health care.

Should All Children Be Immunized Against Childhood Diseases?

Are Chiropractors Legitimate Health Providers?

ISSUE 17

Should All Children Be Immunized Against Childhood Diseases?

YES: Royce Flippen, from "The Vaccine Debate: Kids at Risk?" *American Health: Fitness of Body and Mind* (July/August 1990)

NO: Richard Leviton, from "Who Calls the Shots?" *East West: The Journal of Natural Health and Living* (November 1988)

ISSUE SUMMARY

YES: Health writer Royce Flippen argues that since measles and some other potentially dangerous childhood diseases are making a comeback, all children should be immunized against them.

NO: Health journalist Richard Leviton maintains that many vaccines are neither safe nor effective and that parents should have a say in whether or not their children receive them.

A number of infectious diseases are almost completely preventable through routine childhood immunizations. These diseases include diphtheria, meningitis, pertussis (whooping cough), tetanus, polio, measles, mumps, and rubella (German measles). Largely as a result of widespread vaccination, these once-common diseases have become relatively rare. Before the introduction of the polio vaccine in 1955, epidemics of the paralyzing disease occurred each year. In 1952, a record 20,000 cases were diagnosed, as compared to the last outbreak in 1979, when only 10 paralytic cases were identified.

Measles, which can cause serious complications and death, has also declined considerably since the measles vaccine became available. In 1962 there were close to 500,000 cases in the United States, as compared to under 4,000 cases in late 1980. Unfortunately, measles still kills some children and causes permanent damage to others who have not been immunized. In some parts of the country, particularly in urban areas, measles epidemics rage among nonimmunized children of all ages, who pass the disease along to each other.

Unfortunately, measles is not the only disease making a comeback. In 1983, an outbreak of whooping cough in Oklahoma affected over 300 people. By 1988, nearly 3,000 cases nationwide had been diagnosed. Whooping cough is a serious and sometimes fatal disease, especially among young infants. Although the risks of whooping cough and other childhood diseases are serious, many children remain nonimmunized because their parents either cannot afford vaccination, are unaware of the dangers of childhood diseases, or believe that the risks of vaccination outweigh the benefits—the last of these is the basis for this debate.

The whooping cough vaccine has been the subject of more concern than any other immunization. While almost all of the 18 million doses administered each year cause little or no reaction, about 50 to 75 children suffer serious neurological injury, a few of which lead to death. Although some consider this risk to be too high, before the vaccine was available, nearly 8,000 children died annually from whooping cough. Still, many parents who are concerned about the dangers of the vaccine have chosen not to protect their children.

In the following articles, Royce Flippen argues that vaccines are much safer than the diseases and that parents must continue to have their children immunized. Richard Leviton believes that many vaccines, particularly whooping cough, are not safe or effective and that parents must have a say in whether or not their children receive them.

YES
Royce Flippin

THE VACCINE DEBATE: KIDS AT RISK?

Measles outbreaks swept through the nation last year, leaving more than 16,000 children and young adults feverish and dotted with red itchy spots—up from 3,400 cases in 1988. The numbers are expected to be even higher this year. In 1989, the fretful "whooping" cough of pertussis—the deadly scourge of the '30s and '40s—struck more than 3,700 American children, a rate more than double that of the early '80s. And the number of reported cases is only a small fraction of the actual caseload, health officials fear.

Though these childhood diseases are almost entirely preventable by vaccines, immunization rates in the U.S. have dropped significantly in the past 10 years. Incredibly, more than one in five American two-year-olds now go unprotected against either polio, measles, rubella or mumps. One in seven have never received a full series of shots against diphtheria, tetanus and pertussis (the DTP shot—formerly called DPT). Those are national estimates; in some urban centers as few as 40% of tots are fully immunized. Many of the unprotected children are impoverished. Their parents often can't afford the $80 to $150 per child (plus office fees) for a complete set of shots.

But beyond cost or oversight, there's also genuine concern about the safety of some vaccines—measles, mumps, polio and especially the pertussis shot for whooping cough. Critics especially fault pediatricians for failing to single out children at high risk of being injured by these shots. Now comes news that a vaccine against the varicella virus that causes chicken pox might become available as soon as next year, pending FDA approval. Published studies indicate it's a safe and effective vaccine for normal kids, says the CDC's Dr. Laura Fehrs.

While public health officials push for more immunizations, some parents' groups are charging that many vaccines themselves are unsafe, and that the public hasn't been fully informed about the danger of adverse side effects. Many parents whose children have had severe, sometimes lasting complications from vaccines have joined grassroots organizations such as Dissatisfied Parents Together. This group was formed in 1982 to spread the word about

From Royce Flippin, "The Vaccine Debate: Kids at Risk?" *American Health: Fitness of Body and Mind* (July/August 1990). Copyright © 1990 by Royce Flippin. Reprinted by permission of *American Health: Fitness of Body and Mind.*

the risks of pertussis and other vaccines and lobby for better record-keeping and safer vaccines, as well as compensation for those who suffer vaccine injuries.

Medical researchers, caught in the middle of the debate, have struggled to determine the true risk to kids, while scientists race to produce a new generation of safer vaccines.

A SHOT IN THE DARK

By far the vaccine that has inspired the most fear is the whole-cell pertussis shot (so called because it's made of entire dead bacteria). Linked with complications ranging from fever to seizures, the vaccine is even accused of causing brain damage and death.

Other vaccines have come under scrutiny as well: Measles and mumps vaccines, given as part of the MMR shot (measles, mumps, rubella), can cause fever, rashes and swollen glands in children. (Rubella, the other part of the shot, has been suspected of sometimes causing rheumatoid arthritis when given to adults.) The oral polio vaccine can in extremely rare instances actually cause the disease.

The pertussis vaccine, however—usually given in a series beginning at two months of age—is the subject of worldwide controversy. In the mid '70s fear of adverse vaccine reactions in Great Britain drove immunization rates down to near 30% for pertussis. Several years later, as the "herd immunity" effect of group vaccination wore off, whooping cough cases began to climb. The English reported 66,000 cases in 1978—compared with an annual rate between 2,000 and 17,500 for the years 1969 through 1977. As the disease spread, more and more people opted to get shots.

Today, 75% to 80% of the English are immunized and the case load dropped to 11,700 last year. In 1976, Japan's pertussis vaccination rate dropped to about 10% but now is back up to over 80% in part because of a new, purified form of the vaccine. Sweden, however, hasn't vaccinated against pertussis since 1979, and the disease is prevalent.

Today, some scientists are saying the worst fears about the vaccine simply aren't justified. Last March in the *Journal of the American Medical Association* (JAMA), investigators studying 38,000 Tennessee schoolchildren found no association between the pertussis vaccine and the incidence of serious neurological effects or brain damage (encephalopathy). An editorial in the same issue cited two other recent studies with similar findings and suggested there was no absolutely no doubt of the shot's safety. "It's time for the myth of pertussis vaccine encephalopathy to end," declared Dr. James Cherry, chief of infectious diseases at the UCLA Medical Center.

But Barbara Loe Fisher, executive vice president of Dissatisfied Parents Together, isn't convinced. Fisher believes adverse reactions are underreported: It was only after the passage of the National Childhood Vaccine Injury Act in 1986—an effort spearheaded by her group—that doctors were required to report all reactions.

In her book *A Shot in the Dark*, Fisher and her coauthor describe scores of horrifying accounts of complications among children within hours or days of receiving a DTP shot. Some children recovered, but others were left paralyzed, brain damaged—some even died. Fisher's own son collapsed in shock within hours of a DTP shot, she says, and was left with multiple learning disabilities. "If you

---

MEASLES REDUX

Think you're done with shots? It turns out the measles vaccine given to some baby boomers was less than perfect: Almost one-quarter of the victims in last year's outbreak were college-aged or older. Health authorities are now urging everyone vaccinated between 1963 and 1968 to consider being revaccinated with the more effective "live" vaccine now available. Those born before 1957 probably had the disease and are immune. However, adds George Seastrom, a public health advisor with the CDC, "People born before 1957 who have never had measles should also consider getting vaccinated."

Other preventable diseases pose even higher risks for adults. According to the National Foundation for Infectious Diseases, influenza and pneumonia account for up to 60,000 deaths a year in the U.S., and the 300,000 cases of hepatitis B reported annually cause 5,000 deaths each year. Also, 11 million women of child-bearing age go unprotected against rubella, which is known to cause birth defects, and the vast majority of tetanus and diphtheria cases from 1985 to 1987 occurred in people over 20 who lacked adequate immunization.

However, there is some good news. Confirmed cases of paralytic polio are now so rare in the Americas that international health officials predict they'll have chased the crippling disease from the Western Hemisphere by year's end. With an intensive global vaccination drive, they say polio could be eradicated from the globe—as was small pox in 1977—by the end of the decade.

---

look at these studies, they just don't hold up," she says. "My feeling is that because vaccine manufacturers are involved in the funding of most of them, you're not getting an unbiased opinion." As an example, she points out that Lederle-Praxis, a maker of pertussis and other vaccines, funds Cherry as an independent third-party investigator.

Cherry responds: "I was involved in a recent Denmark study, which found no cause-and-effect relationship between epilepsy and pertussis vaccine, and that was funded by an unrestricted grant from Lederle. This means they had no control over the study. The research was done and peer-reviewed, and published in a respectable journal [*The Journal of Pediatrics*]."

That aside, Dr. Marie Griffin, the Vanderbilt University epidemiologist who led the *JAMA* study, says she wouldn't go quite as far as Cherry's editorial. "Our study is reassuring," she says, "but it was not conclusive. Maybe if we'd looked at 3 *million* children we would have seen a difference. We don't know."

What her study does show, Griffin explains, is that serious complications from the vaccine aren't common. Her group found no cases of brain damage or serious neurological disease within four weeks of receiving DTP shots.

ASSESSING THE RISKS

The situation is complicated by the fact that vaccines are initially given in in-

THE DON'TS OF PERTUSSIS VACCINATION

Most kids who get the pertussis vaccine have no serious side effects. But in rare instances, major complications do arise. The CDC has now developed the following checklist to help identify high-risk kids who should *not* get the pertussis portion of the DTP vaccine.

- Anyone over age seven.
- Children with a fever-related illness.
- Those with a history of convulsions (with or without fever).
- Children undergoing immunosuppressive therapy.
- Children with an underlying neurological disorder, such as epilepsy or infantile spasms.

Children who've had one of the following reactions to a previous DTP shot *should not* receive any more pertussis shots: allergic hypersensitivity; fever of 105° or higher within 48 hours of the shot; a collapse or shock-like state within 48 hours; persistent crying for three or more hours, or unusually high-pitched crying within 48 hours; convulsions (with or without fever) within three days; impaired or reduced consciousness within a week.

The grassroots organization Dissatisfied Parents Together lists the following as high-risk factors *not* officially recognized by the CDC:

- Any illness, including runny nose, cough, ear infection or diarrhea, up to one month prior to a DTP shot.
- A family member who has reacted severely to DTP.
- A personal or family history of severe allergies.
- Premature delivery, low birth weight or birth complications.
- A family history of convulsions.

For other vaccines the CDC recommends: Measles, mumps, rubella and oral polio vaccines should not be given to women who are pregnant or considering becoming pregnant in the next three months. They also should not be given to anyone suffering immune-deficiency diseases, or taking medication that suppresses immunity. People with allergies to neomycin should consult a doctor before receiving measles, mumps, rubella or intramuscular polio vaccine. Those with egg allergies should also check with a doctor before getting measles, mumps and influenza vaccines. Tetanus and diphtheria vaccines should not be given if the patient has had a previous allergic or neurological reaction to the shots. At no time should a vaccine be administered to an adult or child suffering from an illness with high fever.

fancy, when pre-existing neurological illnesses first manifest themselves. For instance, Cherry suspects a form of epilepsy called infantile spasm may be truly to blame in some cases. The condition peaks at three to five months. "Vac-

cines bring it out, but the illness will happen anyway—or perhaps is already happening at the time of the vaccination."

Children are also prone to seizures in infancy. Dr. Gerald Fenichel, a pediatric neurologist at Vanderbilt, says that fe-ver-induced convulsions occur in 4% of all children. "Several articles suggest that in genetically predisposed children seizures can be induced by the fever associated with pertussis vaccine—or measles vaccine, for that matter," he says. Doctors have identified which kids—at high risk for reactions—should not be immunized (see "The Don'ts of Pertussis Vaccination").

Griffin was surprised her study found few vaccine-related seizures. But Danish investigators recently did find a higher-than-normal rate of fever-induced sei-zures in children following their DTP shots; and two large studies reported a slight post-DTP fever in most children, a fever of 105° or more in one out of 330 shots, and convulsions or collapse in one out of 875 DTP vaccinations.

While such relatively common episodes aren't life-threatening, they're frightening, says Dr. Allen Mitchell, associate director of the Sloan epidemiology unit at the Boston University School of Medicine, who publishes a newsletter called *Pediatric Alert*. Mitchell says pediatricians have become sensitive to parental anxi-ety over the shots and their possible complications. "It appears more and more doctors are giving acetaminophen with the DTP shot to prevent high fever," Mitchell says. "This practice may lessen the chance of fever-induced seizures, and also reduce the discomfort that often follows the shot."

DETOXING THE PERTUSSIS SHOT

Meanwhile, scientists say they're closer than ever to a solution—a safer vaccine. In animal studies, a new genetically al-tered strain of "acellular" pertussis vac-cine gave effective protection with no toxic side effects, according to a report in *Science*.

That was achieved by altering two key amino acids in the pertussis toxin, says coinvestigator Dr. Joseph Barbieri of the Medical College of Wisconsin.

Is this the vaccine of the future? "It depends on how it does in clinical tri-als," Barbieri says, adding that such tri-als have begun in Italy. A different form of acellular vaccine, which relies on chemical purification and detoxification, is already being used in Japan.

By most accounts it will be years be-fore a totally nontoxic pertussis vaccine goes mainstream here. Meanwhile, the Department of Health and Human Ser-vices is looking into the issue of adverse reactions to pertussis and rubella vac-cinations. HHS has asked the Institute of Medicine in Washington, DC, to examine the available evidence and present a re-port by next summer.

For the time being, people who choose not to get their kids immunized can be grateful for the generally high U.S. vac-cination rate, which prevents diseases from reaching pandemic proportions. "It's like paying your taxes," says Dr. Charles Gordon, a New York pediatri-cian. "We can survive if a few people don't—but if no one pays, we're all in trouble."

NO
Richard Leviton

WHO CALLS THE SHOTS?

One day in 1980 Barbara Fisher held down her two-and-a-half-year-old son, Christian, so the doctor could give him his fourth DPT (diphtheria-pertussis-tetanus) shot. Neither Fisher nor the doctor knew that Christian, with respect to DPT vaccine, was a high-risk child. He had experienced a violent "local reaction" to his third injection, an experience a physician would diagnose, had one noticed it, as a contraindication against further vaccination.

Within hours of his fourth shot, Christian suffered what his mother now realizes was a classic collapse/shock reaction to pertussis. "I didn't report it to my doctor," says Fisher today. "I had not been informed of what a severe reaction was, and I didn't know I was witnessing one." She thought Christian might be undergoing a relapse of the flu. Fisher didn't want her doctor to regard her as "one of those hysterical mothers who calls up every time the child sneezes."

In the ensuing months it became obvious to Fisher that something had gone wrong with the DPT vaccination. Christian forgot his alphabet. He became hyperactive and emotionally fragile. He had staring spells, lost weight, and developed chronic diarrhea, upper respiratory infections, and allergies. Fisher still trusted her physician, who assured her that Christian was "just going through a stage." "But," says Fisher, "my whole family knew something drastic had happened to Christian, that he had become a totally different child overnight."

Today Barbara Fisher is a much wiser and infinitely better-informed mother. She knows that after his fourth DPT shot her "once precocious" Christian suffered a mild encephalopathy that left him with minimal brain damage, multiple learning disabilities, and an impaired immune system. Fisher, like many mothers, was left raging with many unanswered medical questions.

"Why was I so willing to suspend my common sense and deny reality in order to believe in the infallibility of medicine and my doctor? I believed vaccines were completely safe and effective because that is what I was led to believe by all I had read or heard in the media, by what I had been told by my pediatrician, and because I came from a family full of doctors and nurses and other health professionals who had dedicated their lives to medicine. I had absolutely no idea that a vaccination could result in brain damage or death."

Young Christian Fisher, however, was one of the lucky ones. He is not dead or mentally retarded or suffering from convulsions. There are 67,000 infants vaccinated with DPT every week in America but nobody—not medical professionals, the government, or mothers—has accurate casualty statistics. But that there have been significant vaccine-associated damages is meticulously documented in Fisher's provocative book, coauthored by Harris Coulter, DPT: A Shot in the Dark (Warner Books, 1985).

For Barbara Fisher, educating the public about the dangers of adverse reactions to DPT has become a paramount social responsibility. Christian's experience instantly politicized her. And she cites the familiar equation: Knowledge equals power.

"It is time we as parents begin to take back the right and responsibility for our children's health instead of taking the easy way out and leaving the decisions up to our doctors." Thus in 1982 Fisher founded Dissatisfied Parents Together (DPT) in Washington, D.C., to spearhead the drive for greater public awareness and to initiate legislative change. Fisher's DPT coalition, with chapters in many states, has a huge natural constituency. Each year another 3½ million babies are born in America, who will be legally required to have some ten vaccinations by the age of six.

Barbara Fisher has become a major figure in the controversy over mandatory vaccination policies. On the other side of the controversy are some of the leading policymakers in American medicine—the American Academy of Pediatrics, the federal Centers for Disease Control, and the American Medical Association. They unilaterally endorse vaccination programs. "There is an ineluctable conflict between public health and individual rights and this is a regrettable fact," observes Stanley Plotkin, M.D., chairman of A.A.P.'s Committee on Infectious Diseases and director, Division of Infectious Diseases at Children's Hospital of Philadelphia.

"Public health makes the assumption that the health of a group of people is more important," he says. "When you're dealing with contagious diseases the action of a single individual may impact on others. We do not recognize the right of parents to put their children at risk of developing an infectious disease. We feel that a policy that protects children is superior."

Navigating the waters across which such volleys are fired requires today's parents to be both wary and well-informed.

AN ARSENAL OF VACCINES

The concept behind vaccination is to artificially produce immunity to an infectious disease by introducing a small amount of the disease virus or bacteria into the body. The immune system wages a mini-campaign against the foreign materials and develops antibodies tailored for that disease organism, for future reference, in case the child contacts the pathogens in the environment.

This is called active immunization and theoretically provides lasting, effective protection against specific diseases. "The goal is to mimic the natural infection by evoking an immunologic response which presents little or no risk to the recipient," informs the 1986 *Red Book*, the pediatrician's standard reference work on vaccinations, published by the A.A.P.

. . . Today's vaccines use either live or killed infectious agents, usually a virus or bacteria. They are typically injected; a type of polio vaccine is taken orally. The oral polio vaccine is cultured from the kidney cells of the African green monkey.

In addition to the active immunizing antigen, vaccines contain a suspending fluid (sterile water), trace amounts of preservatives (including formaldehyde and mercury-derivatives), stabilizers, antibiotics, and adjuvants (aluminum phosphate).

While there are no national vaccination laws, the fifty states are fairly uniform in their requirements for mandatory vaccinations as a prerequisite for school admission. Children must be vaccinated against the five traditional childhood diseases of mumps, measles, rubella, diphtheria, and pertussis, plus tetanus and polio.

Mumps is a routine, relatively innocuous viral disease that lasts one to two weeks and requires no medical treatment. Two-thirds of infected children develop a self-limiting illness with swollen salivary glands, fever, headache, and appetite loss, but afterwards they have lifetime immunity. A single vaccination of live virus is given at age fifteen months, usually as part of a triple injection called MMR (measles-mumps-rubella). The mumps component, however, is not required in sixteen states.

Measles is a contagious viral disease that lasts two weeks. Characteristic symptoms are a high fever and a rash of pink spots, but more serious complications include eye and ear inflammations, pneumonia, or, in rare instances, encephalitis. The live virus vaccine was introduced in America in 1963 although the measles mortality rate had already dropped radically from 13.3/100,000 cases to 0.3/100,000 by 1955.

Rubella (German measles) is often a benign disease with symptoms so mild they often escape detection. There is a three-day rash, fever, a slight cold, and sore throat. The principal danger is congenital rubella syndrome (CRS), whereby a pregnant woman can expose her fetus to injury if she contracts rubella in her first trimester. A children's mass immunization program for rubella began in 1969 after a CRS epidemic among 20,000 babies in 1964.

Diphtheria has nearly disappeared from America, where it was once greatly feared as a highly contagious bacterial disease with a mortality rate at 3–10 percent. Medical treatment with penicillin or erythromycin is usually indicated. Although mortality rates from diphtheria had dropped by 50 percent before a vaccine was developed, today three to five doses are required in all fifty states.

Pertussis, or whooping cough, is probably the most virulent of the traditional childhood diseases and it can be life-threatening. The infectious agent, *Bordetella pertussis*, was first isolated in France in 1906. Pertussis vaccination, using whole-cell killed virus, began in 1936 and became widespread by 1957. Pertussis symptoms, including a paroxysmal cough, usually afflict infants younger than two years. Today thirty-nine states require three to five injections, beginning at age two months.

Tetanus, technically not a childhood disease, is a potentially dangerous, sometimes fatal, random bacterial infection. Tetanus infection can produce severe neurologic symptoms and muscular spasms (the spasms in the jaw gave the disease the name of "lockjaw"), and worldwide it has a 30–50 percent mortality rate. It is especially prevalent in tropical countries. A regimen of one to five tetanus inoculations are required by forty-seven states, beginning at age two months.

Poliomyelitis infection actually produces no symptoms in 90 percent of its recipients and only 1–2 percent of children infected develop its classic, virally produced symptoms. Polio vaccine, required at three to four doses nationwide, comes in two forms: Salk killed-virus injection and Sabin live-virus oral vaccine.

BRAVE NEW VACCINES

. . . The A.A.P. is categorically opposed to any kind of optional vaccination approach, states G. Scott Giebink, M.D., professor of pediatrics at the University of Minnesota Medical School and a member of the A.A.P. infectious diseases committee. "This is because the virtual eradication of many of the vaccine-preventable diseases has been based on universal rather than optional, or partial, immunization. All of the programs have been incredibly effective—but not because only a few people had the vaccines."

Childhood diseases are still a significant public health threat, requiring prevention, Giebink stresses. "That's the primary reason for continuing a strong and universal immunization program as these diseases are rampant in the world. I'd place the public health benefits first."

Alan Nelson, M.D., president of the A.M.A., agrees. "The data that support the advantages of vaccinations in terms of neurologic injury or mortality to those unprotected are so clear-cut that our public policy still has to support mass immunization. There are few things in medicine that are totally risk-free. That's why we have to measure the benefits against the risks, but with vaccinations the benefits clearly outweigh the risks."

Nelson cites the example of Britain. "There the choice of parents was expressed and DPT vaccination rates have dropped, but the experience has been bad in terms of epidemics and outbreaks of pertussis ever since."

The primary issue at stake is the communicability of infectious diseases, says Walter Orenstein, M.D., director of the Division of Immunization at the CDC in Atlanta. "It's a community decision. When we have children vaccinated, we not only protect the children, we protect the community at large. Parents who decide not to have their children vaccinated not only are not protecting their children, but potentially their actions are leading to danger for other children in that community. If this happened on a large scale, that would put an entire community at risk." . . .

CONTRAINDICATIONS

Not everyone shares this rosy prognosis for preventive vaccination for nearly all diseases. In the mid-1980s a combination of television documentaries, major newspaper stories, and several books—most prominently, Fisher and Coulter's *DPT*—raised public awareness to a shocked appreciation of problems with the mass vaccination approach. Major fissures in the otherwise solid medical edifice were suddenly revealed. The issues are complex and myriad, and often emotionally tinged.

The DPT shot, among all vaccinations in use, produces the most serious adverse reactions. Before 1985 parents were never adequately advised (if at all) of the potentially harmful side-effects of DPT, state Fisher and Coulter. Even today pediatricians still usually downplay the risks. Adverse reactions, which are medical contraindications against further injections, run the gamut from localized skin reactions to seizure, brain inflammation, and death. In 1988, more than forty years after the DPT vaccine was introduced, no accepted parameters have been developed for prescreening hypersensitive children who might be at major risk from DPT.

Prior to 1988 there was not a nationally mandated reporting system either, one which required physicians or health departments to file reports on adverse reactions. Thus accurate data on the prevalence of adverse reactions is lacking and estimates vary widely. Often pediatricians fail (or refuse) to make the connection between a DPT injection and adverse reactions, even when they occur within hours of each other. Coulter and Fisher did their own calculations, based on the best available published data, and came up with some staggering damage estimates.

They calculated that, based on an infant population of 3.3 million per year eligible for DPT shots, 4,248 children have either post-injection convulsions or collapse, 10,377 have high-pitched screaming within forty-eight hours, and 18,873 infants have some form of significant neurological reaction within two days. Possibly as many as 943 deaths and

11,666 cases of long-term damage are attributable to DPT.

There is also considerable disagreement over the level of efficacy of the DPT vaccine, state Fisher and Coulter. Estimates range from 63 to 94 percent. DPT was never adequately tested for safety, its artificially induced immunity lasts only two to five years, and it is regarded as "one of the crudest vaccines on the market." American medical authorities are inexplicably reluctant to adopt the newer and apparently safer Japanese acellular pertussis vaccine.

Given these conditions, Fisher's DPT coalition is understandably strongly in favor of making vaccinations a voluntary act. Fisher would like the DPT vaccine to function freely in the marketplace, like other consumer goods. "Then you will have the good, safe, effective vaccines used, and the poor ones will be dropped. That will give an incentive to the drug companies and government to come up with the most effective and the safest vaccines possible."

Most European nations now allow optional vaccinations for DPT. Voluntary programs are actually generating "control group" data for natural infection rates in countries without mass vaccination. Communist countries such as the Soviet Union, Poland, and East Germany still require vaccinations.

The examples of Britain, West Germany, and Sweden are often cited on both sides of the DPT debate. In these countries, when vaccination rates plummeted in the 1970s and incidence of pertussis infection climbed, a corresponding higher incidence of infantile complication or death did not occur, as many had predicted it would. In 1984, researchers at London's Epidemiological Research Laboratory concluded, in contrasting twenty-five deaths at an 80 percent vaccination rate in 1974 with twenty-three deaths at a 30 percent vaccination rate in 1977, that "since the decline in pertussis immunization, hospital admission and death rates from whooping cough have fallen unexpectedly."

The A.M.A., however, is not convinced that the European model of optional pertussis vaccination is medically worthy of importation to America.

"The incidence of pertussis is cyclic and the severity could also run in cycles," observes A.M.A.'s Nelson. "It's still a very bad disease, a terrible, tragic disease. The burden is on those who say the disease is not still an extraordinarily bad illness to prove that. I don't think you will find very many physicians willing to say we don't have to worry about pertussis anymore, that its severity has lessened."

Medical authorities contend that the kind of documentation Fisher and Coulter present, culled from interviews with over 100 mothers of presumed vaccine-damaged children, are "anecdotal" and not scientifically admissible.

"Most of the pertussis controversy revolves around observations that are anecdotal and unconfirmed," states Plotkin of the A.A.P. "The value of such anecdotes is very limited. On the basis of the information available, I would think there are only rare reactions to pertussis vaccine."

Extensive studies in the U.S. and Britain, explains Giebink, have shown "quite conclusively that some of the most serious of these nervous system disorders are in fact not caused by the vaccine but are only temporally related with it. We've looked at some of the particular diseases using scientific methods and we have not been able to show a cause-and-effect relationship."

CDC's Orenstein concurs. "These adverse events are so rare that we can't detect them. A lot of the responsibility falls on the parent who has to make the connection and file a report. Some of them may forget in their crisis. Suppose we do get all the adverse events reported? It doesn't mean that any of these events are *caused* by the vaccination."

It is precisely statements like these that have infuriated mothers whose babies have suffered damages "temporally" following DPT injections, whatever the true causality might be. Many mothers say their physicians don't listen to them, caution them against hysteria or making trouble, are complacent or patronizing. Other women contend their doctors lied to them and betrayed their trust. Barbara Fisher excoriates this "cavalier disregard for vaccine toxicity and human life."

"We are so conditioned to the idea that our doctor's word is to be trusted without question," said one mother whose infant died thirty-three hours after a DPT shot. "I am a nurse. I watched my son die that day, and I didn't even know what was happening until it was all over."

Mother-activists like Fisher find something immoral lurking within the risk-benefit equations of medical science, especially in light of the lack of exemption options for parents in many states.

"The epidemiologists look at mass vaccination the way a military general studies a battle. A general knows he must sacrifice men to take a hill. This is how government health officials see mass vaccination. They start getting into the idea that some children are expendable. I cannot think of any other instance in our society where we say it's okay to kill children, to have them brain-damaged, because it's for the greater welfare of society."

As Fisher tersely puts it, "When it happens to your child, the risks are 100 percent."

HOLISTIC IMMUNOLOGY

There might be more reasons than symptomatic contraindications arguing the case against mandatory vaccination. According to a variety of holistic practitioners, including M.D.'s, homeopaths, and naturopaths, the general practice of vaccination may have long-term damaging effects on the vitality of the immune system. One such bold M.D. was the late "People's Doctor," Robert Mendelsohn.

Mendelsohn had very impressive credentials to support his strident criticism of vaccinations. He was a practicing pediatrician for twenty-five years, professor at the University of Illinois Medical School, Chairman of the Medical Licensure Committee for Illinois, author of three popular medical guidebooks, and publisher of a medical newsletter for consumers.

For Mendelsohn, vaccinations were a "medical time bomb," the "most threatening" of which was DPT. "The greatest threat of childhood diseases lies in the dangerous and ineffectual efforts made to prevent them through mass immunization," he said. "Although I administered them myself during my early years of practice, I have become a steadfast opponent of mass inoculation because of the myriad hazards they present."

Vaccinations, said Mendelsohn, are one of the harmful sacraments of the modern religion of medicine. "In the total absence of controlled studies, all vaccines today remain, scientifically speaking, unproven remedies—the po-

lite term for medical quackery. The only proven characteristic of vaccines is their devastating adverse effects." Mendelsohn also suggested there might be a causal link between degenerative diseases and immunizations.

Richard Moskowitz is an M.D., homeopath, and former president of the National Center for Homeopathy, now practicing at The Turning Point clinic in Watertown, Mass. He is one of many holistic practitioners who have corroborated Mendelsohn's early indications. In Moskowitz's view *all* vaccinations may be injurious to the functioning and integrity of the immune system.

Moskowitz argues that vaccination may produce a form of immunosuppression and chronic immune failure. The injected virus, because it has been artificially weakened before injection, no longer initiates "a generalized, acute inflammatory response." Instead, it tricks the body into an antibody response— "an isolated technical feat" and only an aspect of the overall immune ability. Worse, the virus may persist in the blood for prolonged periods, perhaps permanently.

"Far from producing a genuine immunity, vaccines may actually interfere with or suppress the natural immune response," says Moskowitz. "By making it difficult or impossible to mount a vigorous, acute response to infection, artificial immunization substitutes a much weaker *chronic* response with little or no tendency for the body to heal itself spontaneously."

Evidence indicates that the individual vaccinations may each have unique deleterious consequences on the immune system. Tetanus may interfere with the immune reaction. It has been linked with peripheral neuropathy, allergic reactions, and laryngeal paralysis. Rubella has been tentatively associated with arthralgia (joint pain) and arthritis. A 1980 report in *Mutation Research* indicated that children who underwent repeated smallpox vaccinations in Czechoslovakia showed chromosomal aberrations in their white blood cells, indicating a mutagenic effect.

The British journal *Medical Hypothesis* reported in 1988 in a study of 200 patients with chronic Epstein-Barr virus syndrome that the disease was attributable to the live rubella virus found in the vaccine. In 1987 a consultant for the World Health Organization announced in the London *Times* that the prevalence of smallpox vaccinations over a thirteen-year period in seven African nations actually triggered the AIDS virus outbreak in those countries. In 1985 a scientist at Harvard's School of Public Health revealed that STLV-3, an AIDS-type virus, had been found in the green monkey (*Cercopithecus*) whose kidney cells were routinely used to culture oral polio vaccine.

Other anomalous long-term medical trends implicating vaccinations have recently been brought to light. Widespread measles vaccinations seem to be shifting the incidence of the disease into older age groups; 80 percent of cases are now occurring in people aged ten to nineteen and with atypical, often untreatable symptoms. Vaccination immunity is clearly less than complete, as 1988 CDC figures showed that of 795 reported cases of pertussis in infants aged three to six months, 49 percent of them had been fully vaccinated.

While holistic health providers are finding alarming grounds for connecting today's auto-immune anomalies and a weakened immune response with vaccines, Giebink of the A.A.P. states un-equivocally, "Those are all groundless speculations." . . .

IN SEARCH OF WILLING DOCTORS

All fifty states allow a medical exemption for high-risk children. Generally what is required is a written statement by a licensed M.D. indicating that the proposed vaccination is medically contraindicated, based on a previous adverse reaction, a family history of reactions, or a personal history of convulsions, neurological disorders, severe allergies, prematurity, or recent severe, chronic illness.

While individual state regulations vary slightly in terminology, essentially the intention remains uniform, as this excerpt from the New York state regulation makes clear: "If any physician licensed to practice medicine in this state certifies that such immunization may be detrimental to a student's health, the requirements of this section shall be inapplicable until such immunization is no longer found to be detrimental."

Philip Incao, M.D., is a licensed New York state physician with offices in Harlemville, New York, near Albany. Incao has been signing medical exemptions for most of the fifteen years of his family practice. But Incao, who practices anthroposophic medicine (see "The Promise of Anthroposophical Medicine," July 1988 *EW*), as developed by the Austrian philosopher Rudolf Steiner (1861–1925), makes a broader interpretation of "detrimental."

Anthroposophical medicine states that the struggle with childhood infectious diseases is salutary for the child's personal and spiritual development and they should not be suppressed; homeopathic medicines may be used to ameliorate the process, however. In this model the illness is seen as an acute, inflammatory event which mobilizes the immune system. It enables the child's "Ego" (the Higher Self, in other vocabularies) to remodel the inherited body according to its own blueprint.

None of Incao's medical exemptions have been refused. Beginning in 1986, however, his unconventional practice may have provoked New York state health officials to begin what has been a smoldering form of harassment and informal investigation of his anthroposophical procedures. While the medical exemption is nationally available, it shouldn't be surprising to find that most doctors are reluctant to grant it, even in conditions of obvious contraindications—because it bucks too much against the orthodoxy. *DPT: A Shot in the Dark* is full of harrowing examples of distraught families scouring an entire state in search of a sympathetic M.D. to sign their medical exemption.

On the positive side, Washington state recently licensed naturopaths to give vaccinations, which means they can also grant exemptions. In some states, including Florida, chiropractors are allowed to write medical exemptions. The cracks in the orthodoxy may be gradually widening to allow parents more latitude.

BROADENING RELIGIOUS BELIEFS

An exemption from vaccinations based on religious beliefs is permitted in all states except West Virginia and Mississippi. Recent favorable litigation in New York has expanded the legal interpretation of religious beliefs, thereby granting parents further options.

The New York statute defines the parameters for religious exemptions by stating that mandatory vaccination requirements "Shall not apply to children whose parents are bona fide members of a recognized religious organization whose teachings are contrary to the practices herein required." This exemption works fine if a parent in fact belongs to a recognized religion. But what happens if a family has sincere beliefs but is outside the folds of any church? In 1984 a family in Clinton, New York, found out. They refused to have their two daughters vaccinated and took the issue to court. And they won.

Robert and Kit Allanson had initially secured a medical exemption for their daughters Naomi and Marika, but the school rejected it. The girls were expelled from school, their return pending on vaccination. Allanson secured the legal services of Attorney James Filenbaum and they immediately filed a suit in federal court, suing the school district, superintendent, and principal for $2 million. They also demanded a religious exemption for their girls.

The only weakness in the Allanson strategy was that they didn't belong to any church and the nearest recognizable label they had for their convictions was macrobiotics. The prosecutor had a field day with this.

At the trial, however, Filenbaum brought in a minister and the chairman of the religious department at nearby Hamilton College to testify on behalf of the religious authenticity of the Allansons' beliefs, however much those beliefs might lack an institutional context. After five-and-a-half months of testimony, charges of child neglect, and, Robert Allanson says, "hand-to-hand combat with the government," the Allansons prevailed as the U.S. district judge ruled in their favor.

The Allanson case was a valuable precedent for everyone, even outside of New York. Since the 1984 ruling, Filenbaum has argued another dozen religious exemption cases (in addition to advising hundreds of other clients) and has won nearly all of them. . . .

PERSONAL BELIEFS

Probably the best compromise all around is now legally available in twenty-two states. This is a harassment- and red-tape-free exemption on the grounds of personal or philosophical belief.

Vermont is a "triple-exemption" state which approved the personal belief exemption in 1981. According to Bob O'Grady, administrator of the Epidemiology Division in the Vermont State Health Department in Burlington, of Vermont's 98,600 students enrolled in public and private schools (kindergarten through twelfth grade), .5 percent (493 children) take the personal belief/religious exemption and .2 percent (197 students) take the medical exemption. Clearly 690 exempt and unvaccinated students representing about .7 percent of the school population is not viewed as a threat to public health.

All that is required to obtain the joint religious/philosophical exemption in Vermont, says O'Grady, is a written statement from the parent indicating that she has "a religious or moral conviction opposed to vaccination." The exemption is automatically granted. One needn't even specify the nature or details of the beliefs. Since Vermont has one of the highest vaccination rates (at 98.9 percent) in the country, the option of offering medical, religious, and philosophical exemptions for a tiny minority is a satisfactory compromise among conflicting demands,

says O'Grady. "I would have to judge that most people in Vermont feel it is, too."

California also has the personal belief exemption, mandated in 1961 when polio vaccinations were made legally necessary for school admissions. Here a parent must file a letter with the school stating that vaccination is contrary to his or her beliefs, explains Lauren Dales, M.D., chief of the Immunization Unit, California State Department of Health Services in Berkeley.

However, the health officer has the option to "temporarily exclude" a child from school "during the incubation period" if the child is believed to have been exposed to an infectious disease and is still at risk for developing symptoms. Other than that, the California statute "doesn't leave any grounds for a parent's application not to be accepted," says Dales. In his ten years with the department, he's never heard of a complaint from parents.

In California, of 475,000 new pupils each year, about 3,000 take the philosophical/religious exemption and about 1,000 take the medical. "We don't have a problem with these exemptions," says Dales. "We obviously don't want to see disease outbreaks, but when the exemptions are coming in at the low level they are, we don't think they are epidemiologically critical." . . .

WHO DECIDES?

The right of freedom of choice in vaccinations is clearly a difficult one to wrest from the hands of the medical establishment, as Barbara Fisher realizes after six years of strenuous effort.

"We haven't gotten anywhere near as far as we had wanted to. We have tried to be as credible as possible. We did our homework before we went out and criticized vaccines. We're dealing with a very powerful and wealthy pharmaceutical industry, with the government, health agencies, and organized medicine. That's a formidable force we're up against."

The exact nature of this "formidable force" may actually lie below the skin of the vaccination controversy and, as Fisher maintains, it may well touch at the "very heart of what is wrong with American medicine today."

The controversy really comes down to two diametrically opposite medical views. Plotkin of the A.A.P., for instance, does not recognize the right of a parent to subject a child to infectious disease. Anthroposophical physician Incao recognizes the necessity for a child to undergo the maturing struggles of early childhood infectious illnesses whereby "the higher self remodels the body in accordance with spiritual ideals."

This stark contrast raises important questions. Do we have the right to be sick anymore? Have we become overly afraid of being sick? Can illness be legislated out of existence, as something aberrant and unnatural?

The fundamental issue could also be seen as a question of one's rights: Does an individual have the right to oversee his/her own immune system (and his or her children's) and its interaction with the environment and the rest of society?

"We're so afraid of nature," says Incao. "What is the purpose of our life? If this purpose is to allow our individuality to unfold and express itself to the fullest, then this happens through the process of the immune system unfolding and reacting as self meets nonself. We become susceptible to infectious disease when we open ourselves to the world. Then we can become full human beings."

And for that voyage of discovery, concludes Incao, vaccinations are contraindicated.

RESOURCES

DPT (Dissatisfied Parents Together)
128 Branch Road
Vienna; VA 22180
(708) 938-DPT3
DPT: A Shot In the Dark, by Harris L. Coulter and Barbara Loe Fisher, Warner Books, 1985.
Dangers of Compulsory Immunization: How to Avoid Them Legally, by Tom Finn, Family Fitness Press (P.O. Box 1658, New Port Richey, FL 34291-1658), 1987.
Immunization: The Reality Behind the Myth, by Walene James.

POSTSCRIPT

Should All Children Be Immunized Against Childhood Diseases?

Currently, all 50 states require vaccination before school enrollment. However, the safety of various vaccines, particularly the whooping cough (DPT) vaccine, continues to be the subject of debate. Although both the American Academy of Pediatrics and the U.S. Public Health Service continue to endorse the whooping cough vaccine, many parents and health providers feel the risks are too high. Steven Black, codirector of the Kaiser-Permanente Pediatric Vaccine Study Center in Oakland, California, feels that the DPT vaccine is far from ideal. Newer vaccines, he believes, reduce the risks of injury by a significant percentage ("The Perils of Pertussis," *American Health*, June 1991). Unlike the current DPT vaccine, which uses whole, killed bacteria cells to trigger the formation of antibodies, the new immunizations contain materials that produce immunity without as many side effects. The new vaccines, currently available in Japan but not yet in the United States, cause a significantly lower percentage of some side effects, such as high fever and swelling, but whether or not they will reduce the incidence of brain damage is unclear.

Parents of young children are facing two crises relating to immunizations: First, widespread publicity about the genuine but extremely rare adverse effects of the whooping cough vaccine; and second, drug manufacturers' concerns about producing vaccines without the protection from expensive lawsuits brought by parents of injured children. As a result, fewer companies are willing to produce vaccines. This, in turn, will lead to vaccine shortages and higher costs (which will be passed on to the consumer).

Vaccines other than the DPT vaccine are also thought to be harmful. A 1980 article in *Mutation Research* indicated that children who had smallpox vaccinations in Czechoslovakia showed harmful changes in their white blood cells. Also, in 1988 the British medical journal *Medical Hypothesis* reported a study of 200 patients with a chronic viral disease, Epstein-Barr syndrome. The article claimed that the disease was caused by a live rubella (German measles) virus that was found in the vaccine.

The controversies surrounding vaccination continue. The medical community's endorsement of vaccination is evident in the following: "Declining Childhood Immunization Rates Becoming Cause for Concern," by J. W. Zylke, *Journal of the American Medical Association* (September 11, 1991); "Why Aren't We Protecting our Children?" by A. Jurgrau, *RN* (November 1990); and "Complying With Vaccine Law Will Help Prevent Errors," by M. R. Cohen, *Nursing* (August 1990). In *Immunization: The Reality Behind the Myth* (Bergin & Garvey, 1988), Walene James claims that immunization is not the answer to disease control. Barbara Fisher and Harris Coulter echo James in their book *DPT: A Shot in the Dark* (Warner Books, 1985).

ISSUE 18

Are Chiropractors Legitimate Health Providers?

YES: Ellen Ruppel Shell, from "The Getting of Respect," *The Atlantic* (February 1988)

NO: Editors of *Harvard Medical School Health Letter,* from "Low Back Pain: What About Chiropractors?" *Harvard Medical School Health Letter* (January 1988)

ISSUE SUMMARY

YES: Associate professor of journalism Ellen Ruppel Shell maintains that it is in the public's best interest that chiropractors continue to provide care to the millions who have back pain.

NO: The editors of the *Harvard Medical School Health Letter* argue that although some people may be helped by chiropractic treatment, many chiropractors adhere to a philosophy that is unproven at best and harmful at worst.

After nearly a century on the fringes of health care, chiropractic is seeking respectability; in some ways, it is gaining it. Chiropractic now ranks behind medicine and dentistry as the third largest primary health care profession in the Western world. Americans spend over $2 billion on chiropractic care each year, and over 30 hospitals in the United States have chiropractors on staff. And spinal manipulation, the primary therapy practiced by chiropractors, has achieved some recognition as a valid treatment for back pain.

The field of chiropractic was begun in 1895 by D. D. Palmer, a "magnetic healer" and tradesman living in Davenport, Iowa. Palmer allegedly cured a janitor's deafness by pressing on one of the man's spinal vertebrae. Palmer believed that misalignment of the spine, which he called "subluxations," could cause virtually all human diseases. He theorized that when these subluxations irritate the spinal nerves—which exit the spinal cord through openings between the vertebrae and branch off to the body's limbs and organs—diseases and pain would develop. According to Palmer, pressure from nerve irritation could be relieved, and health could be restored, by manipulating the appropriate vertebrae. This manipulation is the basic spinal adjustment practiced by all chiropractors.

Today, few chiropractors—who must attend at least two years of under-graduate school and four years of chiropractic college before they can be licensed by national and state boards—still believe in Palmer's view that subluxations cause nearly all health problems. However, most acknowledge that disease is caused by both infectious agents, such as bacteria and viruses, and health behaviors, such as sedentary life-styles and smoking. Despite these modern beliefs and in accord with Palmer's original theory, chiroprac-tic has remained preoccupied with the spine as the primary factor in health and disease. Chiropractors still subscribe to the theory that misaligned vertebrae impair the nervous system, causing a lowering of the body's defenses and resulting in disease. Good health, they believe, requires that vertebrae be kept in proper alignment, which is achieved only through spinal manipulation.

Spinal manipulation has been used for thousands of years to treat back pain, but there are conflicting opinions on whether or not it really works. Scientists who have evaluated the effects of chiropractic have concluded that spinal manipulation is probably helpful for some patients with back pain, specifically when the pain has been present for three weeks or less and so long as there are no tumors, fractures, or other abnormalities. For other types of back pain, medical experts are divided.

Because of the lack of definitive scientific evidence, and because chiro-practic is strongly identified with spinal manipulation, traditional medicine has, overall, been suspicious of chiropractic and has not considered it to be a legitimate medical treatment. Until 1980, the American Medical Association (AMA) considered it to be unethical for a doctor to refer a patient to a chiropractor; any doctor who did so risked losing his or her membership in the AMA. Although the AMA dropped this position in 1980, many doctors still refuse to refer patients to chiropractors. Despite this view, chiropractors are licensed to practice in the United States, and their services are covered by workers' compensation in all 50 states. Most states also cover chiropractic care under Medicaid and partially under Medicare, although private insur-ance coverage varies by state.

In the following selections, Ellen Ruppel Shell argues that there is a benefit to chiropractic care. She claims that spinal manipulation can relieve back pain for some patients and that it is a cost-effective, beneficial therapy for certain sufferers. The editors of the *Harvard Medical School Health Letter*, representing traditional medicine, acknowledge that some people may be helped by chiropractic treatment, but they maintain that many chiropractors adhere to a philosophy that could be harmful.

YES
Ellen Ruppel Shell

THE GETTING OF RESPECT

As a teenager, I occasionally spent an evening baby-sitting for the daughter of a chiropractor. My father, a pediatrician, dubbed these evenings "a night at the quack's." At the time I thought he was joking, but as it turns out, he was merely spouting the official opinion of his trade organization, the American Medical Association. The AMA had in fact formed a Committee on Quackery in 1963 to deal with what it considered to be the chiropractic problem. Thirteen years later five chiropractors responded by filing an antitrust suit.

Last September the suit was finally decided. A federal district court judge, Susan Getzendanner, found that the AMA was guilty of conspiracy in "restraint of trade" against the chiropractic profession, that it had unlawfully deprived chiropractors of association with medical doctors, and that by calling them "unscientific cultists" it had eroded the credibility of the profession. The Committee on Quackery was disbanded in 1975, but the AMA continued its official anti-chiropractic efforts until 1980. Getzendanner found that the AMA had "never acknowledged the lawlessness of its past conduct" and that to this day "there has never been an affirmative statement by the AMA that it is ethical to associate with chiropractors."

The AMA is appealing this decision. Dr. Alan Nelson, the chairman of the board of trustees of the AMA and an internist in Salt Lake City, contends that chiropractic is not scientifically based and that in some cases it can be dangerous. Meanwhile, more people than ever—something like 11 million a year—are seeking the help of chiropractors, most of them for the treatment of low back pain.

There are hundreds of different causes for low back pain. Tumors, infections, ruptured disks, and fractures are a few of the unhappier possibilities, and all of these require skilled medical intervention. But the vast majority of back-pain sufferers have what is called an idiopathic condition—there is no apparent cause for their pain. No treatment approach for idiopathic back pain can truly be called scientific, and of the so far nonscientific approaches, chiropractic appears to be among the most effective.

CHIROPRACTIC IS BASED ON THE THEORY that many disorders of the body are traceable to a misalignment of the spinal column and a concomitant disruption of the nervous system. This is a very old idea, and intuitively it makes a good deal of sense. The spinal cord is a pathway along which messages are carried to organs throughout the body; altering this pathway could well affect the transfer of information and, subsequently, the health of the organs. Chiropractors claim to be able to feel partial dislocations, or "subluxations," of the joints, which, they say, may be responsible for any number of disorders. The main therapeutic method used by chiropractors is spinal manipulation (they also treat other parts of the body), in which the vertebral segments of the spine are adjusted to correct these subluxations, release compression, and improve nerve transmission. There is no proof that any of this occurs—subluxations do not appear on x-rays, and according to Alan Nelson there is no evidence that subluxations are associated with any underlying illness. Nor is there solid evidence that manipulation significantly alters the spinal pathway. Nonetheless, preliminary clinical evidence indicates that chiropractic is more effective than, say, simple massage for cases of acute back pain. There is also evidence that victims of acute back pain who get the help of chiropractors recover more quickly than those who do not.

Dr. Gerald Leisman, a neurologist who also has a Ph.D. in biomedical engineering, is the chief of the research division of New York Chiropractic College, in Glen Head. Leisman, who is not a chiropractor, says that the process of detecting subluxations is deductive, not scientific, just as is any method of determining a treatment for idiopathic pain. "When I

was playing clinical neurologist, I saw at least three thousand patients who suffered from low back pain," he says. "Generally, the diagnosis was radiculopathy, or irritation of the nerve roots. But there is no scientific way to establish what such a diagnosis means, because irritation, per se, cannot be measured. Subluxation and irritation are not the same, but they are related concepts. There are demonstrable physical states associated with subluxations, and it is possible to show that after a manipulation these states are changed."

Like many doctors sympathetic to the chiropractic approach, Leisman was trained in Britain, where, he says, chiropractors do not compete with doctors and are treated with a good deal less skepticism than they receive in the United States. In Britain chiropractors are an integral part of the national health-care system, and doctors frequently refer patients to them. Until 1980 the AMA deemed it "unethical" for an American doctor to refer a patient to a chiropractor, and any doctor who did so risked losing his AMA membership. The AMA says that its motive for ostracizing chiropractic was a noble one—that it believed that the dangers of chiropractic outweighed the benefits.

"There is no question that our committee [on quackery] tried to educate the public in good faith," says Kirk Johnson, the AMA general counsel. "Our motive was patient care. Our campaign went on too long, and it went too far, but we are not going to apologize for it. It's as old as medicine that unscientific practices are things that doctors will not associate themselves with. The attitude in the early seventies was, Aren't we allowed to have ethical rules regarding the treatment of patients? To the extent that there has been a stigma against chiropractic, many doctors thought that it was probably earned."

The AMA dropped its official position on chiropractors in 1980, four years after the antitrust suit was filed, and referring patients to chiropractors is no longer deemed unethical by the association. Still, doctors generally prefer not to comment on chiropractic, and most of those who would speak to me about it said that they would not refer their patients to chiropractors. Dr. Aubrey Swartz, an orthopedic surgeon and the founding executive director of the American Back Society, says that while chiropractors are generally eager to share information with orthopedists, few orthopedists will cooperate with chiropractors. "Frequently chiropractors and orthopedic surgeons share the same patients, but the surgeon will refuse to recognize the chiropractor," he says. "The doctors are frustrated and angry—they believe chiropractors to be illegitimate. But naturally it is not in the best interest of the patient for the two not to communicate."

ONLY ABOUT A DOZEN HOSPITALS IN THE United States have staff chiropractors. The National Institutes of Health and the National Science Foundation, major funding sources for research in science and medicine, have yet to fund chiropractic research. Hence chiropractors have not had access to the research facilities and funds that would allow their case to be proved or disproved. That problem is being remedied in part by the Foundation for Chiropractic Education and Research, an independent funding organization that has picked up the tab for about seventy studies. One of these is a clinical trial being conducted by Dr. Malcolm Pope, a professor of orthopedic surgery and mechanical engineering and the director of research in orthopedics at the University of Vermont School of Medicine, which has a federally funded center for research on low back pain. Pope is comparing the relative benefits of chiropractic, massage, electrical muscle stimulation, and two types of back braces in the treatment of severe back pain.

"I have looked extensively at the literature on trials of chiropractic and found them to be very poorly done," Pope says. "It is true that the scientific basis for chiropractic is weak, but it is nevertheless a very commonly used therapy. There is no proof that any of the treatments we are looking at are effective in the long-term management of back pain. That's why a well-controlled study is so important."

Dr. Rowland Hazard, an assistant professor of orthopedics who works with Pope, says that most doctors know little or nothing about chiropractors but that this lack of understanding does not keep them from holding a generally negative opinion. "Chiropractic is a very complicated field," he says. "There are many different kinds, not only in terms of the science they believe in but in their styles of practice. Some chiropractors feel manipulation is only for spinal pain, while others believe it can be used to treat colds and diabetes. Any generalized statement about chiropractic will get you in trouble." Hazard says that part of the appeal that chiropractors have for the public may well be in their seeming ability to pinpoint ailments that physicians would not venture to diagnose. "Most chiropractors will tell you they can make a very specific diagnosis," he says. "They'll take x-rays and give you what sounds like a highly technical reason why you need realignment, and why you'll have to keep coming back for alignment for months. What they don't tell you is that there are any number of people walking down the street who would have very similar x-rays and who have no problem."

Hazard observes that orthopedic surgeons are in a similar bind. About fifty years ago a couple of surgeons at the Massachusetts General Hospital, in Boston, discovered the herniated disk. Disks are cushions of a jellylike substance surrounded by fibrous material that keep vertebrae from bumping into one another. As we age, the jelly dries up and can rupture through a crack in the fibrous material, sometimes hitting a nerve and causing serious pain. Generations of surgeons were taught to remove abnormal discs suspected of causing pain. But with the advent of penetrating imaging devices like the CAT scanner it gradually became clear that as many as a fifth of people between the ages of thirty and fifty have abnormal disks, yet most of them do not experience pain as a result. Also, statistics emerged showing that disk surgery was not necessarily successful in eliminating pain and, in fact, could sometimes make matters much worse. There are guidelines but no hard rules for distinguishing those who will be helped by surgery from those who won't—just as there is no certainty that chiropractic manipulation will be effective in a given case. As one orthopedic surgeon told me, deciding whether or not to operate is a matter of judgment.

"The fact is, science is absolutely stretched when it comes to the diagnosis and treatment of back pain," Hazard says. "A lot of people are operating way beyond what they can prove."

TRADITIONALLY, THIS LACK OF HARD DATA hasn't been a problem for chiropractors.

Chiropractic is considered by its practitioners to be a healing art, not a science, and only in the past decade or so have chiropractors themselves come to believe that they need a scientific basis for what they do. According to Stephen Wolk, the director of research for the Foundation for Chiropractic Education and Research, most chiropractors today stick to the treatment of neuromuscular and skeletal disorders, such as joint problems, headaches, and back pain, and no reputable practitioner would attempt to tackle infectious disease, diabetes, or cancer. But this is something of a departure from the not so distant past. At one time or another in its history, which extends roughly a hundred years, chiropractic has claimed to cure almost every condition afflicting man.

"Twenty years ago some chiropractors professed to do more than they could do," says Dr. Michael Pedigo, the president of the International Chiropractic Association, the smaller of two nationwide chiropractic trade organizations, and a plaintiff in the antitrust suit. (Like dentists, chiropractors are legally entitled to call themselves doctors.) "But we've become more realistic. Naturally, one should be leery of a chiropractor who makes outrageous claims—if he says he can cure cancer, go elsewhere. But one should also be aware that the medical establishment exaggerates the number of chiropractors who make such claims. There are medical doctors who make unrealistic claims, but I would doubt that the AMA would appreciate it if we portrayed these few irresponsible physicians as typical of their membership."

Chiropractors are required to attend two years of undergraduate school and four years of chiropractic college before they can be licensed by national and state boards. Nonetheless, the AMA contends that chiropractors are not qualified to diagnose. This is a sticky issue, because chiropractic procedure inappropriately applied can be disastrous. Patients with severe atherosclerosis, congenital hardening of the arteries, fractures of the spine, and rheumatoid arthritis are not candidates for chiropractic. Spinal manipulation could be lethal for them. However, chiropractors are trained to spot these problems and will refer patients to a physician if they do.

Chiropractors do not perform surgery or administer drugs, and therefore have less opportunity to do harm than doctors have. The good ones give advice on exercise and diet (most chiropractors are better versed in the fine points of nutrition than are most physicians), and many offer physical therapy as part of their treatment. Whether there is a scientific basis to chiropractic theory remains to be seen, but the fact is that, for whatever reason, many people are helped by chiropractors, at least over the short term. Despite the efforts of the medical establishment to keep them out, chiropractors are gradually edging their way into the mainstream of health care, thanks mostly, it seems, to popular demand for their services. If, as the medical community claims, the success of chiropractic is due to good politics rather than to good health care, then it is certainly politics of the grass-roots variety. Chiropractic will not go away. Nor does it seem to be in the public's best interest that chiropractic should.

NO

Editors of *Harvard Medical School Health Letter*

LOW BACK PAIN: WHAT ABOUT CHIROPRACTORS?

About one out of every five backs that pass you on the street is causing its owner some distress. Sooner or later almost everybody becomes acquainted with low back pain. Fortunately, painful backs tend to get better by themselves. About two-thirds of cases of low back pain improve within 30 days—regardless of the treatment they do or don't receive. That may seem too long, though, to someone who has to work or wants to play. Rather than wait it out, many people go in search of help. The specialists they turn to most often are orthopedic surgeons; next most commonly they go to chiropractors. Lots of other practitioners are available to treat back pain: internists, neurologists, family physicians, physiatrists, osteopaths, acupuncturists, physical therapists, massage therapists. Why is it that chiropractors get so much of the "back business"?

Two reasons come to mind. The first, which everyone would agree on, is that nobody else is all that effective with low back pain. The second, which is less certain, is that chiropractors have something special to offer their patients.

FACTIONS AND PHILOSOPHY

The field of chiropractic was invented in 1895 by an Iowa grocer, D. D. Palmer. Palmer's notion was that the central nervous system controls all the body's functions—principally through the nerves that come out of the spinal cord. Each of these nerves must pass through a small aperture between two vertebrae. If two vertebrae were improperly aligned, Palmer reasoned, a nerve could become pinched. The nerve would then tend to misfire, and the part of the body served by it would not function well. If this situation persisted, or became severe, illness would result. Palmer wasn't much impressed by the idea that germs, for example, cause illness. He preferred to think that all symptoms were expressions, one way or another, of malfunctioning nerves. Nerves could be made to work better if they were relieved of pressure caused by slight dislocations of vertebrae (termed "subluxations"). Thus, in his view, adjusting the spine was the best possible treatment for all kinds of illness.

Some of the principles underlying chiropractic practice are philosophical or spiritual—not the sort of statements that can be proved or disproved by scientific methods. The basic ideas about subluxations and pinched nerves can be scientifically studied, though. And there's every reason to believe that this body of chiropractic lore is simply wrong. It has been shown that many organs of the body work well enough even if their nerve supply is cut off completely. And subluxations are not abnormal; every spine has slight "misalignments." Nerves are rarely pinched or damaged as a result of these variations of normal anatomy, and specific physical symptoms are not usually associated with irregularities in a particular area of the spine.

One group of chiropractors—known as the "straights"—has continued in the tradition established by Palmer. Identified with the International Chiropractors' Association, this faction continues to see pinched nerves as a cause of dizziness, eye and ear problems, high blood pressure, glandular troubles, skin disorders, hay fever, congestion, low blood pressure, rheumatism, impotence, knee pains, bed wetting, hemorrhoids, and ankle swelling—to name but a few of the conditions that they imply will be relieved by spinal adjustment. (State and federal laws limit how explicit chiropractors can be in stating such claims.)

The majority of chiropractors in the United States, however, are "mixers" and are more likely to be members of the American Chiropractors' Association. They share a general philosophy derived from Palmer: that illness results from a kind of disharmony in the body, a failure of the natural drive to health. But mixers don't make spinal manipulation the end-all and be-all of their practice. Mixers may attempt to treat their patients by modifying diet, giving vitamin supplements, or offering counseling and education. However, by law and as an aspect of their philosophy, chiropractors do not use medical treatments, such as prescription drugs or surgery. Virtually all chiropractors do take x-rays (occasionally a great many x-rays) to examine the spine.

Finally, there is the National Association for Chiropractic Medicine, which is a minority voice in the field. According to its president, the NACM is "an organization that was formed specifically to reject and renounce the untenable historical chiropractic theory." Chiropractors associated with the NACM limit their practice to treating joint conditions that may be relieved by mobilization or manipulation, and they advocate basing chiropractic practice on research that meets accepted scientific standards. This group is seeking to become more closely allied with regular medicine in a cooperative relationship.

MANIPULATION AND BACK PAIN

If you ask whether chiropractic treatment of low back pain works for some people some of the time, the answer is yes. So do all types of therapy, including placebo treatments against which potentially more effective treatments are often tested. Nevertheless, studies suggest that chiropractic adjustments provide more immediate reduction of pain than placebo treatments, and they often appear to produce speedier improvement than standard medical approaches.

Few well-conducted trials have compared chiropractic to other forms of therapy. But, although neither plentiful nor perfect, some studies of chiropractic approaches to low back pain have been carried out. Manipulation is the best studied.

Manipulation is a hands-on therapy that is not well standardized. The term may be applied differently in different settings. Chiropractors often use the term "spinal adjustment" for their procedure. In any case, the patient with low back pain is often placed on his or her side while the practitioner grasps the uppermost shoulder and a hip or bent knee for leverage. The shoulder and pelvis are then pressed in opposite directions, so as to rotate the torso. This maneuver sometimes produces a cracking sound that seems to emanate from the spine. This sound has been attributed to the sudden release of gases dissolved in the joint fluid; it may signal what is probably a temporary change in the relative positions of some vertebrae. Skilled practitioners seem able to apply pressure to, and "crack," a single intervertebral joint.

Trials conducted under varying conditions and using practitioners with various kinds of background have demonstrated that manipulation is indeed better than nothing at relieving back pain for a short while. An acute episode of back pain in someone who does not have a long history of the problem seems most responsive to this form of treatment. After a few weeks, though, manipulated backs appear to be no better or worse off than backs that have been left to their own devices. It is, thus, unlikely that chiropractic treatment is making some fundamental or "curative" change in the spine. There is less support for the use of manipulation to treat established, chronic low back pain, although some sufferers do experience transient relief from manipulation.

One quite well-designed study of manipulation used massage as the control therapy in order to test the possibility that personal touch is more important than the specific technique. The therapists in this study were both chiropractors and physicians trained in manipulation or massage. The subjects, who had never before undergone manipulation, were unable to guess accurately which treatment they had been given, and thus their prejudices presumably did not affect their perception of relief obtained by one treatment or the other. The efficacy of therapy was evaluated both by asking patients whether they felt better and by testing to see whether they had gained flexibility. By both criteria, manipulation reduced pain immediately after treatment more effectively than massage. Six to seven weeks later, however, neither group was significantly more free of pain than the other.

The outcome of this study is, on the whole, typical. When compared with other nonsurgical treatments, such as anti-inflammatory drugs, pain killers, heat treatments, and so forth, manipulation often appears to have a short-term advantage but loses its edge in the long run. None of the trials has been perfect, so there is plenty of opportunity for debate and difference of opinion (and for taking refuge in claims of "clinical experience").

WHY THE CONFUSION?

Studies of manipulation for back pain are not very satisfactory, but neither are studies of many other treatments. The hurdles to designing and executing good research on pain of any kind are many and large.

To take just one example, it can be very difficult to test alternative treatments on comparable groups of subjects. British researchers sought to compare patients reporting to a chiropractic clinic with others who went to a hospital clinic. Half of each group was to be referred to the other treatment center, but over a third of the chiropractic patients refused to enter the study for fear that they would be sent to a hospital for conventional treatment, whereas only 6 percent of the hospital patients refused to have chiropractic manipulation. Likewise, keeping subjects "blind" to the therapy they are receiving (as was achieved in the study of manipulation versus massage) often is not feasible.

A real possibility, suggested by the trials of manipulation, is that the treatment works well for some people with low back pain and poorly for others. The problem is to know in advance which will be which.

PROS AND CONS OF CHIROPRACTORS

Manipulation is not the exclusive "property" of chiropractors. Doctors of osteopathy, who have training quite similar to that of medical doctors, apply a form of manipulation, as well as prescribing drugs and performing surgery. Some other health professionals outside chiropractic are also trained in manipulation. But the majority of experienced practitioners are chiropractors. New York Chiropractic College, to give an example, allots 15% of its students' classroom time to courses in technique, including manipulation. The curriculum, which continues for 10 trimesters, also includes courses in anatomy, physiology, biochemistry, microbiology, and pathology. Practical experience in internships consumes another 20% of the students' time. Manipulation then becomes a significant component of the chiropractor's daily work.

Chiropractors emphasize that their approach to treating disease is "drugless" and "natural." These may or may not be virtues, depending on the condition that is being treated. But a consequence is that chiropractors spend a lot of time in developing a relationship with their patients and often see their patients with considerable frequency. If a warm and supportive association is developed, a sense of well-being may be promoted in nonspecific but nonetheless important ways.

In treating back pain, chiropractors often stress education about the back and its care. This may appeal to patients and, if well done, is very helpful. On the other hand, many chiropractors adhere to a philosophy of disease and treatment that at best is unproven and at worst is wrong. To the extent that a chiropractor encourages patients to avoid effective treatment, he or she is doing them a disservice. But chiropractic and regular medicine do not appear, in practice, to be mutually exclusive. A Canadian survey found that 97% of chiropractors refer patients to physicians for care and that 84% also had patients referred from physicians. It appears that patients generally use chiropractic care in addition to, not instead of, regular medical care. Chiropractors are licensed to practice in most states, though state licensing laws vary in the scope they grant to chiropractors.

Whatever the realities of referral back and forth between chiropractors and physicians, the American Medical Association has called chiropractors "unscientific cultists," has resisted licensing of chiropractors, and has opposed any professional interaction between them and physicians. As of last August, however, this policy was found by a Federal district judge to violate antitrust legislation.

In 1968 the Department of Health, Education, and Welfare recommended that chiropractic not be included in the Medicare program. A law passed 4 years later allowed some chiropractic services to be covered. The policies of private insurance companies may extend coverage to chiropractic treatment, but there is considerable variability, and most seem to be quite restrictive with respect to the conditions they cover.

A patient need not accept Palmer's views of disease and health to accept manipulation as a potential avenue to relatively rapid relief of low back pain. On the other hand, anyone willing to wait it out is likely to find that there is no need to seek intervention at all.

As a rule of thumb, it seems fair to say that if manipulation is going to help, the benefit should be evident after no more than half a dozen treatments. Repeated manipulations over a prolonged period without significant improvement are seldom worthwhile. Spinal disorders are not the only causes of back pain. Manipulation therapy without a proper diagnostic work-up (not just x-rays) is ill-advised and may even be disastrous for patients whose back pain is due to abdominal disease, osteoporosis, cancer, or other metabolic diseases.

POSTSCRIPT

Are Chiropractors Legitimate Health Providers?

Currently, 1 in 20 Americans visits a chiropractor each year. This visit is, generally speaking, not enthusiastically endorsed by traditional physicians. Chiropractic has not yet become mainstream despite the large number of people who use this service. The reasons, chiropractors claim, is that spinal manipulation is more an art than a science.

Gerald Leisman, a neurologist (not a chiropractor), is the chief of the research division of New York Chiropractic College. He claims that the process of subluxations is deductive, not scientific, as are most methods of determining an unknown cause of pain. Leisman believes that for most back pain sufferers, there *is* no scientific way to establish a specific diagnosis, since back pain often does not show up on an X ray or produce abnormal blood or fluid values. This lack of scientific evidence in chiropractic, he maintains, does not negate the benefits of spinal manipulation.

Scientific research into the benefits of chiropractic care is still limited. The National Institutes of Health and the National Science Foundation, both primary funding sources for research in medicine and science, have yet to fund chiropractic research. Chiropractors, thus far, have had limited access to funding and research facilities, which would allow them to scientifically evaluate the effectiveness of chiropractic treatment.

The evaluation of chiropractic treatment is also difficult because of the diversity of chiropractic practices. Different chiropractors believe in a variety of ideologies and practice in many different ways. Some chiropractors feel that spinal manipulation should be used only for back pain, while others believe it can benefit certain illnesses, such as high blood pressure and the common cold. Most chiropractors, however, treat only muscle and bone disorders, headaches, and back pain. Also, the majority of reputable chiropractors do not attempt to treat infectious diseases or other illnesses and are trained to spot these conditions and refer patients to a physician.

While chiropractors do not administer drugs or perform surgery, they often supply good advice on diet and exercise along with spinal manipulation. Whether or not there is a valid scientific basis for chiropractic treatment is unclear, but for whatever reason, chiropractors seem to help some people, at least in the short term. While the medical establishment continues to question the legitimacy of spinal manipulation, chiropractors are making their way into mainstream medicine, usually at a lower cost than traditional treatment. As medical costs continue to rise in the United States, chiropractic care may claim a valid place in the health care system. This cost factor is discussed in "A Low Cost Cure for Back Pain?" *Kiplinger's Personal Finance* (February 1992) and in "Does Anything Work for Back Pain?" *Consumer's Reports on Health* (February 1992).

For additional reading on chiropractic and other alternative health care, the following are suggested: "Beating Back Pain," *McCall's* (June 1991); "New Age Meets Hippocrates," *Newsweek* (July 13, 1992); "Big Claim, No Proof," *U.S. News & World Report* (September 23, 1991); "Executive Board Debates Chiropractic," *The Nation's Health* (May 1983); and "Why New Age Medicine is Catching On," *Time* (November 4, 1991).

For the 30 million Americans who suffer from back pain, chiropractic care may be a beneficial, lower-cost alternative to traditional medicine. For some members of the American Medical Association, chiropractic treatment is not scientific and may do considerable harm if treatable conditions are managed with spinal manipulation rather than with modern medicine and/or surgery.

CONTRIBUTORS
TO THIS VOLUME

EDITOR

EILEEN L. DANIEL, a registered dietician with the state of New York, is an assistant professor in the Department of Health Science at the State University of New York College at Brockport. She received a B.S. in nutrition and dietetics from the Rochester Institute of Technology in 1977, an M.S. in community health education from SUNY College at Brockport in 1978, and a Ph.D. in health education from the University of Oregon in 1986. A member of the Eta Sigma Gamma national health honor society, the American Dietetics Association, the New York State Dietetics Society, and other professional and community organizations, she has published over 20 articles on issues of health and health education in such professional journals as the *Journal of Nutrition Education,* the *Journal of School Health,* and the *Journal of the American Dietetics Association.*

STAFF

Marguerite L. Egan   Program Manager
Brenda S. Filley   Production Manager
Whit Vye   Designer
Libra Ann Cusack   Typesetting Supervisor
Juliana Arbo   Typesetter
David Brackley   Copy Editor
David Dean   Administrative Assistant
Diane Barker   Editorial Assistant

AUTHORS

BRUCE AMES, a genetic toxicologist, is a professor of biochemistry and molecular biology and the director of the National Institute of Environmental Health Sciences Center at the University of California, Berkeley, where he has been teaching since 1968. He has authored or coauthored over 300 publications, and he has received the General Motors Cancer Research Foundation Prize, the Tyler Prize for his work in environmental science, and the Gold Medal Award of the American Institute of Chemists.

MARCIA ANGELL is a pathologist and the executive editor of the *New England Journal of Medicine.* She graduated from Boston University School of Medicine and did postgraduate work in internal medicine as well as in pathology. She is also a lecturer in the Department of Social Medicine at Harvard Medical School, and she frequently writes on ethical issues in medicine and biomedical research.

WILLIAM M. BROWN is a director emeritus of energy and technological studies at the Hudson Institute. Since retiring from the Hudson Institute in August 1988, he has been an independent consultant on policy research and has been involved in studies on the long-term future and on revitalizing education in U.S. schools. He received a Ph.D. in theoretical physics from the University of California, Los Angeles, and he has taught at UCLA and at the New York Polytechnic Institute.

B. BRUCE-BRIGGS is an independent policy analyst and a 30-year smoker.

DANIEL CALLAHAN, a philosopher, is the cofounder and director of the Hastings Center. He received a Ph.D. in philosophy from Harvard University, and he is the author or editor of 31 publications, including *Ethics in Hard Times* (Plenum Press, 1981), coauthored with Arthur L. Caplan, and *Setting Limits: Medical Goals in an Aging Society* (Simon & Schuster, 1987).

MICHAEL A. CARRERA is the Thomas Hunter Professor of Health Sciences at Hunter College of the City University of New York. He is also the director of the National Sexuality Training Center for the Children's Aid Society, a multiservice, nonprofit child and family care agency in New York City. He has served as the president of the board of directors of the Sex Information and Education Council of the United States and as the president of the American Association of Sex Educators, Counselors, and Therapists.

PATRICIA DEMPSEY is an assistant professor of social work at the Hunter College School of Social Work and the training coordinator for the Children's Aid Society's National Training Center for Adolescent Sexuality and Family Life Education. She is a specialist in child welfare and family issues and serves as a consultant to the New York City Human Resources Administration.

RICHARD J. DENNIS is the president of *New Perspectives Quarterly* magazine, a publication of the Center for the Study of Democratic Institutions; president of the Chicago Resource Center, a grant-making foundation concerned with civil liberties; and the chairman of the advisory board of the Drug Policy Foundation. He also serves on the boards of the CATO Institute, the Reason Foundation, and the Chicago Council of Foreign Relations.

JASON DePARLE is a former editor of *Washington Monthly*.

BERNARD DIXON, an editor of *Medical Science Research* and a European contributing editor of *Bio/Technology*, is the vice president of the General Section of the British Association for the Advancement of Science and the chairman of the Programme Planning Committee of the Edinburgh International Science Festival. He is a fellow of the Institute of Biology and a fellow of the International Institute of Biotechnology. His publications include *Health, Medicine and the Human Body* (Macmillan, 1986).

HERBERT FINGARETTE is a professor emeritus of philosophy at the University of California, Santa Barbara. He has also served as an alcoholism and addiction consultant to the World Health Organization.

ROYCE FLIPPIN is a free-lance health and science writer living in New York City. He writes on a variety of health issues, including physical psychology (how the body affects the mind) and exercise and fitness, and he is a former senior editor of *American Health: Fitness of Body and Mind*.

MICHAEL FUMENTO, a former AIDS analyst and attorney for the U.S. Commission on Civil Rights, is the science and economics reporter for *Investor's Business Daily*. He has written two books, *The Myth of Heterosexual AIDS* (New Republic Books, 1990) and *Science Under Siege* (William Morrow, 1993), and he is the author of numerous articles on AIDs that have appeared in publications worldwide.

SARAH GLAZER is a researcher and author.

ROBERT E. GOODIN is a professor of political and moral philosophy in the Research School of Social Sciences at the Australian National University in Canberra, Australia. He is also the founding editor of the new *Journal of Political Philosophy*, to be published by Basil Blackwell, Inc., starting in March 1993, and he is the author of numerous books on political theory, public policy, and applied ethics, including *Motivating Political Morality* (Basil Blackwell, 1992).

LENN E. GOODMAN is a professor of philosophy at the University of Hawaii. He received the Baumgardt Award of the American Philosophical Association and is the author of nine books, including *On Justice* (Yale University Press, 1991). He and his wife, Madeleine

Goodman, often collaborate on research in the areas of bioethics and biophilosophy. He received a B.A. from Harvard University and a Ph.D. from Oxford University.

MADELEINE J. GOODMAN is a professor of human biology and a senior vice president of academic affairs for the University of Hawaii. She received a B.A. in zoology from Barnard College, a diploma in human biology from Oxford University, and a Ph.D. in human genetics from the University of Hawaii School of Medicine. A Sigma Xi national lecturer in science, she has published prolifically on her research on women's health issues.

MARY GORDON is a novelist and short story writer. She is the author of *Men and Angels* (Ballantine Books, 1986) and *The Other Side* (Viking Penguin, 1989).

JOEL GURIN is the science editor of *Consumer Reports* magazine. A Harvard University graduate in biochemistry, he has covered science and medicine as a journalist since 1975. He has won several national awards for his work, including the top science-writing awards of the American Association for the Advancement of Science and the National Association of Science Writers.

NAT HENTOFF, a former board member of the American Civil Liberties Union, is a writer and an adjunct associate professor at New York University. He is a regular contributor to such publications as

The Washington Post, The Progressive, The Village Voice, and *The New Yorker,* and he is the author of several books on public policy, including *The First Freedom* (Delacorte Press, 1980).

ALBERT L. HUEBNER is a professor of physics at California State University, where he has been teaching since 1975. He has completed more than 15 years of industrial research on energy and environmental science, and his current research interests focus on energy, the physics of the environment, and biophysics. He is a member of the American Institute of Biomedical Climatology, the American Association of Physics Teachers, and the American Association for the Advancement of Science.

JOHN K. IGLEHART has been the national correspondent for *The New England Journal of Medicine* since 1981. During that same period, he also founded and served as editor of *Health Affairs,* a quarterly policy journal published in Washington, D.C. He has been a member of the Institute of Medicine, National Academy of Sciences, since 1977.

JAMES A. INCIARDI is a professor in the Department of Sociology and Criminal Justice and the director of the Center for Drug and Alcohol Studies at the University of Delaware. He is also an adjunct professor in the Comprehensive Drug Research Center at the University of Miami School of Medicine and a member of the South Florida AIDS Research Consortium. He has published 24 books and more than 100 articles and chapters on substance abuse, criminal justice, social policy, and the law.

TIMOTHY JOHNSON is a lecturer in medicine at Harvard Medical School, a clinical associate in medicine at the Massachusetts General Hospital, and the medical editor of ABC News on such programs as "World News Tonight," "Nightline," and "20/20." He is also the founding editor of *The Harvard Medical School Health Letter*. He received an M.D. from Albany Medical College in Albany, New York, and an M.P.H. from the Harvard School of Public Health.

LEON R. KASS is the Addie Clark Harding Professor in the College and the Committee on Social Thought at the University of Chicago and an adjunct scholar at the American Enterprise Institute. A trained physician and biochemist, he is the author of *Toward a More Natural Science* (Free Press, 1985).

RICHARD LEVITON, a health journalist, is a senior writer for the *Yoga Journal*, published in Berkeley, California, and a regular contributor to *The Quest*. A professional, published journalist for 15 years, he has written over 150 feature articles, many of which have been reprinted in Canada, Germany, Australia, and many other countries throughout the world.

JON R. LUOMA is a widely published environmental writer and a regular contributor to such magazines as *Audubon, Wildlife Conserva-*tion, *The New York Times Magazine,* and *Discover*. His publications include *Troubled Skies, Troubled Waters* (Viking Penguin, 1984) and *A Crowded Ark: The Role of Zoos in Wildlife Conservation* (Houghton Mifflin, 1988).

DUANE C. McBRIDE is a professor in and the chairman of the Behavioral Center of the Institute of Alcoholism and Drug Dependency at Andrews University in Berrien Springs, Michigan. Active in a variety of drug abuse and crime and drugs research projects funded by the National Institute on Drug Abuse and the U.S. Department of Justice, he has authored or coauthored 2 books and over 40 monographs, articles, and chapters in the substance abuse field.

THOMAS J. MOORE is a journalist and the author of *Heart Failure* (Random House, 1989).

LAWRIE MOTT is a senior scientist with the Natural Resources Defense Council. Active on a variety of pesticide issues at both the state and national levels, she is a member of the advisory board for Americans for Safe Food, the board of directors of the Pesticide Education Center, and the advisory board of the Environmental Media Association. She was also appointed to the EPA administrator's Pesticide Advisory Committee and the University of California's Advisory Committee for Public Education on Food Safety.

TIMOTHY F. MURPHY is an assistant professor of philosophy in the Department of Biomedical Sciences at the University of Illinois College of Medicine in Chicago, Illinois. His publications include *Writing AIDS: Gay Literature, Language, and Analysis* (Columbia University Press, 1993), coedited with Suzanne Poirier.

VICENTE NAVARRO is a professor of health at Johns Hopkins University in Baltimore, Maryland. He is also the president of the International Association of Health Policy and the editor in chief of the *International Journal of Health Services*.

LINUS PAULING is a chemist at the California Institute of Technology, where he has been teaching since 1931. He is one of the few recipients of two Nobel prizes, having received the Nobel Prize in chemistry in 1954 and the Nobel Peace Prize in 1962. He is also well known as an active proponent of disarmament and an advocate of the use of chemotherapy for mental diseases.

TIMOTHY E. QUILL is an associate professor of medicine and psychiatry at the University of Rochester School of Medicine in Rochester, New York, and the chairman of the university's Program for Biopsychosocial Studies. He is the author of numerous publications on physician-patient communication and end-of-life decision-making, including *Death and Dignity: Making Choices and Taking Charge* (W. W. Norton, 1993).

ELLEN RUPPEL SHELL is an associate professor of journalism and the codirector of the Program in Science and Journalism at Boston University. Her publications include *A Child's Place: A Year in the Life of a Day Care Center* (Little, Brown, 1992).

KAREN SNYDER is a pesticide researcher in the San Francisco office of the National Resources Defense Council, which addresses almost every major environmental issue facing the United States, including air and water pollution, energy use and development, wilderness preservation, nuclear armament, and control of toxic substances.

HENRY A. SOLOMON is a clinical associate professor of medicine at Cornell University Medical College, and he maintains a private medical practice in New York City. A fellow of the American College of Physicians and the American College of Cardiology, he is also a columnist for the *Tampa Tribune* newspaper, the medical director of Health Education Technologies, Inc.

GEORGE E. VAILLANT, a recipient of the Jellinck Prize for alcoholism research, is the director of adult development at Harvard University. He received an M.D. from Harvard Medical School in 1955 and has taught at Tufts University, Harvard Medical School, and Dartmouth Medical School. He is also the author of *The Wisdom of the Ego* (Harvard University Press, 1993).

INDEX